Mad Tuscans and Their Families

Mad Tuscans and Their Families

A HISTORY OF MENTAL DISORDER
IN EARLY MODERN ITALY

Elizabeth W. Mellyn

PENN

UNIVERSITY OF PENNSYLVANIA PRESS *Philadelphia*

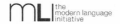

THIS BOOK IS MADE POSSIBLE BY A COLLABORATIVE GRANT
FROM THE ANDREW W. MELLON FOUNDATION.

© 2014 University of Pennsylvania Press

Published by
University of Pennsylvania Press
Philadelphia, Pennsylvania 19104-4112
www.upenn.edu/pennpress

Printed in the United States of America on
acid-free paper

10 9 8 7 6 5 4 3 2 1

A Cataloging-in-Publication record is available from
the Library of Congress.

ISBN 978-0-8122-4612-4

For Albert Mazza

CONTENTS

A NOTE ON DATES AND MONEY

DATES

Until 1751, the Florentine year was reckoned to begin on March 25 (Annunciation) rather than on January 1. Thus, the date March 23, 1536, corresponds to March 23, 1537, by our system of dating. I have made all dates consistent with the modern style.

MONEY

In the fifteenth century, Florence operated on two monetary standards. One was based on the gold florin and the other on the silver lira. During the ducal period in the sixteenth century the two units of account were the florin and the scudo. The florin was divided into 20 soldi of 12 denari. The scudo was worth 7 lire, which was also divided into 20 soldi of 12 denari. The exchange rate between the lira and florin constantly varied, for which see Richard Goldthwaite, *The Building of Renaissance Florence: An Economic and Social History* (Baltimore: Johns Hopkins University Press, 1980).

Mad Tuscans and Their Families

Introduction

The Tales Madness Tells

Ajax, so long as the mad fit was on him,
Himself felt joy at his wretchedness,
Though we, his sane companions, grieved indeed.
But now that he's recovered and breathes clear,
His own anguish totally masters him,
While we are no less wretched than before.
Is not this a redoubling of our grief?

—SOPHOCLES, *Ajax*

Many books have been written about men and women like Ajax and the madness that gripped them; fewer have been written about the companions who watched them suffer, cared for them, and grieved over their condition. This book is not so much about people like Ajax as it is about those companions who watched, cared, and grieved. It takes as its starting point not the commonly asked question of how a past Western society represented madness, though it is certainly an important part of the investigation. Rather, it asks first and foremost what families, communities, and civic authorities *did* to address the disorder or, in its worst manifestations, the chaos that it visited on their households or unleashed in their streets.

The focus on action rather than representation is meant to capture, to the extent that it is possible, the lived experience of madness in a specific time and place. Such an endeavor rests on three assumptions. First, madness, or in current terms, mental disorder, is a universal and persistent feature of human history. Every society, past and present, struggles to make sense of it; every society, past and present, struggles to address it. Second, madness is at once biological and social. As a failure of a person's internal mechanisms it can produce cognitive, emotional, and behavioral states that lie outside the bounds of what a society generally considers reasonable.[1] At the same time, it is a society's values and attitudes that mark out the bounds of the reasonable in the first place. Third, madness is a powerful category of historical analysis.[2] Every society defines it in its own terms and tackles it with a contingent range of institutional strategies.

And its reverberations run deep. In the words of one scholar, "madness is the most solitary of afflictions to the people who experience it; but the most social of maladies to those who observe its effects."[3] It undermines the conventions of thought, feeling, and behavior that bind people together as members of families, neighborhoods, cultures, and communities; it strains the foundations of social and civic life. Because it radiates so deeply and broadly, the study of madness as a social reality in search of a pragmatic solution offers historians an especially sharp lens onto the past.

For the richness of its archival material, the stage on which this particular drama is set is the city of Florence and its Tuscan domains from the mid-fourteenth to the mid-seventeenth century. Evidence from Florentine judicial records recalls the circumstances that led nearly three hundred men and women from all walks of life before civil and criminal courts for being allegedly mad. Some were brought there by family members trying to protect the economic and social stability of their households; others were summoned by magistrates seeking to maintain public order; still others went before the courts of their own accord to defend their sanity or even to declare their own insanity. In many of these cases, petitioners had benign intentions; they sought only to arrange long-term care for vulnerable kin. But sometimes their ends were predatory: to exploit helpless relatives, to overturn a contract, or to escape punishment for a criminal offense.

These cases uncover the complex networks of people and institutions that lived with, cared for, and in some cases cast off or exploited the mentally impaired. But they offer, too, a unique view onto great changes unfolding in late medieval and early modern Europe. Together they tell a larger story that begins in the fourteenth century when the allegedly mentally disturbed first trickled into the records of Florence's civil and criminal courts. At this point, the only long-term custodial institution was the family; hospitals generally administered acute care to the sick poor; monasteries and convents were reluctant to admit potentially dangerous or disruptive people into their communities; and the courts were just beginning to provide families with guardians for vulnerable kin.

By the seventeenth century, the social, cultural, professional, and institutional landscape of Tuscany had significantly changed. First, medical language and ideas had entered the courts. Petitioners and magistrates had come to explain madness in organic terms and the disease melancholy was recognized as the most common cause of abnormal thought and behavior. Second, learned medical practitioners in Italy and France had begun to write treatises touting their skill in resolving legal questions that involved the body in court. Their medical expertise was crucial, they maintained, in helping judges determine when, how, and in what situations particular types of madness were likely to express themselves and what that meant for the law. Finally, the mentally disordered began to move from household to hospital. In 1643, Florence established Santa Dorotea, its first institution devoted solely to the care of the severest cases of madness. About forty years later, the famous old Florentine hospital of Santa Maria Nuova followed suit, creating the "pazzeria," a mad ward for poor and indigent mad men and women. Simply put, the Tuscan who wondered what to do with a mad relative in the seventeenth century had more institutional options than his or her fourteenth-century counterpart. But what do these changes mean and how should they be interpreted?

Such transformations might inspire the telling of origins stories—the medicalization of madness, the foundation of legal medicine, the birth of the clinic, the rise of the early modern state, the roots of European penal institutions, or the formation of state or elite programs of discipline and social control. Indeed this is how many scholars have framed similar developments. Histories of psychiatry, for example, have praised the triumph of modern psychiatric practice and institutions over the superstition and barbarism that supposedly characterized the treatment of mentally disturbed men and women during the European Middle Ages. Despite considerable evidence to the contrary, this view unfortunately persists. A textbook frequently assigned in American colleges and universities still claims that the "Middle Ages in Europe were largely devoid of scientific thinking and humane treatment for the mentally disturbed," a point this book categorically rejects as another example of the "enormous condescension of posterity."[4]

Florentine society, like other late medieval and early modern European societies, like our own society, grappled with how to care for people who, on account of mental disorders, could not care for themselves or who wrought havoc in households and communities. Like us, they struggled to arrive at concrete if imperfect and shifting solutions for dealing with disturbed men and women within a society that had limited public and private resources. Given the state of their medical knowledge, the remedies available to them through the courts, and the availability—or lack thereof—of private or public custodial institutions, Florentines and their European counterparts often did the best they could with the knowledge and institutions they had.

Of course, psychiatry has had its critics. But even the most vociferous among them did little more than exchange a narrative of triumph for one of oppression or decline. Scholars in this camp claimed that the medicalization of madness and the birth of the asylum were disastrous, signaling little more than the pernicious growth of society's mechanisms of social, professional, and political control.[5] The most famous and influential of these critiques remains that of Michel Foucault, who imagined the countryside of Renaissance Europe dotted with mad men and women, its seas speckled with ships of fools.[6] In his vision—more provocative than accurate—townsfolk drove the mad from their gates, consigning them to lives led wandering terrestrial or watery spaces along the fringes of civil society. As objects of historical analysis, they were not so much individuals as bearers of their society's obsession with sin and the impossibility of true knowledge and the fear of God's wrath, the devil, and death. The only reasonable thing to do was to push them to the margins of society. But exile on land or sea was better than what was to come.

Foucault's real target was late seventeenth- and eighteenth-century Europe, his real goal to expose the Age of Reason as an age of confinement in which a new bourgeois ethic came to associate morality with labor and diligence, madness with unemployment and idleness. Europeans hauled madness from the margins to place it at the center of society; they locked up the mad—unemployed, idle, and poor—and dissected their disease in institutions devoted to their physical treatment and moral reform.

This book tells a story of a very different kind and one that builds in no small part on historical scholarship that has exposed the limits of teleological thinking and the deceptive linear narratives it tends to generate.[7] Through a stunning array of new sources—the casebooks of mad doctors, patients' narratives, asylum registers, a range of legislative and administrative documents, and, more recently, judicial records—a number of historians have reexamined the role families, civic authorities, and professional groups played in the care and confinement of the mad.[8] Michael MacDonald's classic study of the casebooks of a seventeenth-century astrological-physician and R. A. Houston's social history of madness in eighteenth-century Scotland have shown the persistent role ordinary men and women played both in defining madness even in official arenas and in caring for or abusing the mad despite the growth of a medical profession and the foundation of mental hospitals well into the eighteenth century.[9]

Furthermore, mental hospitals were by no means a late seventeenth-century innovation or uniformly mechanisms of control in the hands of repressive social and political regimes.[10] The first European institutions that cared for the mentally disordered appeared in Spain as early as the beginning of the fifteenth century.[11] Over the next two centuries and beyond, similar institutions emerged throughout Europe. As Lisa Roscioni has cautioned, there is not one history of European mental institutions but many. Each institution recalls a custodial experiment whose nature was shaped largely by its immediate context. Sometimes the foundation of institutions that took on the care of the mad offered desperate families compassionate care options outside households; at other times their foundation signaled the tightening mesh of political or professional power over certain social groups or types of behavior; sometimes well-intentioned institutional missions failed in one generation, succeeded in another, only to fail again.[12]

The three hundred or so cases that make up this study show that the practical and sometimes highly adversarial arena of the courts was also an important site of social experimentation. In the Tuscan context, conflicts and collaborations between petitioners and their officials over what to do about the mentally impaired or criminally insane generated new social, legal, and institutional remedies. They also provided predators with opportunities to exploit the vulnerable for their own gain—something that did not escape the notice of attentive magistrates. But herein lies both the creative and destructive potential of what Olwen Hufton called "the economy of makeshifts" and Nicholas Terpstra the "politics of makeshifts," that constant and opportunistic grasping for solutions to intractable realities be it a poor person trying to make ends meet, an entire society at work on providing social welfare, or families and courts tackling the problems madness posed.[13]

Historians like neat paradigms; human experience resists them. As Terpstra has elegantly shown in his recent book on poor relief in

Renaissance Bologna, the sweeping linear drive of history papers over the complex shifting dynamics that characterize a society's efforts to confront its challenges. It is that spirit of experimentation, dynamism, dialogue, and exchange that I invoke here.

THE LEGACY OF CULTURE

Although historians have brought the seventeenth- and eighteenth-century experience of madness more sharply into view, the social reality of madness has been harder to capture for medieval and early modern Europe because of the fragmentary nature of the period's archival records and, perhaps counterintuitively, because of the extraordinary richness of its cultural tradition.[14] Decades of excellent scholarship have shown that medieval and early modern Europeans thought a great deal about behavior that defied their sense of what it meant to be rational. During this period, the European intellectual and cultural elite contemplated madness in art, literature, philosophy, and theology, passing on to posterity moving visions of mad lovers, melancholy artists, brooding scholars, frenzied heroes, courtly fools, and the divinely or demonically possessed.[15] The mad and their madnesses were living symbols of the wages of sin, the consequences of immoderate passion, and the vanity of earthly life.

And indeed such representations of madness have important and revealing histories. As the fifteenth century drew to a close, for example, personifications of folly captured the European imagination with renewed vigor.[16] From Sebastian Brandt's (1457–1521) ship of fools to Erasmus's (1466–1536) drunken trollop Stultitia to Cervantes's (1547–1616) addled knight Don Quixote, artists and authors invoked folly simultaneously to entertain their audiences and to remind them of the fragility, uncertainty, and wretchedness of the human condition and the glory of the kingdom of God.[17]

Tuscans also availed themselves of folly's symbolic potential. On June 22, 1514, the first day of the celebrations for the festival of Florence's patron saint John the Baptist, one of the floats that appeared along the procession route was a *fusta piena di matti*—a ship of fools. Prancing along behind it were about thirty men dressed as devils, holding hooks and bells. At one point they grabbed someone from the crowd and tossed him in the ship, barring his escape unless he paid a bounty.[18] But these topsy-turvy, carnivalesque performances of folly that entertained as much as they challenged social norms bear little resemblance to the men and women who appear in court records. They tell us a good deal about how madness was imagined, little about how it was lived.

As the sixteenth century progressed, melancholy, at once a physical disease, mental disposition, and potentially perilous spiritual condition, became all the rage among Europe's elite. For historians of northern Europe, melancholy's heightened profile was an expression of deep psychological anxiety triggered by the turbulent era of religious reform in western Christendom. In England, Michael Mac-Donald connected the melancholy vogue to sectarian conflict and the fanaticism it inspired.[19] During the English Revolution, various sects used madness to describe a world beset by demons and sin on the one hand and, on the other, humankind's troubled path to righteousness. Falling into the ditch of despair along the road to right belief was just as dangerous as falling prey to unbridled religious exuberance. Fueled by achievements in physical science and anatomy as well as their "orthodox hatred of religious enthusiasm," elites rejected religious views about madness and melancholy to embrace instead more level-headed secular, medical explanations.[20] In Germany, melancholy begins its sixteenth-century career as a Lutheran obsession with sin and the devil to find itself on the eve of the seventeenth century recast as mental illness—the result of both spiritual exhaustion after more than a century of sporadic but devastating religious warfare throughout Europe and the fruits of the medicalization of European society.[21]

Tuscans did not suffer the same religious turmoil as their northern neighbors, but they shared early modern Europe's fascination with melancholy. It was, after all, a number of famous Tuscans often in dialogue with other Italian philosophers and literati who helped originate and spread ideas about melancholy throughout Europe. The three crowns of Florentine literature, Dante, Petrarch, and Boccaccio, spoke of the physical and spiritual perturbations that gripped the melancholy lover; Marsilio Ficino (1433–1499), a famous medically trained Neoplatonist from Florence in his influential work *Three Books on Life* (1489), and Angelo Poliziano (1454–1494), a Neoplatonist among Ficino's set who hailed from the Tuscan town of Montepulciano, popularized the idea of melancholy genius.[22] Lodovico Ariosto (1474–1533), one of Emilia-Romagna's if not Italy's most famous Renaissance poets, drew heavily from these sources to shape the character of Orlando Furioso, the hero driven mad by obsessive and pathological love.[23] These works in turn nourished a broader fascination with melancholy and its many manifestations.

Larger-than-life characters fascinate, but they also mislead. Literary invention should not—must not—obscure the lives of mentally disturbed individuals and the people who lived with and around them. Some of the men and women who populated Florentine court records were said to have been melancholic, but they remain far removed from the likes of Ariosto's mad Orlando. The three hundred cases that make up this study push beyond the heady realm of high culture to recapture those decidedly unromantic, day-to-day experiences of madness that, in some cases, measured themselves out in interminable moments of stress and anxiety for everyone involved. As one petitioner told a Florentine court in the sixteenth century, "the care of a mad man is a heavy burden." Madness for him and his family was not symbolic; it was real. How it was experienced, how it was addressed, by whom and with what results—these are the questions that open new windows onto the social and institutional history of a late medieval and early modern society.

The goal of catching Tuscans in the act of dealing with madness has shaped this book. We begin not with the evocative representations of madness in medieval and early modern art and literature but with Tuscans in their households as they tried to figure out—sometimes desperately—what to do with their mentally impaired or criminally insane kin. Chapter 1 examines cases emanating from civil courts. Accounting for a little less than half of the three hundred sample cases, they show families asking judges for help assigning legal guardians to mentally incompetent kin. This was ordinarily done to protect them from exploitation and abuse by other family members or to protect the family itself from financially reckless behavior. Chapter 2 addresses the remaining half of this sample, which appeared in criminal courts where Florentine families strategically and effectively employed categories denoting madness to negotiate sentences, mitigate punishments, or get relatives released from prison.

Florence underwent far-reaching constitutional changes during the period covered by this book. From the thirteenth century to 1494, the Florentine polity was communal with a republican form of government. By 1532, after four political revolutions and significant constitutional reform, the republic finally gave way to a regional duchy with a Medici once again at the helm. Like the early Medici and their partisans who came to exercise extraordinary executive power beginning in 1434, the Medici dukes and their administrators saw legal institutions, particularly those with criminal jurisdiction, as important mechanisms for legitimating, maintaining, and exercising political power.[24] The ducal system of justice was highly centralized and absolutist relative to the one it replaced. It did not, however, significantly imperil the mentally impaired as some historians have suggested.[25]

Even as the size and reach of the government grew, private strategies employed by families in pursuit of long-term custodial arrangements often trumped legal norms. Far from revealing expanding mechanisms of control in Florentine government and society, these cases illustrate the limited (though not unimportant) role that public institutions played in the care of those who could not care for themselves. In all of these cases, the spirit of compromise and negotiation reigned; judges were willing to take into account the needs of families as long as there was no threat to public order and as long as the courts were not being abused for personal gain—a likelihood in some cases. The thorniest of questions was what to do with the mentally disturbed. To that question, there was no easy answer. Care of mad men and women was more often than not an *ad hoc* arrangement of uncertain duration, utterly contingent on the presence, willingness, and ability of relatives to bear the inconveniences associated with tending to their incapacitated kin.

To put it another way, this book is not merely a "bottom-up" corrective to histories that have taken madness in medieval and early modern Europe for a cultural artifact or a lever of social control. It argues, too, that social ordering from household to street was a collaborative affair in which petitioners and civic authorities mutually worked to find solutions to the practical problems madness created with a view to serving both private and public interest though balance between them might not always have won the day.

Chapter 3 puts households in dialogue with Tuscan society's values more broadly. The civil and criminal cases that make up this study show in particular its changing attitudes to wealth and consumption. From the fourteenth through the seventeenth century, in pace with the rise of a consumer society and a constantly changing economy, petitioners and officers of the ducal administration came more and more to apply an economic definition of mental incapacity to regulate financial behavior in Tuscan households and invalidate contracts made by reckless kin—a tactic that was used by individuals to protect family patrimony and by ducal administrators to police transactions in the marketplace. Petitioners and magistrates alike explicitly linked prodigality and madness—in Roman law two categorically distinct states—on the principle that only a truly mad person would throw money away to the detriment of his or her family. To put it differently, in the fourteenth century, Christian values of poverty, humility, and renunciation shaped attitudes to spending and consumption. By the sixteenth century, attitudes to money and its uses had shifted so as to foreground what I call patrimonial rationality, an ethical bent that considered the relative appropriateness of material expenditure in the context of a web of social relationships and obligations. In the fourteenth century, the spendthrift was a sinful man. By the sixteenth century, he was a patrimonial saboteur; he was a mad man.

Chapters 4 and 5 address the organic or medical turn that the history of madness in Florence took in the mid-sixteenth century. Prior to the reforms of the 1540s, traditional Roman law categories for incapacity sufficed; the mentally impaired were generically referred to as *furiosi*, *mentecapti*, *fatui*, and *dementes* in Latin, and, in Italian, *pazzi*, *matti*, and *mentecatti*. After 1540, lay petitioners began for the first time to put learned medical ideas that originated in professional or pedagogical settings in the service of the complex social realities of their households. By the sixteenth century, madness had become more explicitly an illness and one thought adversely to affect proper brain function.

The learned medical tradition offered several ways of resolving legal ambiguities in cases of alleged mental illness. Physicians had made an art of reading the signs of the body on the assumption that madness was a disease of the brain with physical manifestations. The Roman doctor-jurist Paolo Zacchia (1584–1659) argued forcefully in favor of medical expertise in certain types of cases, including those involving mental incapacity. Between 1621 and 1659, he issued the *Quaestiones Medico-Legales*, a monumental analysis of medico-legal topics and case studies that would continue to appear in multiple editions throughout Europe until 1789.[26] In light of these developments, historians have spoken of the emergence of "legal medicine" in seventeenth-century continental Europe.

But the focus on the doctor in court has obscured other key players in the history of medico-legal relations. Lay litigants and their witnesses were far more central than historians of medicine and law have led us to believe. This shift in thinking and talking about mental incapacity is part of the history of the medicalization of European society, that long and complex process by which medicine was increasingly woven into the social, cultural, institutional, and legal fabric of European life. Until relatively recently medical practitioners took center stage in the history of the medicalization of European society. By contrast, new scholarship has refocused the spotlight on patients/consumers as key players in molding the growing market for health care during the later Middle Ages and early modern period.[27]

Building on these studies, the principal *dramatis personae* here are lay petitioners who successfully used medical language in court—often without the help of medical practitioners. Formal medical-legal writing that privileged the expertise of the physician in cases of mental illness echoed a conversation that had already been taking place in the households and courts of Florence for at least a century, and one that was not necessarily driven by physicians, lawyers, judges, or magistrates. What is more, lay petitioners advanced medical explanations for madness in court and courts tended to accept them without recourse to medical testimony or explicit certification by a medical practitioner.

The book closes with the opening of Santa Dorotea and Santa Maria Nuova's "pazzeria" in the mid- to late seventeenth century. These institutions could not house large numbers, but they provided a new answer to an old question: what on earth should we do with our severely disturbed kin? These new answers were not crowning moments in state-building or professional progress narratives. They were rather the culmination of a long and dynamic sociocultural process that saw ordinary Tuscans struggling sometimes with and sometimes against professional and civic authorities to find long-term care solutions for their vulnerable or unmanageable kin. At no point did learned men operating in their professional milieux enjoy unique authority in describing madness specifically and incapacity more generally. The categories of madness were instead hammered out in practical arenas like the courts where litigants and judges together forged pragmatic solutions to the range of problems madness visited on their households and communities.

As the title suggests, *Mad Tuscans and Their Families* tells a Tuscan story. But Tuscany shared with the rest of Italy and Europe common legal and medical traditions and, until the cataclysmic religious upheavals of the sixteenth century, a more or less common theological tradition as well. In this respect, the history of madness told here reflects larger European trends. Though other regions may follow the same general patterns of thought and action, the particular contours of the political, economic, and institutional history of Florence and her Tuscan domains distinguish her from her Italian and European counterparts who had different institutional and governing arrangements as well as different experiences of sixteenth- and seventeenth-century religious reformations. Variations in frameworks of care existed throughout early modern Europe. The history of madness in Spain, for example, would perhaps begin rather than end with the foundation of hospitals devoted to the care of the mad. It is for this reason that *Mad Tuscans* is *a* rather than *the* history of mental disorder in early modern Italy. It is intended not as a universalizing narrative but one that forms a base from which other Italian and European comparisons can be made.

Some may take issue with the use of the phrases "late medieval" and "early modern" to refer to the period covered by this study, from roughly the mid-fourteenth to roughly the mid-seventeenth century. Other historians have used the category "early modern" to cover the period beginning in the mid-fifteenth century and extending as far as 1789. This book does not set out to solve what Randolph Starn called the "early modern muddle."[28] The term remains an awkward and imperfect solution to the problem of periodizing the time between medieval and modern history without falling back on restrictive and value-laden categories like Renaissance and Reformation that limit a study's temporal and regional scope. Where the term "Renaissance" suggests the literate, classicizing, urban-based culture of lay elites, the term "early modern" is socially inclusive. Most of the families who went to court were from elite or at least middling backgrounds, but the whole social spectrum appears. This reason warrants its use here.

WAYS OF SEEING

In *The God of Small Things* Arundati Roy speaks of an old, abandoned place that her characters call the History House. The fleshy, life-worn Chacko explains to his young niece and nephew that "history [is] like an old house at night. With all the lamps lit. And ancestors whispering inside." "To understand history," he tells the children, "we have to go inside and listen to what they're saying. And look at the books and the pictures on the wall. And smell the smells."

"But," he admits, "we can't go in because we've been locked out. And when we try and listen, all we hear is a whispering."[29]

Social historians have long tried to gain entry to the History House. They have used tax records to re-create the structure of families.[30] They have rifled through letters, diaries, day-to-day domestic scribbling, and court records to conjure up the beliefs and practices that animated social life in the home and public square.[31] They have examined or imagined the furniture, *objets d'art*, textiles, jewelry, trinkets, and baubles that people from the past made or purchased to furnish and decorate their rooms, to dress and adorn their bodies.[32] They have pored over recipe collections, medical books, and self-help manuals that were stashed in drawers or sat on shelves in private households in order to observe men and women in the act of caring for and treating their bodies, minds, and souls.[33]

This book also endeavors to cross the threshold of Tuscan households to try to observe what families did when faced with a mentally impaired relative. The documentary record, however, tends to confront the historian with a grimy if not completely shuttered window. Histories of madness are in some respects histories of invisible people. Seldom do mad men and women appear, for example, in the stemma that the great nineteenth-century Italian genealogists Pompeo Litta and Luigi Passerini made of Italy's oldest families. The three mad Martellis that we meet in Chapter 1 are invisible boughs on these celebrated ancestral trees. One wonders how much fuller the foliage would be if all of the invisible people came into view.

Social historians have typically sought information about family life in the account books and family journals (*ricordanze*) that many Tuscans left behind. On the subject of their mad relatives, they are practically mute. In a rare entry of 1466, Domenico Cambini spoke of a cousin who asked that he assume the care of his sister Caterina who "had a lack of mind and intellect."[34] He tells us that she stayed in his house for three years before moving in with her brother Berto. What those three years were like he did not say. In 1522, the notary Piero Bonaccorsi mentioned an "infirm and mad" sister whose care he and his brothers took turns assuming. She seems to have been a handful. She made a mess of the house he kept her in so much so that he would not bring his family there and kept her locked up.[35] Except for these brief mentions, I know of no private accounts written by mentally incapacitated individuals, their caretakers, or their abusers.

In the absence of direct access to the social experience of madness, we must proceed obliquely. In the absence of a coherent demographic, we must seek sources that open up a broad catchment area.
The entry point for this study is the civil and criminal courts of Florence from roughly 1350 to about 1670, our principal (though by no
means only) sources, the legal records that these institutions produced
in the course of daily practice and the statutes that regulated them.
The mentally disturbed first appear in the records of the civil and
criminal courts of Florence in the fourteenth century. At this point,
they are few, far between, and buried in the heavy caseloads of several different courts whose jurisdictions overlapped. In order to proceed as systematically as possible, I took two-year soundings of the
Podestà and Capitano del Popolo, republican Florence's principal civil
and criminal courts, for every decade beginning with 1350 until 1502
when these courts were abolished.

After 1502, the Otto di Guardia e Balia picked up the criminal
jurisdiction in Florence; it is this court that supplies the bulk of
criminal cases. Although many of these records have succumbed
to time, a fairly regular document run can be put together from
1470 to the 1680s with occasional lacunae of a year or two. By
contrast, the records of Florence's main prison, the Stinche, provide some additional examples, but they are not as revealing as
one might hope. The entry and exit registers refer in the briefest
of terms to people who ended up there *per pazzo* (for being mad).
The records of the Stinche's infirmary are similarly reticent. Unless
an inmate appeared also in the Pupilli or the Otto, there is simply
no way of giving these men and women personalities or back stories. Whether the charge that someone was *pazzo* stuck or merely
marked the beginning of litigation arguing the contrary remains
obscured from view.

The records of Florence's court of wards (the Magistrato dei Pupilli
ed Adulti) have furnished the largest sample of civil cases. With the
exception of some missing registers, I was able to consult most of the
extant records of the Pupilli from its foundation in the 1390s through
the 1670s when the mad become less numerous in the documentary
record. I cannot account for this diminution except to say that it corresponds with the reign of the penultimate Medici duke, Cosimo III
(r. 1670–1723), who reconfigured and expanded the Tuscan system
of justice.[36] The mad resurface in the Pupilli during the 1720s, but by
that point the context has changed markedly.[37]

For ducal Tuscany, there are examples of mentally disturbed men and women in the records of an executive council established in 1532 called the Magistrato Supremo. Composed of a *luogotenente* chosen by the duke and four counselors who were elected every three months, this magistracy served also as a tribunal of first instance and appeal.[38] The Magistrato Supremo directly controlled the Pupilli, which could not declare a person mentally impaired without its consent.

On the whole, the courts of the Capitano and the Podestà for the republican period and those of the Pupilli backed by the Magistrato Supremo and the Otto for the duchy were the legal arena in which petitioners and authorities met to deal with the practical problems that severe mental or physical incapacity generated in their households and on their streets. All told, these sources yield about three hundred cases in which a term indicating mental impairment was pinned onto a person by a civic official, a petitioner, an accuser, or, in rare instances, by the very person him- or herself.

Cases of mental and physical incapacity are rare relative to the usual business of Florence's criminal and civil courts. Surely there were a good deal more than three hundred mentally disturbed men, women, and children in Florence and its Tuscan domains between the mid-fourteenth and mid-seventeenth centuries. That number reflects only the number of times Tuscan families went to court or ended up there. Allegedly mad men and women tend to leave archival traces only if they posed a serious threat to their families or communities. To put it another way, these three hundred or so cases generally show families and communities in desperate situations using the courts to restore or maintain order. Without a doubt a great many more lived in obscurity behind the closed doors of households, some may have been lucky enough to secure temporary beds in hospitals, others may have ended up in foundling homes, monasteries, or convents, or, having been turned out, some likely joined the ranks of the homeless poor.

Whether or not we "hear" a case involving madness seems to have been contingent on regime. The great bulk of the three hundred cases were prosecuted between 1540, when the newly fashioned ducal system of justice was fully operational, and about 1609, when power devolved to Cosimo II (r. 1609–1621), who, owing to ill health, left much of the administration of the duchy to his ministers. Beginning around 1610, cases involving mental and physical incapacity grow less numerous. After the 1650s they fade yet more until the second quarter of the seventeenth century when they break the documentary sound barrier again. The instability of the record particularly after 1650 made the foundations of Santa Dorotea and the mad ward at Santa Maria Nuova good notional end points for this study. After 1670, some of our best evidence for the lived experience of madness in Florentine society comes from Santa Dorotea itself, but there begins a very different play acted on an alien stage. It is a tale worth telling but a different tale from the one I tell here.

Making these cases speak is also difficult. If history is an act of translation involved in making the objects, images, and texts created and used by past peoples intelligible in the here and now, court records are written in a queer cipher. Their decoding warrants a good deal of care. Historians have long warned of their power to fascinate and mislead. As Arlette Farge and Trevor Dean artfully put it, judicial records create a "reality effect," that is, the false sense that we have direct access to the experiences of real people and their real problems or struggles.[39] But court records are artifacts of the courts that produced them. The interpretation of judicial documents must begin with an understanding of the formal apparatus and language of the courts that necessarily shaped and limited the way parties could present and argue their cases. The structure, procedure, and language of Florentine justice changed a great deal between the fourteenth and seventeenth centuries. Each chapter establishes the institutional context in which cases were argued with particular attention to what type of language petitioners used to frame their arguments and judges drew on to make their decisions.

There is also the problem of what Sara Tilghman Nalle has called the "negative spaces of the historical text." Sometimes it's not so much what was documented but what was not recorded—those important details that were too obvious, too mundane, or perhaps too dangerous to write down—that holds the key to understanding a family's situation. I have tried where possible to include peripheral documentation to add further layers to a family's story. For the most part, though, what we have here are the tantalizingly imperfect records from courts.

It is worth pausing for a moment to consider language, the most obvious and problematic of transformations that took place in Florentine courts for the "reality effect" it introduces into judicial sources. Republican courts operated in Latin, ducal courts in Italian. Prior to the 1530s, when petitioners and litigants brought cases to court, lawyers or recording notaries had to translate the vernacular words they used to describe the mental state of their relatives into preexisting legal categories and concepts as they existed in Latin—a task that necessarily involved linguistic distortion. Jurists and magistrates plucked these terms from Justinian's sixth-century compilation of Roman law, the *Corpus iuris civilis*, where the opinions of a range of Roman jurists on the problem of mental incapacity and its legal consequences were scattered throughout.[40] This was no easy task.

Roman jurists recognized that madness did not reside only on the outer extremes of human behavior. They acknowledged that its manifestations stretched across a spectrum, ranging from immaturity and foolishness to complete mindlessness, and that these internal conditions produced a range of different behaviors. They captured the breadth of this spectrum in terms and phrases that generally described the lack of reason (*intellectus*) and intent (*animus, voluntas, affectio*).[41] The mad were likened to children, a person who is asleep, and a person who is absent or not properly present in mind. Roman jurists called states of madness *furor, dementia, insania*, alienation of mind (*alienatio mentis*), to lack one's senses (*intellectu carere*), and not being in possession of one's mind (*non suae mentis* or *non compos mentis*). Those suffering from these impairments they called *furiosi, dementes, insani, mentecapti*, and *fatui*. The term *furiosus* generally referred to an unaccountably violent or wild person while *demens, mentecaptus, insanus*, and *fatuus* usually suggested a nonviolent but feebleminded person. These were not hard and fast distinctions; categories often overlapped.[42]

Learned legal ruminations on the matter by medieval jurists did little to clarify the situation. The famous Italian jurist Bartolus da Sassoferrato (1313–1357) systematically analyzed Roman law categories for mental incapacity in a treatise in which he listed the qualities a witness necessarily had to possess for his or her testimony to be considered valid. Like his Roman counterparts, Bartolus broadly distinguished between the *furiosus* who raved and the *mentecaptus* who showed an innocuous inability to make sense of or judgments about the world. *Dementes, insani, fatui*, and *stulti* were specific types of *mentecaptus*. Bartolus went to some length to make finer distinctions between these states in an attempt to link abnormal thought and its consequent behaviors more accurately.[43] But he did not ultimately change the categories handed down by Roman law or do much to solve the problem of ambiguity between them in the courts.

After the 1530s, Italian replaced Latin as the language of legal record. Florentines did not abandon Roman law vocabulary; they Italianized it to create the terms *furioso*, *mentecatto*, *insano*, *dementia*, *fatuità*. They added colloquial vernacular terms like *pazzo* and *matto*, both roughly meaning a person out of his or her senses with *pazzo* on the more aggressive and *matto* the more docile sides of the spectrum, though again, these generalizations often overlapped. Both sets of terms, the technical Latinate and colloquial vernacular, were effective in court.

Freed from restrictive Roman law terminology, petitioners in ducal Tuscany also employed a rich array of terms and modifying adjectives to identify as precisely as possible the particular nature of the mental disturbance at hand. They described their incapacitated kin as being completely out of mind ("non in cervello," "non sta in cervello," "non in sè," "mancamento di cervello"); of limited or tending toward bad judgment ("poco cervello," "poco ingegno et cervello," "pochissimo cervello," "debol mente," "poco capacità d'intelletto," "difecto di mente," "mezzo matto"); or having a childlike commerce with the world around them ("scemo di cervello," "semplice," "leggier di cervello," "semplice che altro," "uccellabile,"). There are also many examples of people who were called by terms that generally suggested mental incapacity but who also seem to have had accompanying sensory or motor impairments. Muteness and stuttering were commonly thought to indicate mental as well as physical disability. Tuscans also described the mental states and explained the unaccountable behavior of their impaired relatives by drawing on vocabularies of honor, economy, and medicine.

Fine categorical distinctions were important in cases where a petitioner may have wished only to excuse strange or unruly behavior without depriving a person of legal agency once and for all. In other words, linguistic shading gave magistrates and laypeople a way to accommodate a broad spectrum of incapacity as they experienced it in the hopes of achieving the legal outcome they sought. For historians, such distinctions are slippery. It is imperative to try to establish whether what looks like a real transformation in the ways Florentines talked about their mentally disturbed kin were the result of substantive social or cultural changes or merely an unveiling phenomenon attributable to changes in the way the courts operated and the language they employed. It is, in part, for this reason that I have left many terms in their original Latin or Italian. The purpose is to invite the reader to experience the fluidity, malleability, and subtlety of language—in this case, I think it fair to use the term "discourse"—as Tuscans struggled to explain mental, emotional, and behavioral states that made little sense to them.

It is also for this reason that I use the term "madness" throughout the book. Like Erik Midelfort, whose lead I follow on this point, there is a certain methodological utility in the ambiguity of the term precisely because it forces historians to pay close attention to the language historical actors used to describe people whose thoughts, feelings, and actions seemed unreasonable. Readers will also notice that I sometimes refer to physical disabilities. This study is full of examples of people who were called by terms that generally suggested mental incapacity but who might also have had accompanying sensory or motor impairments as well.[44] Disability is a capacious category of historical analysis; in modern usage it includes a range of mental, cognitive, sensory, and physical impairments. Madness here functions as a subset of disability, referring specifically to the impact abnormal cognitive, emotional, and behavioral states had on families. Moreover, in Florentine courts, the ability to exercise reason was the *sine qua non* of legal agency. The mad may have suffered from some kind of physical impairment, but the physically impaired were not necessarily considered mad.

I have also used the term "mental" in combination with incapacity, impairment, and disorder to describe instances in which families believed sickness, injury, or some external cause had adversely affected brain function and consequently a person's rational faculties. This is not a modern but a late medieval and early modern distinction. It is also not meant to evoke a philosophical notion of mind. In the twenty and twenty-first centuries, the problem of madness has raised a host of questions about the relationship between mind, soul, and body, competing biological and psychological theories about the brain, the nature of selfhood, consciousness, and identity that lie outside the purview of this study. Medieval and early modern Europeans, who had a worldview that incorporated philosophical, medical, and religious ways of thinking about the relationship between mental and physical states, found these modern problems less discrete.

As for numbers, I have analyzed these cases qualitatively rather than quantitatively, but some important patterns emerge. Mad men and women constituted a complex, heterogeneous population that defies easy categorization. They were young and old, male and female, rich and poor. They also exhibited varying degrees of incapacity. Some never developed the rational faculties of adults while others matured more or less in line with social expectations but repeatedly made poor or disastrous decisions. Some were chronically vegetative or wild while others swung in and out of lucidity, wavering between periods of high and low functioning.

Many of them were not marginal but deeply networked. As carriers of patrimony, husbands and wives, fathers and mothers, sons and daughters, kith, kin, and neighbors, they were entangled in the social, economic, and political webs that bound society together. They were not universally considered "bambini innocenti," or innocent babies as Enrico Stumpo called them.[45] Most of them were not children but adults for whom there were no obvious custodial institutions. In other words, these were not necessarily people who had slipped through holes in the social web. In many cases, they were the threads that constituted it.

Broadly speaking, a little less than half of the three hundred cases that make up this study are civil suits, a little more than half are criminal. Since the Pupilli was a patrimonial court, civil suits tended to involve people who had property to protect. That said, where well-heeled families tend to make up the bulk of civil cases prior to 1540, after that point, people from middling and even humble backgrounds availed themselves of the courts in greater numbers. A larger cross-section of the social world appears in criminal courts. The poor and socially unconnected tended, as they typically do, to fare worse than their wealthier neighbors in criminal cases. They were, for example, more likely to be sent into penal servitude or exiled; they generally tended to pay for their crimes with their bodies rather than their purses.

Numbers are most revealing when we consider gender. From 1540 to roughly 1600, men are identified as mad in 84 percent of civil cases and women 16 percent. Similarly, men appear as mad in 89 percent of criminal cases and women only 11 percent. Where were the mad women in medieval and early modern Tuscany? Surely they existed. They are underrepresented there because Roman and Florentine law considered sex a limiting factor on legal status. A woman, by virtue of her sex, enjoyed the same privileges and limitations as a minor even after she had attained her majority.[46] Men were the primary social, political, and legal actors in their communities, the primary guardians and transmitters of patrilineage, and the principal bearers of honor. A man's descent into madness threatened to send shock waves through his family especially if he were the head of the household. The implications of a woman's madness were much less significant.

The courts tell us little about the madness of women but rather a lot about how it affected them since their social and legal vulnerability made women big stakeholders in the problem of male madness. They were the primary caretakers of mad kin; and, like children, they tended to suffer the most when a man could not perform his occupation or manage patrimony. That said, vulnerability did not mean automatic victimhood. Where women were rarely brought to court for being mad, they frequently appeared in court records as petitioners. In civil cases, male kin accounted for 46 percent of the petitioners named in civil cases and female kin made up 42 percent, roughly the equivalent.

Of the 42 percent of female petitioners who brought civil cases, the great majority were widowed matriarchs—mothers and aunts—who, in the absence of a strong male presence in the household, often policed the social and economic behavior of their sons and nephews. Practically speaking, the loss of a husband was not universally a bad thing. It left some women with liberty and leverage to manage their estates or meddle in the estate management of their relatives. In cases involving madness, we are just as likely to see women acting as guardians of patrimony, savvy navigators of the courts, and even shameless exploiters of vulnerable relatives as we are to see them as victims. Here a woman's ability to act was determined more by her socioeconomic status than her sex.

This is an important point to make because some historians might interpret what I call patrimonial rationality in Chapter 3 differently. In a recent study of gender and charity, for example, Philip Gavitt spoke of lineage ideology, by which he meant a rigidly patriarchal view of the Tuscan household that came to prominence in the fifteenth and sixteenth centuries. The culprit, according to Gavitt and historians of similar mind, was a profound economic crisis that reshaped the system of inheritance especially to the detriment of women. To soften its effects, elite families vigorously promoted the patrimonial interests of their eldest male heirs.[47] As a result, boys and girls who might dilute a patrimony were sent to foundling homes, orphanages, and convents. Women had little chance of marrying out of this system and increasingly came to spend their lives in institutions that were not originally meant to house them. To add insult to injury, these

institutions fashioned themselves according to the domestic meta-
phors that shaped lineage ideology. In other words, they foisted onto
their wards the very ideals that had marginalized them in the first
place.

While lineage ideology is a useful concept for thinking about the
poor and poor relief, it tends to break down in the face of the intractable realities or golden opportunities that madness brought to better-
off Tuscan households. The maintenance of patriarchal inheritance
schemes was counterproductive in the extreme if the person diluting
or dissipating patrimony was the man controlling the family's purse
strings. The case studies that appear throughout this book do not necessarily demonstrate the immiseration of relatives, especially women,
at the hands of male heads of households. Rather, they tend to show
the unseating of those addled heads in the interest of the family as a
whole. To put it another way, patrimonial rationality was simultaneously a standard against which people measured a person's spending
habits and a practical strategy that we see in action when the material
integrity of a line was in peril. Unlike lineage ideology, patrimonial
rationality could empower women. Through it we see the society of
makeshifts at work.

The title of this book is meant to evoke David Herlihy and Christiane
Klapisch-Zuber's revolutionary study, *Tuscans and Their Families*, a
massive analysis of the Florentine population as seen through the lens
of the 1427 tax census known as the *Catasto*. I could not have written this book without that monumental work and the scholarship it
inspired. According to Herlihy and Klapisch-Zuber, the *Catasto* had
the power to "scan the land like the rays of the summer sun," so rich
was it in demographic and social detail.[48] The cases that form the
basis of this study are more akin to three-hundred-odd spotlights of
varying strength and breadth flickering across Tuscan domains over
a three-hundred-year period. In some cases, the spotlight centers on
a person while also capturing a complex network of relatives, neighbors, and civic authorities as they interacted at home, on the streets,
and at court. In other cases, the light is narrow and dim, making a
person seem like an inscrutable glow surrounded by darkness.

But the situation is not as grim as that. Generations of scholars
have shed light on the social, political, economic, and cultural landscape of medieval and early modern Italy. This book helps populate
that already bountiful space with a group of people who are usually

invisible in the histories of premodern European societies, not just the mentally and physically impaired but those who watched, cared for, and struggled with or near them.

Used properly, legal sources have a great deal to tell, not least of all that late medieval and early modern Europeans did not routinely, as it was once claimed, push the mad outside of cities and towns. They were not shut up in prisons, hospitals, monasteries, or convents or crammed onto fictional ships of fools. Far from being marginal or merely satirical in medieval and early modern Tuscan society, they lived in households; they inherited property that had to be managed and passed on; they had legal rights and obligations that they may or may not have been competent to exercise. They did not live as cultural artifacts but as parents, siblings, neighbors, citizens, and subjects. When they appear in court records, they are often at the center rather than on the fringes of family struggles over property, patrimony, and household management. Perhaps there were some, perhaps many who wanted to cast their disturbed relatives out, throw this one in jail, send that one off to a convent—in other words, make a mentally disturbed person someone else's problem. Surely that happened. It happens now. Archival records tell a more complex and compelling story.

CHAPTER I

Incapacity, Guardianship, and the Tuscan Family

The care of a madman is a heavy burden.

—ASF, MPAP 2276, fol. 6r

In the late summer of 1560, a widow named Monna Francesca went before the Magistrato dei Pupilli ed Adulti, Florence's court of wards, to arrange for the guardianship of her young relative Francesco. At nineteen, Francesco was a year past the age of legal majority, yet Monna Francesca still "treated him like a child." "Mute" and "impaired," the boy "did not speak or understand anything." Several years before, the Pupilli had entrusted his care and the management of his estate to Monna Francesca, an arrangement that was meant to be temporary. When Francesco turned eighteen, his care was to shift to his closest living male relative on his father's side.[1]

That person happened to be his brother Lodovico, whom Monna Francesca considered unfit for the job. After some investigation, the Pupilli agreed. Lodovico, they discovered, was not a suitable guardian: "he spent the greater part of the year in a villa, he had his own wife and children, and he had rather diminished his own wealth." Moreover, he stood to inherit Francesco's modest income after he died, adding between thirty-four and thirty-six ducats a year to his own pocket.[2]

Florentine law prevented Monna Francesca from appointing a guardian she deemed appropriate on her own. That privilege was the sole province of relatives who could exercise paternal power, namely, fathers and grandfathers.[3] She was not without recourse, however. Through the Pupilli, she could invite magisterial intervention to try to protect Francesco from abuse or the plunder of his estate by a relative on the make. In response, and wishing "to avoid every sinister

suspicion" of fraud resting on the improvement of Lodovico's fortunes should his brother die, the Pupilli assumed Francesco's care.[4]
They would manage his property and see to it that he was properly
fed and clothed until his death when the remainder of his estate would
revert to Lodovico through the established legal path of succession.
With that the record falls silent; we have no sense of where, how, and
with whom Francesco measured out the rest of his days. Still his case
brings to light the anxieties that relatives and magistrates alike shared
about the fate of vulnerable kin and the property attached to them.

We catch glimpses of people like Francesco and hear the reverberations they sent through their families in cases that involved guardianship. Legal guardianship aimed, often missing its mark, to solve two
perennial problems. On the one hand, it sought to protect vulnerable kin from exploitation and abuse by predatory or negligent family
members. On the other hand, guardianship endeavored to protect the
family as a whole from the kind of social and financial anarchy that
mental or physical incompetence of whatever type threatened to visit
on a household. A person like Francesco disrupted the safe passage of
patrimony from one generation to the next—one of the most important obligations a man of property owed the future of his lineage. He
was simultaneously a mark for grasping relatives and a menace to the
social and financial stability of his family.

Cases in which families sought guardianship for impaired relatives reveal the complex blend of conflict and negotiation, sentiment
and interest that existed within and between Tuscan families. They
bear witness to how families cooperated with each other, often reaching across lineages to provide care for those who could not care for
themselves. By contrast, they show that men and women like Francesco could be staging grounds for battles over the control of property
and patrimony between maternal and paternal kin. In such cases, the
allegedly mentally incapacitated person was incidental, more akin to
an object of value, not unlike a piece of real estate, returns on shares
in the public debt, or a disputed claim on rental income, than a person needing care.

These cases also show the instrumental use of legal institutions and
the limits of their intervention. Although family strategies and legal
institutions directed toward such care existed, neither families nor the
courts had worked out a surefire way to ensure the long-term supervision and protection of the impaired. Legal norms could not always
be made to fit the complex vicissitudes of family life. Parents and

caregivers died, lived far away, or were absorbed in their own affairs. Eligible candidates for guardianship often renounced their responsibility and those deemed responsible for providing care were not always equal to the task. The question of who ultimately bore responsibility for incapacitated adults had no easy answer. It was a burden often left at the door of others. In its worst instances, it was an opportunity seized by those who preyed on vulnerable relatives for profit.

It has long been the practice of social and political historians to use the law and its application in the courts and magistracies of Florence to reveal mechanisms of social and political control in Florentine government and society. Disorder caused by cyclical recurrence of plague beginning in 1347, the costs of warfare, and struggles for political supremacy have all been cast at one time or another as stimuli for the "centralizing administrative tendencies" of Florentine governing institutions in the late fourteenth and fifteenth centuries. The problem of finding long-term care solutions for the mentally or physically impaired complicates this story.

Whether the courts helped families make or imposed on them arrangements for the long-term care of their impaired kin, in the end, the relative comfort of mentally disturbed men and women depended wholly on the web of family they had the fortune or misfortune to find themselves entangled in. Quality of care and supervision depended as much on family resources—wealthy families with capital and connections had more care options at their disposal than did the poor—as on the will of relatives to bear such a burden day to day, year to year.

THE ORIGINS OF LEGAL GUARDIANSHIP

When Monna Francesca petitioned the Pupilli during the summer of 1560, she drew on a long tradition of guardianship first established in Roman law as a way of protecting patrimony from the ineptitude or imprudence of kin on account of age, gender, illness, mental incompetence, physical impairment, or moral laxity. Roman law and its antecedents left the task of making such determinations in the hands of families, neighbors, and judges.

With the recovery and revival of Roman law in medieval Italy, Italian jurists adopted and adjusted the Roman institution of guardianship to fit the social realities of Italian cities. In Florence, jurists enshrined these ideas for the first time during the mid-1320s in the statutes of the courts of the Podestà and the Capitano del Popolo.[5]

Under these laws, Florentines could seek legal guardianship for relatives who lacked the ability to manage their estates or care for themselves. Moreover, at the request of relatives, judges could both appoint guardians and scrutinize their conduct.[6]

In the Roman tradition, guardianship rested on the idea that sons and daughters were subject to paternal power (*patria potestas*), the legal authority of their fathers, which limited their freedom to perform legal transactions. This practice was meant to protect patrimony from the inexperience of youth. But fathers often died before their children came of age, leaving them *sui iuris* or not in the power of another. On their own, the young were thought to be targets for fraud or liable to make poor financial decisions. Thus all persons *sui iuris* who, for reasons of mental or physical defect, age, or gender, could not assume the management of their own affairs were put under one of two kinds of guardianship, *tutela* or *cura*.

Tutela referred to the guardianship of adult women and children under the age of puberty.[7] Gender was an important factor here. Roman law considered women equal in status to minors. It was only through the activating force of a man that a woman could exercise legal rights.[8] Thus women always required guardianship—*tutela* during their minority and *cura* during their majority. All Florentine women were similarly required by statute to have a male—a father, brother, husband, uncle—assist them in their legal transactions. This guardian, the *mundualdus*, was not of Roman but Lombard origin, and Florence was unique among the Italian city-states in maintaining this term to refer to the guardianship specifically of women. The *mundualdus* gave women the legal capacity otherwise lacking in their sex to make contracts and in general perform legal actions. The *mundualdus*'s duties were in large part identical to that of the Roman *curator*.

Tutors were appointed in several ways. In Roman law, the nearest agnates according to degree—a ward's grandfather, paternal uncle, brother by the same father, paternal cousin, and so forth—automatically and without court intervention assumed the role of guardian under the category of statutory guardian (*tutor legitimus*). A father or a person who had paternal power over a minor could also nominate a tutor in his will as a testamentary guardian (*tutela testamentaria*).[9] If no statutory tutor existed and no testamentary appointment had been made, a magistrate could appoint a *tutor* called the magistrate-appointed guardian (*tutor dativo* or *tutela a magistratu dativa*).[10]

In the minds of early Roman jurists, the mentally incapacitated were on equal footing with minors; they required guardians, namely the nearest agnate, who could provide for their creature comforts as well as manage their property.[11] Later law extended this provision to the deaf, mute, feebleminded (*mentecapti*), and those laboring under perpetual illnesses.[12]

The main work of the *tutor* was to administer the ward's patrimony and manage his or her affairs.[13] For this reason, the *tutor*'s first task was to make an inventory of the estate.[14] Thereafter, he carried out the business of the ward, recovered and paid debts, brought and defended actions on the ward's behalf, and, if need be, represented the ward in litigation.[15] During the empire, Roman law had come to regard *tutela* as a public service (*munus publicum*).[16] As a result, anyone appointed a *tutor* was required by law to serve unless he was formally disqualified or excused.

Tutela ceased once a ward reached the age of puberty—in the Roman system eventually established at fourteen for males and twelve for females. Nonetheless, since Roman law did not consider minors capable of administering their own affairs, minority lasted until the age of twenty-five.[17] Between the ages of eighteen and twenty-five, a minor could apply for a *curator* in order to perform specific legal acts that normally required full legal majority. Guardianship of the mentally and physically impaired fell under the category of *cura* rather than *tutela* since it extended beyond the age of majority, though minors who were mentally incompetent had protection in the form of a *tutor*. At majority, their care transferred to a *curator* whose obligation applied not only to the patrimony but also to the health and well-being of the *furiosus*.[18]

Florentine statutes of the 1320s for the most part adopted these provisions. The judges of the Podestà were granted the authority to appoint *tutores*, *curatores*, and guardians for unmarried women, widows, and minors under the age of twenty-five without a formal court proceeding. All a petitioner need do was have a notary draft a petition in the proper form, deposit it in the official acts of the curia, and give it to another notary to make copies for any and all other interested parties so that it would be a matter of public record.[19]

But medieval and early modern jurists and judges were not slaves to their Roman counterparts. The Pupilli's decision to appoint Monna Francesca as a guardian and later to accept her petition against the guardianship of Lodovico, the next agnate, demonstrates their willingness to adjust Roman institutions to better address moral and practical concerns raised by the practice.[20] Early in Roman law, *tutela* favored the *tutor* who stood to receive the property under his care should the ward die. In this line of thinking, guardians next in the order of succession and cognizant of their own direct interest would ensure the preservation and enlargement of the ward's estate since they would eventually enjoy its fruits. That was the hope anyway.

Experience revealed that guardians, particularly paternal uncles, were not always so generously disposed toward their wards. Thus legislation of the fifth century CE made protection of the ward rather than enrichment of the *tutor* the main goal of *tutela*.[21] To this end, cognates or relatives on the mother's side could also serve as guardians since they could not inherit from their ward.[22] This legislation also named grandmothers and mothers provided they did not remarry after their husband's death.[23]

Competition of interests between guardian and ward and conflicts between maternal and paternal kin over guardianship was a recurring theme in legal thought and practice. After the revival of Roman law in Italy, it became a legal commonplace that some guardians were no more than wolves in sheep's clothing.[24] In his treatise on the guardianship and care of minors, the sixteenth-century jurist Vincenzo Manzini played on the phrase used to describe guardians to capture the reality of their service; he changed the words "tuitores ac defensores," protectors and advocates, to "tollitores," thieves.[25] English common law took a similarly dim view of guardianship, believing that assigning a guardian to a minor was like handing a sheep over to a wolf to be devoured.[26]

Florentine judges and magistrates increasingly favored paternal grandfathers and then widowed mothers and grandmothers as guardians since they had little to no hope of inheriting a ward's property over paternal uncles who benefited from the ward's untimely death.[27] Some medieval jurists argued that maternal affection was a powerful force against interest; love for their children might not put mothers and grandmothers beyond reproach as guardians, but it made them more attractive candidates for the role than other family members, agnate or cognate.[28]

Practice bears out this shift in thinking. Late fourteenth-century statutes for the Pupilli rank statutory guardians in order of preference as "paternal grandfathers, mothers, paternal grandmothers, paternal uncles, brothers by the same father, and paternal cousins."[29]

Testaments from the fourteenth through sixteenth centuries also reflect this trend; widows and kinsmen related by marriage were frequently assigned as testamentary guardians for minors.[30] By the mid-seventeenth century, mothers were the guardian of choice. Giulia Calvi has observed that between 1648 and 1766, of 614 guardianships assigned in the city of Florence, mothers accounted for 75.4 percent and paternal uncles only 22.6 percent; out of 880 guardianships outside of Florence between 1652 and 1733, mothers accounted for 69.7 percent, paternal uncles, 28.5 percent.[31]

In the eyes of the Pupilli, Monna Francesca was a safe bet. Because she could not inherit from Francesco, she was presumed likely to act on his behalf out of affection rather than interest. The opposite applied to Francesco's brother, whose financial problems seemed to tip the scales in favor of interest. Even if Lodovico had the best intentions in the world, it was the worst scenario the Pupilli wanted to avoid.

THE IDEAL GUARDIAN

The trouble with Lodovico underscores one of the most nettlesome problems of guardianship: who was, in practice, the most suitable candidate for providing responsible and benevolent long-term care? Precarious though it might be, minority was a temporary state. Minors grew up. In Florence, boys achieved majority at eighteen, assuming some measure of control over their lives and estates. Girls reached majority at marriage when they passed into the legal power of their husband, at monacation when they passed into the care of a convent, or at twenty-five when they could contract with the help of a *mundualdus*.[32] By contrast, the severely mentally and physically impaired might spend their entire lives in perpetual minority, forever existing at the mercy and pleasure of someone else.

But suitability was a two-way street. Archival evidence shows that care of the impaired was as important as the proper devolution of his or her property. The ideal guardian saw to it that patrimony was not derailed as it traveled from one generation to the next. The courts tried to add transparency to this process by making the assignment of guardians highly publicized events so that any and all legitimate property claims came to light before judges made their final decisions.

The suitability of a guardian was the paramount concern in the first petition seeking guardianship for a mentally incompetent person that I know of in the Florentine courts. On December 10, 1348, a notary submitted a petition to the court of the Podestà on behalf of one Giovanni de' Bandi, who claimed that his sister Tessa was "*fatua, demens*, et *furiosa* and that she conducted herself and managed her estate poorly."[33] Giovanni asked the court to assign a *curator* to manage her affairs and care for her person. Arnaldo degli Altoviti of Florence, Tessa's paternal cousin, was presented as a suitable candidate. Giovanni argued that Arnaldo was prudent, conducted his own affairs well, and was a man of standing in Florentine society. More to the point, he was wealthy and so thought unlikely to despoil Tessa's property for his own gain.[34]

Summarily and without formal court proceedings, as statute allowed, Giovanni conveyed the management, administration, and governance of the affairs and property of Domina Tessa, again referred to as "furiosa," "demens," and "mentecapta," to Arnaldo.[35] In order to legitimate the instrument of guardianship he produced a public document drawn up by a notary, which he then deposited with another notary charged with making copies for any interested parties. A herald of Florence read out the terms of the guardianship at Tessa's house so that her relatives and neighbors had ample opportunity to air any grievances or reservations they might have about it in court.[36]

There is no evidence that anyone came forward to challenge the petition. It is likely, in fact, that Tessa's relatives and, most important, her heirs had all agreed that Arnaldo was, for whatever reason, the right man for the job. Moreover, his alleged prudence, distinction, and independent wealth served to dispel doubts a judge might have that personal gain was the underlying intent of the petition.

Without more evidence, Giovanni's motives for petitioning the court are unknowable. His intentions could have been purely benevolent (the care of his sister and the orderly devolution of her estate); they could have been mercenary (the unlawful appropriation of her estate through some private agreement with Arnaldo). The record does not beat a sure path to either conclusion. What it does show is that the courts were sensitive to the possibility of fraud and had put in place safeguards against it.

The problem of a guardian's suitability was sometimes solved by assigning two or more guardians from different sides of a family who, in principle, balanced competing interests. This strategy gave the impression that a family was concerned for the care of a vulnerable relative, had no designs on his or her property, and sought the smooth legal transfer of property from one generation to the next. In October 1410, for example, one Giusto from the neighborhood of San Niccolò in the Oltrarno of Florence went before the court of the Podestà to claim that by the time of his petition it had been over a year that his maternal aunt Pasqua was "in word and deed manifestly *mentecapta*, not of sound mind, and lacking in intellect."[37] He petitioned the Podestà's court to assign Pasqua a *curator* or *curatores* who could manage her affairs, protect her rights, and care for her person by making sure she was clothed, housed, and fed. He nominated Bartolo, Pasqua's nephew through one of her brothers-in-law (Giusto's paternal cousin), and Miniato, her nephew through one of her sisters (Giusto's maternal cousin), as suitable candidates for guardianship. Thus Giusto offered a relative from the paternal and maternal sides of his family or, in other words, the two lineages brought together by the marriage of his parents. [Fig. 1]

Flow of patrimony shaped this arrangement. According to the record, Pasqua's parents were dead. She shared their estate with her two married sisters. The record implies that she never married and had no children of her own. Marital status was a crucial piece of information since it necessarily added another group of players to the field of interests. If there had been a husband still living Pasqua would have been under his legal control. If she had been a widow with or without children, her dowry would have been entangled in the patrimony of her marital family.

Without a husband or children to claim rights to her dowry and in the absence of male agnates, her sisters were her heirs. If Pasqua died her sisters would inherit equal portions of her part of their parents' estate. If her sisters then died their estates plus equal shares of that of Pasqua's would pass to their children, namely, Miniato and Giusto. A petition from Miniato and Giusto seeking sole or joint guardianship of Pasqua might raise eyebrows since her property would eventually devolve to them. Thus Bartolo, who could not inherit from Pasqua, was a good choice for co-guardianship; he brought to the arrangement what appeared to be disinterested participation.

The outcome is not revealed. Barring any challenges in court, which do not appear in the record, Bartolo and Miniato likely undertook Pasqua's care without opposition.[38] In this case, maternal and paternal families collaborated to arrange care for a mentally incapacitated woman in such a way as to avoid suspicion that any one person or lineage would benefit unduly at her expense.

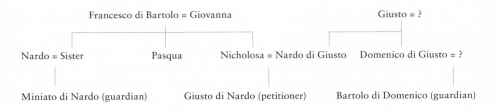

Figure 1. Partial reconstruction of Pasqua's family. From ASF AP 4210, fols. 16v–17v.

In some cases, guardianship arrangements required a considerable amount of good faith on the part of natal and marital families whose interests might be in conflict. The character, means, and intentions of the person chosen to serve as guardian were particularly important in such instances. In a case of 1439, for example, finding long-term care for a severely impaired woman was just as important as ensuring that her estate eventually found its way intact to its rightful heirs.

In March of that year, a notary petitioned the podesterial court for an investigation into the case of one Appollonia. Although it is not stated, the occasion of the petition was in all likelihood the death of her father and the rightful devolution of his estate. Several factors conspired against easy resolution. First, according to the record, for more than twenty years, Appollonia "was and continued to be *demens* and *mentecapta*, and without the least bit of rational sense." She was so impaired that "she could not understand what things remained to her nor was she or did she continue to be of sound mind, nor could she take care of herself." To put it differently, Appollonia lacked the ability to understand what she inherited from her father as well as the capacity to manage and pass it on. To make matters worse, she "had no father or uncle or any other agnate to assume her care," and "her father had died without having given her any *curator*."[39] Appollonia was *sui iuris* and so a perceived target for grasping relatives.

But she was not alone in the world. The record also states that she was living in the house of her maternal half brother, Cristoforo, together with their mother. This arrangement complicated the situation. Cristoforo and her mother were Appollonia's closest living relatives by blood, not by law. It was her paternal cousin, Caterina, who was the more proximate kin since she and Appollonia were related to each other through their fathers. As such, Caterina and her children were Appollonia's legitimate heirs. Herein lies the crux of the matter.

Appollonia lived with and presumably received care from her mother and her half brother. While she lived, her estate was attached to her. But by right of succession, it would eventually have to pass back to the patriline through Caterina. Could Caterina and her family count on Cristoforo, the likeliest candidate for guardianship, responsibly and honestly to manage property that was not ultimately his?

Appollonia's case uncovers the kinds of complex relationships that lie buried in the legal language of these texts. Webs of relations and paths of succession became yet more tangled when women and men remarried. In principle, when a Florentine woman married she left not only the household but the lineage of her natal family to enter into the household and lineage of her husband. She was emancipated from the legal control of her father to come under the legal control of her husband. She brought with her a dowry, a portion of her father's estate that helped sustain the newly forged marital household.[40] Her dowry, now embedded in her husband's patrimony, entered his line of succession. If she had children but predeceased her husband, her dowry passed to their children (excluding children the husband had from a prior marriage). If her husband predeceased her, however, she returned with her dowry to the household and lineage of her father, perhaps to be married again. If a woman remarried she entered yet another household. Although her dowry followed her to the second marriage, her children from the first marriage did not.

At times these practices engendered conflict, namely, the battles waged by natal families to recoup dowries from marital households or the strategies employed by marital households to stall or prevent the restitution of a woman's dowry.[41] In numerous studies, Christiane Klapisch-Zuber has plumbed the depths of these conflicts. Her evocative description of women as "passing guests" in patriarchal households has left an indelible mark on how we understand the shape of Florentine families.[42] Struggles over dowries were common between a woman's natal and marital families. It often happened that young widows were pressured by their natal families to leave the marital household and reenter the marriage market. In this case, she left her children behind, leading the famous orphan Giovanni Morelli (1371–1444) to accuse his mother of being "cruel."[43]

Historians have given Morelli a disproportionate amount of press. To be sure, women caught between natal and marital households or maternal and paternal households were in a difficult position. Yet Appollonia's case illustrates that affective ties often remained where legal ties had been severed. Where some remarriages may have fomented conflict between lineages, others occasioned collaboration. Appollonia's mother, for example, actively remained in the lives of her children from different marriages. Her relationship to Cristoforo did not end with the end of her marriage to his father or her remarriage to Appollonia's father. Nor did the death of Appollonia's father cause her to abandon Appollonia, a severely incapacitated young woman with no marriage prospects.

Whatever suspicions may have existed between Appollonia's maternal and paternal kin, both sides seem to have arrived at a workable solution so long as everyone's concerns were addressed. For her part, Caterina needed assurances that if Appollonia were to remain in her mother's household with her half brother acting as guardian, her claims as legitimate heir to the estate were publicly recorded and recognized. The podesterial court offered the two families a legal mechanism both to provide care for Appollonia and to observe the proper path of succession. It investigated and confirmed Appollonia's mental incapacity, it scrutinized Cristoforo's candidacy as guardian, and it publicized the proceedings.[44] The petition was read aloud in the piazzas of San Giovanni, Or' San Michele, and the old and new markets of the city of Florence, as well as affixed to the door of the municipal palace.[45] Anyone who wished to oppose, challenge, or express opinions about it was invited to do so before the judge of the podesterial court within three days of the original citation. Finally, if Cristoforo was to become Appollonia's legal guardian he had to make an inventory of her estate, swearing before the court that it was accurate and that he would execute all of his duties faithfully and legally. This arrangement seems to have appeased Caterina and her kin. They launched no countersuit and Cristoforo was sworn in as Appollonia's guardian in June 1439. From that point on, the case falls silent.

In the fourteenth and fifteenth centuries, formal guardianship arrangements that won the court's imprimatur were public and publicized events. They required by statute the consent and approval of all relatives and the notification of friends, neighbors, and acquaintances. In many respects the decision to petition necessitated collective social action, that is, the agreement of a whole network of relations before it could be acceptable to and accepted by the court. Heavy procedural framework hung around cases like Appollonia's and for good reason. In the best of circumstances it protected vulnerable people while simultaneously championing the patrimonial interests of legitimate heirs.

   Attention to collective interests involving economic matters as well as a deep sense of family solidarity in the broadest sense that the term "family" allows in this context were both elements of the social physiognomy of medieval and early modern Florence.[46] At the same time that there were poisonous relations between and within families, there were also sincere bonds of affection and solicitude across patri- and matrilines. Cases like Pasqua's and Appollonia's show relatives reaching beyond the confines of one's lineage strictly understood to care for mentally or physically incapacitated kin. They show, too, how the courts—again, in the best of circumstances—provided mechanisms for restoring stability to tense moments within and between Tuscan families. Maintaining social order was a collaborative process that involved families, neighbors, and civic authorities in households, streets, and courts.

GUARDIANSHIP IN A DIFFERENT KEY

Guardianship in the courts of the Podestà and Capitano was a legal remedy for families. By the end of the fourteenth century, a different type of guardianship appeared in Florence. Beginning in the 1370s, the Florentine government connected guardianship to the fiscal structures of the city by entrusting the care of minors and widows to the Monte comune (the public debt), the central institution of Florentine public finance.[47] Wards received interest on the purchase of Monte credits, but the initial goal of the scheme was to service the state's increasing debt obligations. In 1393, the Monte comune passed its authority and prerogative to the newly established Magistrato dei Pupilli, an independent six-man magistracy charged with appointing guardians to minors whose fathers had died intestate.[48] After 1502, when the courts of the Podestà and Capitano del Popolo were abolished, cases involving guardianship became almost exclusively the Pupilli's domain until it was dismantled in 1808.

   The origins of the Pupilli remain somewhat obscure. It has been argued that the Signoria, Florence's main governing body, created the Pupilli at the request of elite families who increasingly laid their concerns about disruptions in the flow of patrimony from one generation to the next at the door of their civic authorities, urging them to play a greater role in aspects of household management. The Signoria

reluctantly responded by creating a state-sponsored form of guardianship.[49] This argument rests on the fact that in the latter half of
the fourteenth century certain Florentines of the ruling class made
the Signoria testamentary guardian of their minors. In 1368, twenty
years after the first catastrophic visitation of plague in Florence, the
Count Palatine of Tuscany did just that. Five years later, a Florentine
wool merchant, Francesco Giraldi, also entrusted the sizable estate
of his children to the Signoria. After some deliberation, the priors
passed the guardianship of Giraldi's children to the officers of the
Monte comune. In the hopes of making government wardships profitable, they invested cash from wards' estates in the public fisc. But
Monte officials quickly found their new role too burdensome; in 1393
the Signoria created the Pupilli, which took up where the Monte had
left off.[50]

Like the officers of the Monte comune, the Pupilli assigned legal
guardians to minors whose fathers had died intestate and whose family members had not already assumed their care. They were not to
intervene if a legitimate guardian were available. Furthermore, like
the Monte comune, the Pupilli purchased and sold wards' properties as circumstances demanded, micromanaging estate expenditure
down to the smallest detail. The remainder of the estate, after all
expenses had been paid, was used to purchase shares in the public
debt at the rate of 5 percent interest (in the 1420s closer to 3.75 percent; by the end of the fifteenth century closer to 2 or 2.5 percent)
accrued annually and collected once the minor reached the age of
majority.[51]

There is no way of knowing for certain why elite families chose
to hand wardships to the Signoria rather than make arrangements in
the court of the Podestà. Impossible to deny is the fact that the Pupilli
developed at the tail end of a series of dramatic crises. Cyclical recurrence of plague beginning in 1347, popular rebellion and political
tensions of the 1370s, and the rising costs of warfare and communal
debt provoked a wide array of institutional adjustments to Florentine
governing arrangements.[52] Fiscal concerns were at the center of these
developments and fiscal innovation was directed primarily toward
paying the costs of war.[53]

When the management of enormous patrimonies fell into its lap,
the Signoria used income from these estates to help defray the carrying charges of the public debt. This scheme benefited wards as well
as the state since they could expect an annual return on their initial

purchase of Monte shares. Prior to large-scale judicial reforms of the 1470s, the Pupilli tended to favor wealthy, well-heeled wards who resided in Florence, sometimes though not always opting to reject the care of more modest wardships that promised little return for the public fisc. This strategy gave the Florentine government a way of tapping into the wealth of its elite families without taxing them directly or resorting to forced loans, the preferred way of compensating for shortfalls from indirect taxes. But preference for golden-egg wardships did little to make the Pupilli a reliable instrument of state debt reduction. For much of the fifteenth century, the office could barely cover its own operating costs.[54]

The judicial reforms of the 1470s drastically changed the size and composition of the Pupilli's clientele and its prerogative. It no longer catered solely to elite clients living in or around Florence but extended its services to every corner of the Florentine dominion, accepting wardships that represented even modest holdings. Moreover, in an attempt to solve the problem of overlapping and competing jurisdictions, the Florentine commune reconstituted the Pupilli as a judiciary directed toward resolving patrimonial conflicts.[55] The abolition of the Podestà and the Capitano del Popolo and the dissolution of those courts in 1502 further fed the Pupilli's caseload. As a court of wards with a clearly defined jurisdiction, the Pupilli offered Tuscan families a centralized and well-articulated arena in which to settle disputes over patrimony, oversee domestic affairs, or defend vulnerable relatives.

Petitions seeking guardianship for the allegedly mentally and physically incapacitated increased at the turn of the sixteenth century in response to these reforms. The Pupilli heard only four guardianship cases involving mental or physical incompetence between 1387 and 1500. By contrast, around ninety such cases went before the Pupilli between 1500 and 1600, 80 percent of them taking place after 1540 when political and institutional stability had returned to Florence after thirty years of civil war. Furthermore, in the fourteenth and fifteenth centuries, petitioners seeking guardianship for the mentally or physically impaired in the Pupilli were usually residents of Florence.[56] After 1550 mad Tuscans join the ranks of mad Florentines.

By 1550, the Pupilli had become a court with a significant amount of power to intervene in family affairs. Already in the 1470s the Florentine government ceded to the Pupilli greater powers of intervention in cases of guardianship. The Pupilli was no longer required to wait until families petitioned its office to have guardianships assigned, nor did it recognize arrangements that families made for guardians if they did not conform to its statutes. New statutes allowed the Pupilli to assume unclaimed wardships after six months if statutory guardians were slow to accept their obligations for whatever reason.[57] Those statutory guardians would then have to petition the Pupilli to reclaim wardships from the state. By the end of the fifteenth century, the Pupilli had begun to play an unprecedented role in the management of Tuscan households.

For some families, the Pupilli's newly established authority to deprive certain legitimate guardians of wardships or to assign wardships to candidates they believed were the most suitable was a great boon. The Pupilli could help relatives protect their kin against neglect or abuse. In the petition that opened this chapter, Monna Francesca tried to anticipate what she believed to be the probable mistreatment or exploitation of her developmentally impaired relative, Francesco. She successfully petitioned the Pupilli to have Francesco's legitimate guardian denied that post. Motivated by similar concerns, in 1586 one Monna Susanna went in person to the Pupilli on behalf of her youngest son, Jacopo. Her husband had "died around fourteen years earlier, leaving her with two sons, Jacopo now thirty-four years old, and his older brother Pandolfo." Jacopo, she claimed, was "rather simple in mind." Moreover, he "had never known nor did he know [then] how to manage his affairs and had always been supervised." What was worse, his brother Pandolfo "had always treated him quite badly." Monna Susanna doubted "that after her death [Jacopo] would not be mistreated and forced to beg or come to some bad end." To "unburden her conscience" she asked that the Pupilli deprive Pandolfo of Jacopo's care and undertake it themselves. After hearing the testimony of Jacopo's relatives in support of her claims, the Pupilli informed the Duke that they believed their intervention was warranted; they should indeed take up the care of "this Jacopo *mentecatto*." The Duke agreed.[58]

In cases like those of Francesco and Jacopo, the Pupilli dissolved legitimate guardianships in order to protect severely impaired men and women. In response to the petitions of concerned family members, Pupilli officers marshaled the full power of the ducal state to play a significant administrative role in households.

GUARDIANSHIP WARTS AND ALL

Access to the Pupilli and its more interventionist prerogative did not make guardianship an easier business. Cases from the sixteenth and seventeenth centuries attest to the persistent problems plaguing the supervision of impaired people. Scrupulous legitimate guardians were not always available. Distance, death, age, and business obligations often prevented relatives who could act as guardians from being able or inclined to provide even the rudiments of care to a person who needed long-term protection. In 1571, for example, one Monna Costanza, seventeen years a widow, asked that the Pupilli take on the care of her son. He was thirty years old but "weak in mind and prevented from speaking," presumably from some physical impairment. Monna Costanza had taken care of him since he was a child. At the time of the petition she was seventy-two, "old, infirm, and unable to help him any longer." The Duke's office instructed the Pupilli to grant the petition.[59]

The nature of one's occupation or obligations sometimes made the care and management of a relative and his or her property if not impossible then very difficult. Even if family members were on hand, practical realities might bar them from serving as guardians. In January 1554, one Fra Girolamo, a cobbler's son, asked the Pupilli to assume the care of his brother Stefano, who was and had been for some time "vexed by maninconic humors [which] drew him out of his mind." Girolamo had put his brother in the hospital of San Paolo on the condition that the hospital receive a subsidy and Stefano's goods. There was no one capable of following through on this agreement save Fra Girolamo himself, who, being a monk and having taken a vow of poverty, was not able to enter into contracts. Fra Girolamo asked that the Duke commit Stefano to the care of the Pupilli or any person or institution he deemed appropriate, including Fra Girolamo, who could, in turn, make the necessary arrangements with the hospital of San Paolo or another place where Stefano would be well treated. The Duke's office left the final decision at the discretion of the Pupilli, instructing them to do whatever seemed best to them.[60] Although the final outcome of the case remains unknown, the problem that Fra Girolamo faced is clear. He was Stefano's only surviving relative, but religious proscriptions prevented him from caring for his brother except by special dispensation from the Duke.

Some relatives were simply too busy to take care of their mentally or physically impaired kin. The *mentecatto* Girolamo Passerini,
for example, had a surfeit of suitable guardians in his family, but he
ended up stowed away in one of the family's country villas with little supervision. When Girolamo's father, Niccolò, the previous Captain of Cortona, died in September 1578, his five sons inherited equal
shares in a sizable estate.[61] Debate over how to divide the shares led
to arbitration the next year. Girolamo was a phantom in these proceedings. While his brothers, Valerio, Silvio, Fulvio, and Pirro, stood
on their own authority, confirming their acceptance of the final settlement with their own signatures, Girolamo's interests were represented by his *curator*, an associate of the Passerini family.[62]

In May 1579, Fulvio and Valerio asked that Girolamo "be put as
a *mentecatto* in the care and protection of the Pupilli." They claimed
that he was "disabled [*inhabile*] and in need of a curator for his person and property." In less than a month's time and at the request of
the Duke, Pupilli officials investigated these claims and drew up a
report.[63]

The Pupilli wrote first to the current Captain of Cortona asking
for information about the case. He could tell them little. He could not
interview Girolamo himself because "he had been locked up again as
a *mentecatto* by his brothers in a room of one of their palaces far from
Cortona."[64] The Captain sent a judge and a notary to visit Girolamo
there. When they arrived, he was alone. The judge and notary chat-
ted with him, trying to divine his state of mind. As they spoke to him,
"he stood there terrified, his hands trembling all the while, speaking
almost as if he were being forced. Although he gave no sign of being
pazzo," still they found him to be "completely unfit for the governance of himself and his property." He was, in their estimation, "a
fool [*balordo*] and out of his senses [*insensato*]." They further claimed
that melancholy humors were likely at the root of the problem. When
the Pupilli relayed this information to the Duke, his office instructed
them to undertake his care.[65]

The bulk of the responsibility for Girolamo, however, seems to
have fallen to his brother Valerio. A document drawn up on July 5,
1579, states that Valerio had been "appointed Girolamo's *attore*."[66]
An undated inventory, presumably submitted by Valerio, outlining the divisions among the brothers of the Passerini estate follows
this document. Prior to enumerating the movable and immovable
goods acquired by each brother, Valerio maintained that he had been

charged with protecting the interests of the "unhappy Girolamo." Those interests were imperiled by litigation involving a claim made against Girolamo's property. In his statement, Valerio described his brother as being unhappy (*infelice*), wretched (*meschino*), and unfortunate (*desgratiato*), suggesting that Girolamo was not just ill-favored by fortune but struck by particularly cruel adversity.[67] He was in no way capable of handling encroachments on his properties by his neighbors.

In January 1580, all the Passerini brothers got together to submit a petition asking that the Pupilli revisit the case of their troubled brother. Valerio could no longer "attend to this duty" since he had been called into the "service of the most illustrious and reverend Cardinal de' Medici."[68] With Valerio in Rome there was no one to see to Girolamo's daily care, to manage his estate, or to deal with litigation attached to it. The decision to petition as a group was itself a communication; Girolamo's brothers were too busy to take care of him. The Pupilli would have to find someone else.

The Pupilli turned to the Captain of Cortona for help, though his advice was not without its own problems. Girolamo had a maternal uncle, Montino, who, in the Captain's view, was "very suitable" as a candidate for guardianship but was "not a subject or resident of the happy states," governed by the Duke of Florence. Although he was family, because he was a foreigner the Pupilli could not appoint him guardian. Still Girolamo's brothers asked that the Duke grant Montino special permission to take on the task. The Pupilli were willing to go along with the arrangement provided the Duke agreed and Montino himself went to Florence to "give appropriate surety that he would render good account of his administration to the Pupilli as other guardians [are] accustomed to do."[69] The Duke's office granted the petition.

The coming months brought more trouble. On February 24, the Pupilli reported to the Duke that Montino had pulled somewhat of a fast one. Instead of coming to Florence himself to give an account of his administration of Girolamo's estate, he offered Girolamo's brother Pirro as his guarantor. Perhaps bristling a bit at Montino's reluctance to comply with their statutes, the Pupilli informed the Duke that they "were not resolved to accept or repudiate Pirro as guarantor" without the Duke's express permission. The Duke's office answered that this arrangement "did not seem reasonable."[70]

Less than two months later, Montino petitioned the Pupilli for permission to give an account of his administration at Cortona rather than Florence. The Pupilli held fast to their position. They told the Duke that "they had difficulty accepting this surety at Cortona because the grace granted him of being able to be guardian was contingent on him giving surety in Florence and the Pupilli could not alter the Duke's rescript without his permission." Perhaps to avoid a situation in which bureaucratic rigidity conspired against resolution, the Duke granted Montino's request.[71]

This compromise did little to improve Girolamo's circumstances. On September 3, 1580, the Pupilli informed the Duke that they had received bad news from the city of Cortona. Without someone to manage his estate, Girolamo's affairs were faring poorly.[72] Even worse, the Pupilli had an imperfect understanding of what constituted Girolamo's estate in the first place. Their first choice of guardian, Valerio, "had renounced his guardianship although he had never rendered an account of his administration."[73] Girolamo's next guardian, Montino, dedicated his energies to avoiding rather than fulfilling his duty of submitting an updated inventory of Girolamo's estate. No one had kept track of Girolamo's property and not one of his brothers came forward to assume his care.[74] The Pupilli asked that the Duke allow them to search anew for a suitable guardian, a request his office granted.

The books close on Girolamo's story in May 1583 when one Giuliano Gondi petitioned to collect money owed him by the Passerini.[75] What happened to Girolamo, where and with whom he lived, who fed and clothed him, and who managed his estate remain unknown. He likely continued to languish in the family *palazzo* perhaps with a skeleton crew of servants to tend to his basic needs. If that is the case, he languished for a long time. Girolamo died in 1601, twenty-two years after his case was first introduced to the Pupilli. There is no evidence that his case was ever resolved. He never married, had no legitimate children, and enjoyed none of the honorifics that adorn the names of his more illustrious brothers.

Lest we assume that the Passerini family's decision to keep Girolamo hidden away in one of their country estates was cruel, callous, or "medieval" in the pejorative sense, it is instructive to consider the circumstances of his social exile. No one who knew Girolamo, not his brothers or the arbiters who valuated and divided the Passerini property, considered Girolamo mentally fit to participate in the proceedings. Furthermore, in their report to the Pupilli, the judge and notary from Cortona painted a grim picture. Social interaction and financial management were beyond Girolamo's abilities.

In more concrete terms, the petitions submitted by Girolamo's brothers and his maternal uncle to the Pupilli demonstrate that they tried to arrange care for him even if it was clear that none of them wanted to take on the burden themselves. The Passerini of Cortona were well connected and active on the Italian political and diplomatic scene. Girolamo's oldest brother, Valerio, was a knight in the military Order of Santo Stefano and eventually a councillor in the court of Ferdinando I, Grand Duke of Tuscany. His brother Fulvio was secretary to Cardinal Ugo Boncompagni and then continued in this service when Boncompagni succeeded to the papal throne as Pope Gregory XIII (1572–1585). Fulvio would go on to be governor of Foligno, bishop of Avellino, and finally bishop of Pistoia. Silvio had an equally brilliant career, serving as papal *nunzio* to the Holy Roman Emperor on behalf of Gregory XIII and was eventually named archbishop of Cosenza.

Where none of these brothers had legitimate children, Girolamo's brother Pirro continued the line. He was a soldier like his father, who spent much of his early life abroad on military campaign. He returned to Cortona in the midst of the Pupilli's vexed search for a guardian for Girolamo to embark on a long and distinguished political career and start a family of his own. Although he was willing to serve as guarantor for Montino's guardianship of Girolamo, he was not himself willing to take on the task.[76]

The Passerini brothers were by no means the only Tuscan relatives to renounce the care of severely incapacitated kin. One Jacopo Barbelli, for example, was similarly reluctant to shoulder the care of his brother. In 1573 he asked the Pupilli to undertake care of Antonio, who was "not of sound mind due to the incurable sickness that continues to afflict him and which takes him out of his senses." Witnesses confirmed these claims. Although Jacopo was Antonio's only family, he claimed that "he could not attend to [his brother's] daily business affairs." In their report of Jacopo's supplication, the Pupilli informed the Duke that Antonio's estate was in peril. His movable property as well as his personal care had been entrusted to his servants "to his own detriment and to the detriment of his creditors." The phrasing of the response from the Duke's office is somewhat ambiguous but suggests that the Pupilli had been instructed to "take care of the matter themselves."[77]

The cases of Girolamo Passerini and Antonio Barbelli bring to light the kind of practical realities that conspired against long-term care for those considered mentally or physically impaired. A host of wealthy and influential relatives did not guarantee protection. Even the existence and intervention of the Pupilli offered no assurances against neglect or abandonment. Care of relatives was traditionally the province of the family. By law, the Pupilli could not intervene in these cases if a legitimate guardian was there to take up the reins until at least one month had elapsed. Where there were questions or conflicts about guardianship in cases involving mental and physical incapacity, the Pupilli still tried to assign the most appropriate, available family member or members to the task.

But long-term care was a demanding job. It meant ensuring that a person was housed, fed, clothed, and, if necessary, supervised. It included managing someone's finances, namely, selling property to pay debts, paying taxes assessed on the value of the estate, and defending the estate in preexisting or future litigation. Family members selected by the Pupilli to discharge these duties were sometimes unwilling or unable to comply. Fra Girolamo could only serve his brother if the Duke granted him special permission. The Passerini brothers were busy men whose lives of civil and military service often took them abroad. They were content to impose guardianship duties on others while Jacopo Barbelli seemed desirous of avoiding involvement in his brother's financial entanglements altogether. From this angle, these cases demonstrate that the practice of caring for the impaired in Florence could amount to the interminable passing of responsibility between families, courts, and Duke. In the meantime, the life of the impaired man or woman dragged on.

MARTELLI V. MARTELLI

What the madness of a relative meant for a family was to a certain extent in the eye of the beholder. For devoted caretakers, it was a source of anxiety about the prospects of stable, benevolent, and reliable long-term care. For those with more predatory or pragmatic ends, it was an opportunity to wrest property or money from a vulnerable person or perhaps to reunite property that the practice of partible inheritance had spread across households over generations. For most families, severe mental impairment was a chaotic force that threatened to destroy lineages. In the case of the *mentecatti* Martelli, it set a withering cadet branch of an otherwise celebrated family against each other in a decades-long battle over patrimony. In the end, they all lost. The last surviving male heir died a childless cleric; his patrimony passed to a more fecund and fortunate line.

We begin our story *in medias res* when one Filippo Martelli urged the Pupilli to assign him a suitable guardian sometime in November 1579. According to his petition he was "incapable of taking care of himself on account of a wound in the head . . . that impeded his memory." His mother, Margherita Pandolfini, had originally served as his guardian, but she had died four years earlier. His care and the management of his estate had since passed into the hands of his brothers, Andrea and Giovanni. If Filippo's allegations are to be believed, these two were dubious characters: "he was ill treated by these brothers [who failed] to feed and clothe him." But Andrea and Giovanni showed themselves willing to fulfill their obligations. When the Pupilli interviewed them they insisted that "they intended to settle the affair in a friendly manner."[78]

On January 10, 1580, the Pupilli informed the Duke of the case. The news was not promising. Over a month had passed and discord still reigned between the brothers. The Pupilli called Filippo before them only to discover that "in appearance and as far as one could see from his clothing and his speech, he had not been treated particularly well by his brothers and needed someone to care for him and manage his property." Two days later, the Duke's office granted the petition, saying that the Pupilli should indeed assume his care and attend to his needs.[79]

That year ended with another Martelli case. On November 30, the widow of Alamanno Martelli, Maria Corsi, asked the Pupilli to sanction a guardianship arrangement she had made with her nephew regarding the care of her mentally incapacitated son Francesco. Maria had acted as Francesco's guardian and caretaker (*tuttrice e governatrice*) since her husband's death in 1533, nearly fifty years earlier. By the time of her petition, she was in her seventies and Francesco in his early fifties. The record does not spell out the exact nature of Francesco's disability, but it is clear that he had never been able to take care of himself. His only brother, Sigismondo, had died in 1547 at the tender age of twenty-five, forcing Maria to look farther afield for a suitable guardian who could assume his care after she died.

Determined not to leave such an important choice to chance, Maria enlisted the Pupilli's help. She was concerned, she told them, that "after her death Francesco might come into the care of someone who would treat him badly." She wished, then, "to provide Francesco

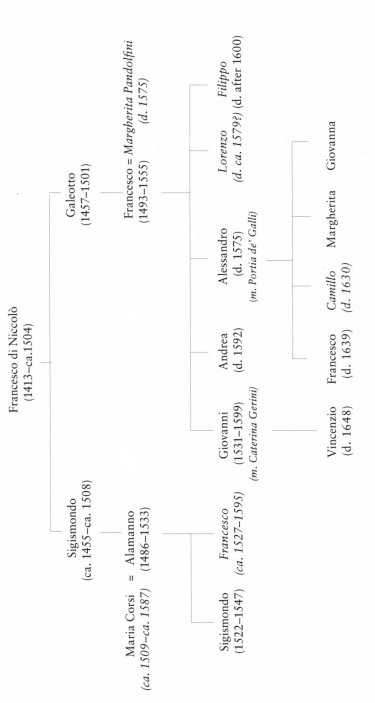

Figure 2. Genealogy of the Martelli: Branch of Francesco di Niccolò. Based on Pompeo Litta, *Famiglie celebri italiane*, vol. 4 (Milan: G. Ferrario, 1833–36) and Alessandra Civai, *Dipinti e sculture in casa Martelli: Storia di una collezione patrizia fiorentina dal Quattrocento all'Ottocento* (Florence: Opus Libri, 1990), 120–21. Names and dates in italic have not appeared in published genealogies.

with security against damage or loss, care and supervision while she still lived." If she had her way, Francesco's care would pass to her sister's son, Francesco di Lapo Vespucci. To sweeten the deal, Maria gave Vespucci the right of "enjoying and holding her estate in usu-fruct" during his service as Francesco's guardian. All he had to do was "keep two maidservants and one manservant and provide Fran-cesco with food and clothing and any other necessary thing during his life." These incentives would hopefully assure Vespucci's cooperation. This arrangement seemed reasonable to the Pupilli and the Duke's officers who granted it.[80]

Two petitions. Two Martelli. Two *mentecatti*. A lot of animosity. Filippo's case was about conflict. He accused his brothers of neglect, implied abuse, and asked that the Pupilli find someone more appro-priate to replace these legitimate but unsuitable guardians. Maria's petition, by contrast, expressed fear of an unspoken though immi-nent threat to her severely impaired son after her death. She hoped to persuade the Pupilli that Francesco was better-off in the hands of a cognate relative who could not inherit from him to circumvent more rapacious guardians who could.

Of real interest here is what Maria left unsaid in that petition. Those rapacious guardians that she suggested were waiting to pounce on her unfortunate son were none other than Filippo's brothers Giovanni and Andrea, the very same men accused of neglect and abuse. Here is where the plot thickens.

Maria's son Francesco and Filippo were second cousins, connected by lines of succession. If Francesco and his brother, Sigismondo, died without heirs, their property passed to the line of Francesco di Galeotto, Filippo's father.[81] Filippo had four brothers: the maligned Andrea and Giovanni as well as Alessandro and Lorenzo, who later documents revealed was also said to be *mentecatto*. Since Francesco di Galeotto died in 1555, these brothers were Francesco *mentecatto*'s universal heirs. In other words, Maria submitted her petition know-ing that those who had the greatest interest in Francesco's property had the least interest in caring for his person.

PATRIMONIAL WARS

What was going on in these two connected Martelli households? What created such tense situations? Thanks to a richer cache of legal, judi-cial, and census documentation than usually survive for these cases, a good deal of the back story can be filled in. What these records show are the death throes of a cadet branch of an elite family. Over three generations, untimely death, mental incapacity, and childlessness stripped the branch until it finally died. It was no coincidence that Filippo and Maria petitioned the Pupilli in November 1579. Whether Francesco was aware of the situation or not, both he and his second cousin Filippo found themselves at the center of a complex multigenerational dispute over patrimony worthy of Charles Dickens and the interminable litigation plaguing the characters of *Bleak House.*

To understand the circumstances that produced the battle for the family's limited patrimonial resources in the 1580s, it is necessary to go back several generations. By the time Filippo and Maria petitioned the Pupilli, the Martelli were a family of distinction and wealth. The eponymous founder of the line first appeared in Florence in the early fourteenth century and matriculated in the Arte di Calimala, the city's guild of cloth finishers and merchants of foreign cloth. On the eve of the fifteenth century, the family was poised to enter Florence's commercial and political elite. Niccolò Martelli (1372–1425) eventually managed to hitch himself to the rising star of the Medici.

In 1472, the "new" Martelli family were counted among Florence's wealthiest families.[82] From that point on and until the turbulent period between 1494 and 1530, Martelli sons enjoyed commercial and political careers full of honors and offices. Like other men of their rank, they also became patrons of art and culture.[83]

Francesco di Niccolò, the great-grandfather of the two *mentecatti,* was similarly wealthy. He matriculated into the silk guild in 1439 and served several times on the Signoria. His eldest brother, Ugolino, would enjoy the special favor of Cosimo *pater patriae* until his death in 1482. Roberto served the Medici bank of Florence with great success, while Antonio (d. 1480), Alessandro (d. 1465), and Bartolomeo (d. 1472) worked in the bank's Venetian branch. Influenced by Leon Battista Alberti's treatises on architecture, Roberto also built a family palazzo in via degli Spadai (now via Martelli) in imitation of the Palazzo Medici that rose a stone's throw away in via Larga (now via Cavour) in 1444. Domenico (d. 1476) became a lawyer at the University of Bologna and an important player in Florentine politics and diplomacy.

At the close of the fifteenth century the Martelli family had amassed patrimony to match their prestige. But relations between the lines had been deteriorating since midcentury. In 1453, a division of patrimony

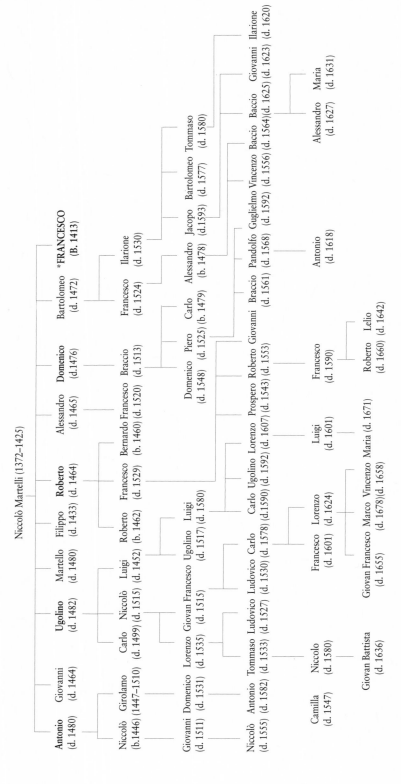

Figure 3. Genealogy of the Martelli. From ASF, Martelli B 232. Names that Civai did not include in her reconstruction appear in italics.

created three new families in three different households. Ugolino, Bartolomeo, and Martello (d. 1480) remained in the paternal household
in via degli Spadai; Roberto, Antonio, and Alessandro acquired a new
house next to the old one; Francesco, great-grandfather to Filippo
and Francesco d'Alamanno, moved in with Giovanni (d. 1464) and
Domenico (d.1476) in the palazzo near Canto alla Paglia (off of the
present-day via Cerretani) a street away from the Piazza del Duomo.
This earlier division set the lines on different paths so that by the sixteenth century they were largely independent of each other.[84]

By the 1530s, ownership of the palazzo at Canto alla Paglia had
passed into the hands of Francesco's (b. 1413) two grandsons, Alamanno di Sigismondo Martelli and Francesco di Galeotto Martelli.
This was prized real estate. Only the archiepiscopal palace separated
it from Florence's cathedral and baptistery, the spiritual center of the
city. But it was still marginal to the more illustrious Martelli households, which were situated in two large palazzi on one of Florence's
most affluent and celebrated thoroughfares.

Alamanno died in 1533, leaving his portion of the palazzo to two
young sons, Sigismondo and Francesco. At roughly twelve and seven
years old, respectively, the boys were in a precarious position. But
their mother, Maria Corsi, and the Pupilli stepped in to protect their
interests against those of their father's cousin.[85]

Tensions mounted over the next decade. In 1544, Sigismondo had
a will drawn up that suggests his brother Francesco's fate weighed
heavily on his mind. He named Francesco, whom he called "mentecapto della mente," his universal heir.[86] He added that should neither
he nor Francesco have children, their estate, including their share of
the palazzo at Canto alla Paglia, would eventually pass to Francesco
di Galeotto Martelli and after him his sons. So far so good.

However, although he was content to let his patrimony pass to the
line of Francesco di Galeotto, he was less comfortable entrusting that
side of the family with his brother's care. It is perhaps for this reason
that he made special provision in his will for his mother despite the
fact that she had remarried. The will states that "in the event that
his mother, Monna Maria, former wife of Alamanno Martelli, now
married to Antonio di Filippo Corbiri, Florentine citizen and banker,
find herself again a widow she will hold all the goods of the testator in usufruct so long as she remains a widow and leads an honest
life."[87] But Sigismondo didn't stop there. After his death, Francesco di
Galeotto and his heirs would indeed own the entire palazzo at Canto

alla Paglia. They were not, however, to throw Maria and her charge Francesco out. If Francesco di Galeotto or his sons wished to live in that residence or hold it in any way that reduced the circumstances of Sigismondo's mother, they had to compensate her to the tune of twenty-five scudi every year that she held his portion in usufruct. This was not an insignificant amount, accounting for roughly a third of the total value of the palazzo.[88]

Sigismondo's will suggests that he knew only too well how vulnerable his younger brother was. Francesco *mentecatto* was a legally dead carrier of property. He held it but could not manage it. His only function in terms of succession was to pass what patrimony he received on. While alive he was worth a good deal to those who controlled his estate; dead, he was worth more. Through his property, Francesco di Galeotto could consolidate an estate that time and the Florentine practice of partible inheritance had split into more and smaller portions among legitimate heirs. With Francesco under his control, he could pass on a reunited estate that included a well-situated palazzo in the center of town and respectable agricultural holdings in the surrounding countryside. The only people standing between him and this happy eventuality were Sigismondo, a sickly young man, and his mother.

Sigismondo died a mere three years later, leaving no legitimate children. Control of his estate passed to Maria Corsi, who held it in usufruct. For the moment, Francesco seems to have had sufficient care. Francesco di Galeotto died in 1555, leaving his estate to his sons. This occasion, too, was cause for compromise rather than conflict. According to the 1561 tax census, Maria Corsi shared ownership of the palazzo at Canto alla Paglia together with Giovanni and Alessandro. Rather than living there, they rented out the residence and an attached *bottega* at the healthy rate of eighty-six scudi a year. By that point, Maria had repaired to via Larga where she leased a residence next to the convent of Santa Caterina on the Piazza San Marco for thirty-one scudi a year. Two females, servants perhaps, and two males, one of whom was surely her impaired son Francesco, lived with her.

The same records place Alessandro next door, leasing a residence for eighteen scudi a year. He shared this house with two males—possibly his young sons—and four women—certainly his wife and likely his two young daughters. Curiously, Filippo lived toward the eastern outskirts of the town nowhere near his family where he leased a residence for eighteen scudi a year.[89] The records do not say where Giovanni and Andrea lived, but it would seem that for the moment they were comfortable and at peace. It was not to last.

If Maria's petition of 1579 suggests that Francesco *mentecatto*'s heirs were waiting in the wings to claim his property for their own uses, Margherita Pandolfini's will of 1570 confirms it. This document unearths longstanding conflicts between her sons that would last well into the next generation. Margherita took up the banner of her sons Andrea and Giovanni. As the eldest of five legitimate heirs, she left Andrea with ultimate authority to execute her will.[90]

Margherita was not well-disposed toward all of her sons, being especially cool toward to Alessandro. She named Andrea, Giovanni, Lorenzo, and Filippo universal heirs of her estate but demanded that Alessandro and his son Francesco receive a "quantità certa," a specified quantity in the amount of five hundred florins to be paid to Alessandro after her death.[91] He would also receive a fifth part of all household goods and a fifth part of all Monte comune credits.[92] She added acidly that Alessandro should "remain quiet and content with the portion assigned to him and not trouble or harass his other brothers on account of his inheritance."[93]

Margherita made special provision for Filippo "in his sickness" and Lorenzo, who was also considered *mentecatto*.[94] Her eldest son, Andrea, had already been taking care of these two and was to continue to do so once his mother died. In order to ease the financial burden of caring for his brothers she left Andrea the inheritance she had received from her mother.[95] Andrea had apparently already used this estate to cover the expenses of care for Lorenzo and Filippo, but he would have full access to it once his mother died.

In addition to the estate of his maternal grandmother, Andrea also acquired control of Filippo and Lorenzo's properties, which included responsibility for paying taxes assessed on the holdings and managing rental agreements and incomes.[96] If Andrea predeceased Filippo and Lorenzo, Giovanni would assume their care; were Giovanni then to die, Margherita asked "for the love of God that the [Pupilli] undertake the protection, guardianship, and care of these poor *impediti* and of their goods and wealth." What she wanted to avoid was guardianship by Alessandro. Her will expressly ordered that "Alessandro, her son can never have nor can he try to have or ever be given by the Pupilli the care of Lorenzo and Filippo or of any of their goods." Margherita, like Maria Corsi, left nothing to chance. Her will stipulated that if Andrea and Giovanni "were negligent or if they misused the guardianship of their poor *impediti* brothers" (a thing she did not believe could happen), she invited the Pupilli to intervene and deprive them of guardianship.[97]

Alessandro died in 1575, the same year as Margherita, but squabbles over patrimony did not end. Rather Alessandro's sons, Francesco and Cammillo, together with their widowed mother, continued the battle. From this point on, the care and property of the three *mentecatti* were at the center of hostilities. In that fateful November 1579, the very same month that Filippo accused his brothers Andrea and Giovanni of neglecting him and Maria Corsi made alternative arrangements for the care of her impaired son, the heirs of Alessandro initiated litigation against Andrea, Giovanni, and Filippo.[98] The guardian of Alessandro's sons claimed that these uncles owed them upward of 569 florins.[99] Litigation centered on the dispersal of the *mentecatto* Lorenzo's estate, suggesting he had recently died.

In April 1587 Maria Corsi, Francesco's mother, died. Her death revived the question of who should care for Francesco *mentecatto*, which, in turn, revived disputes about the control of Martelli patrimony. Her death also prompted Vespucci to go quickly to the Pupilli to assume the guardianship of her *mentecatto* son and claim rights of usufruct to his estate. Vespucci reminded the Pupilli that "part of the goods of the *mentecatto* were left to him by [Maria Corsi] because," he elaborated, "the care of a *mentecatto* is a heavy burden."[100] He further stated that he would submit an account of expenditures pertaining specifically to the care of Francesco *mentecatto*, but nothing else.

Enter Francesco *mentecatto*'s second cousins, Andrea and Giovanni, who, as Maria Corsi suspected, had waited a long time for this day to come. They made a counterclaim, stating that "it did not seem reasonable that this Vespucci should enjoy Francesco's estate in a way that prejudiced them." For their part, Vespucci as an outsider (*estraneo*) had no legitimate claim on Francesco's property. Andrea and Giovanni, as "the closest Martelli [agnate] relations to the *mentecatto*," had rights to his patrimony, which was, after his death, theirs anyway. In response, the Duke's office revoked what it had granted in 1579 since it "seemed to the Duke more appropriate that this *mentecatto* be a ward of the Martelli and that the Pupilli make sure he is treated well"—a strange comment considering proximity in the very recent past had not ensured the good treatment of Filippo by these very men.[101]

Fifteen days after her death, Maria Corsi's fears had come true. The dubious Andrea and Giovanni assumed the care of her impaired son. Getting their hands on Francesco meant that they now had access to what was left of the Martelli estate passed down from their great-grandfather Francesco di Niccolò, which included shares in the house at Canto alla Paglia in Florence as well as holdings in Prato and the Florentine countryside.

By 1600 litigation over the estate had finally shifted to the last generation of this Martelli patriline. The battle lines were the same, the heir of Giovanni Martelli against the heirs of Alessandro, the brother who had been spurned in Margherita Pandolfini's will of 1570. Andrea Martelli had died in 1591, leaving the care of the two *mentecatti*, Francesco and Filippo, in the hands of his brother Giovanni. Francesco died in 1594 followed by his guardian Giovanni five years later. Three potential Martelli guardians could have taken over Filippo's care: Vincenzo, Giovanni's son, or Francesco and Camillo Alessandro's sons. One might assume that Vincenzo would have inherited Filippo's wardship from his father. Pupilli records show rather that Francesco d'Alessandro Martelli quickly won the role perhaps with the collusion of Filippo himself.[102]

This litigation accused Andrea and Giovanni of mismanaging the estates of their incapacitated wards, Lorenzo, Filippo, and Francesco. At no point, so the record goes, did Andrea or Giovanni ever submit an account of the goods and properties they managed for the three *mentecatti*. What was worse, Francesco d'Alessandro accused his uncle Giovanni of having misappropriated Filippo's resources so that he was, by the time of his death, in debt to Filippo's estate.[103]

Vincenzo and his guardian fought Francesco d'Alessandro's claim on Filippo and his property. In October 1600, they urged the Pupilli to deprive Francesco of Filippo's wardship, alleging that "Filippo was poorly treated and poorly governed." "Filippo himself," they maintained, "called himself dissatisfied with Francesco." They added that "it was declared on a previous occasion that Francesco cannot keep Filippo in his house and is prohibited expressly in the will of Monna Margherita their paternal grandmother." Finally, they claimed that Francesco's guardianship was not properly publicized, that is, "it was created without notifying anyone."[104]

Bitterness between Francesco d'Alessandro and his cousin Vincenzo did not end there. Hostilities seem to have reached a fever pitch when the Pupilli records report that in December 1601 Monna Caterina Gerini, Vincenzo's mother, who had been paying rent to live at the Martelli palazzo at Canto alla Paglia, had petitioned the Pupilli in desperation. Francesco d'Alessandro "had changed the locks to the main door so that Monna Caterina . . . could not enter the house."[105] As she saw it, Francesco d'Alessandro wanted to be "padrone assoluto" over his own interests and those of Filippo.

These machinations may have deprived Vincenzo of a sizable portion of the Martelli estate, but he had the last laugh. Francesco d'Alessandro died in 1639 and left the better part of his estate to the only living heir of his patriline, his cousin Vincenzo. Vincenzo had no legitimate children and so the line of Francesco di Niccolò died with him. Thereafter, his estate passed to a more robust Martelli branch.

To the descendants of Francesco di Niccolò Martelli, a withering cadet branch of an otherwise wealthy, respectable, and durable family, property was key. Those who were competent plotted and schemed to wrest property from vulnerable relatives. Those who held property, but could not manage it, were pawns in a long and vitriolic series of patrimonial disputes. But exploitation was not the only choice on the menu. The mothers of the mentally incapacitated men, Maria Corsi and Margherita Pandolfini, were determined to provide care for them: Maria by describing to the letter how Francesco was to be cared for, by whom, and with what funds, Margherita by explicitly excluding one of her sons from guardianship—though, as subsequent litigation demonstrated, perhaps her choice of Andrea and Giovanni was not so well-advised. In the end, Maria and Margherita's dying wishes could not withstand the stratagems of the living.

Guardianship existed as a normative construct that jurists debated, courts adopted, and the Florentine government used to play a role in the management of Tuscan households. By statute, custom, and practice, however, guardianship in Tuscan society was and remained above all the prerogative of the family. Given the small number of cases involving mental and physical incapacity that actually made it to court, we can assume that most families quietly made their own arrangements for good or ill. Archival evidence suggests that families generally turned to courts only when there was some confusion about who should act as guardian, when a large or important slice of an estate was at stake, or when private networks failed them. When a court or magistracy was involved, it worked together with families, monitoring their efforts to provide care of vulnerable kin and their property. Civic officials and judges could intervene in conflicts between relatives over who should or should not act as a guardian, but, for the most part, they sanctioned arrangements that families had already made and favored more proximate over more remote heirs as guardians as a way of protecting legal paths of succession.

It would be wrong to assume that the lead actors in these family dramas were always male. Women, in fact, played a central role in guardianship cases. In the same way that opportunistic male heirs used law courts to exploit vulnerable kin, mothers, aunts, and other female relatives often used the same courts to protect them. The limiting factor on their success was often death rather than gender. But the march of time was a challenge to everyone, relatives and magistrates included. Even under what seemed like the best of circumstances, the care of a mad man or woman was indeed a heavy burden.

CHAPTER 2

"Madness Is Punishment Enough"

The Insanity Defense

Most esteemed and merciful Signore, so many are the favors that I have had from you in these my troubles that I don't know another person more obligated to you than I am, and, especially with your help, it seems to me that where I had a senseless woman for a wife, now she has soundness of mind and intellect . . . at present we remain in good hope that she will never err again. Moved by this hope based in the grace of God I would wish, if it is pleasing to Your most Illustrious Excellency, that you would willingly return her to me so that I may bring her home. [I give] assurance to the Office of the Magnificent Lords of the Otto that she will not harm anyone. If I obtain this from your mercy it would seem like I'm getting out of a hell, the consumption of my resources, and penury.

In May 1549, two years before Paolo da Falla sent this petition to Florence's Otto di Guardia, his wife, Piera, killed her seven-year-old daughter and four-year-old nephew with a hatchet.[1] According to the record, "had she not been held back, she would have slaughtered another."[2] The criminal authorities immediately put her in prison for life as a mad woman (*pazza*). Once there, regardless of her status, she joined the women's ward, where lowly prostitutes rubbed elbows with more favorably born ladies.[3] In accord with its usual practice, the prison would not pay for her upkeep. The costs of food, clothing, and, should she need it, medical care fell instead to Paolo.[4]

Piera had only been in prison one month when her name appeared on the list of forty-four inmates who were to receive special amnesty on the feast day of St. John the Baptist. Yet it would seem that she was not among the group of thieves, murderers, arsonists, debtors, fraudsters, sodomites, and general public nuisances who processed to freedom that June. Paolo's six petitions to the Otto in four years, arguing that her prison costs were too high, suggests rather that she remained in prison.[5]

He appealed to them first in November 1550. Piera "was not particularly sound of mind," he said, but she was not "furiosa." He assured them that if they let her go she would be locked up in a room he built specially for her confinement in his house and supervised by a guardian. The secretary of the Otto passed the case on to the Duke, who ordered that, for the time being, Piera remain in prison.[6]

Paolo made the same request in April 1551. This time he told the Otto that "she was almost cured." Piera, he said, "shows sign of remembering the crime she committed, repents of it, and regrets it greatly." Again he reminded them that supporting her in prison was beyond his means and that he had made necessary preparations at home to protect his family and the community from any lapse back into madness. But the Duke remained unmoved. "Almost cured" was not good enough; remorse and regret were not sufficient safeguards against another attack of madness. Paolo should not, he replied, seek her release again.[7] Undeterred, Paolo petitioned the Otto a third time that October in much the same terms. He asked yet again that the Duke release Piera into his care. Yet again the Duke replied that her return to her right mind was of no consequence. In prison she stayed.[8]

The fourth petition was the charm. In November 1552, Paolo offered a new solution to the problem of Piera's care, while making a more forceful appeal to the Duke's sense of compassion. The years in prison away from her family had begun to take their toll. Paolo could no longer support Piera in prison, but he also did not want her "to lose heart [believing herself to have been] abandoned by all her relatives and children." Since hiring a guardian had not passed ducal muster, Paolo asked that the Otto instead allow Piera to enter a convent in Arezzo where one of her daughters resided. Failing that, Paolo told the Duke that he would "have her locked up in a room where he could at least supervise her and she would sometimes have the pleasure of seeing her children, her husband, and her relatives so that she will not live in despair as she does in prison."[9]

These appeals finally won for Paolo more than automatic refusal. The Otto took up the case anew, interviewing Piera's prison guards. For two years, they claimed, Piera "remained senseless and idiotic," to such an extent that everyone considered her "simple minded (*mentecapta*)." She groundlessly despised everyone, fled all conversation, and lived like a wild person (*frenetica*). But then she seemed "to get better." By the time of Paolo's fourth petition, prison personnel agreed that she had regained her senses. When the Stinche guards asked her to talk about her crime, she said that "she did not recall ever having done such a thing. She was saddened by her miserable lot and every hour thought about her husband, children, and relatives, crying and despairing because she could not speak to them." The guards claimed, too, that she fretted over the morals of the other women in prison: "whenever any of the prostitutes who are imprisoned there say something dishonorable, Piera chastises them, urging them to adopt good habits, work, and do good."[10] These new findings coupled with Paolo's plan to outsource her care to a convent pleased the Duke. After spending more than three years in prison, Piera was released.

But Paolo's plan foundered. Upon her arrival at the convent, the nuns turned her away and she had to be hastily placed in the house of a relative who lived nearby. These circumstances are the backdrop for the petition that opened this chapter. By this point, Paolo was desperate; his wife's anguish as well as the cost of her care threatened to ruin him. This time the Duke through the Otto responded with compassion. He would be content, he replied, so long as Piera was kept in someone's house and was not permitted to venture outside.[11] After three years, Piera finally returned home.

In September 1554, Paolo sought the court's mercy one last time. Piera had been in his house "for twenty months without ever going outside." Since she did nothing crazy during that whole time, Paolo insisted that "she had made a full recovery." "Might then the Duke," he asked, "be persuaded to let her leave the house to attend mass and do some other things?" The Duke was well-disposed, responding simply, "She may."[12]

Piera's case is an excellent albeit gruesome window onto the landscape of criminal law in late medieval and early modern Florence. It shows first that Florentine courts were not vindictive toward the mad; they did not hold an offender who could be shown to lack intent or understanding liable for his or her actions no matter the crime. The dilemma in cases of criminal insanity was not how to punish people like Piera but how and who was to care for them. The problems households and courts confronted in these cases was really another facet of guardianship and the *ad hoc* nature of that institution.

Civic authorities had to do something about violent offenders like
Piera, but they had not figured out what that something was. Even
the most violent among them tended to end up in the custody of their
families. What happened next was entirely dependent on the constitution and disposition of that network. Paolo's petitions to the Otto
suggest that she was fortunate in her kin. Whether he was genuinely
concerned for her comfort or acted on her behalf for some less honorable reason the record does not reveal. Surely other mentally disturbed offenders—some of whom we see dimly through court documents but most of whom we do not see at all—were not so fortunate.

Like civil cases of guardianship, the series of back-and-forth nego-
tiations that engaged the energies of Paolo, the court of the Otto, and
the Duke for four years show the society of makeshifts at work. The
goal of the family was the protection of honor, stability, and patrimony
while that of the republican and ducal justice systems was to maintain
or restore public order. These goals were at times in common, at others in conflict. But neither the ambitions of an ever-expanding state
nor the instrumental use of criminal proceedings by litigants determined the fate of the criminally insane. To put it another way, neither
a purely top-down nor bottom-up model captures the spirit of negotiation that animated cases of criminal insanity as petitioners and
civic authorities met in the arena of the courts to hammer out some
workable solution to the problem of what to do with mad offenders.

If there was one overarching principle guiding the Florentine justice
system it was that everything was negotiable. Like their civil counterparts, Florentine criminal courts were, above all, arenas where magistrates and families collaborated to address the practical problems
caused by mental incapacity or criminal insanity and, in so doing,
to establish some balance between private and public interest. These
joint efforts represent the kind of collaborative social ordering that
took place in Florentine and, on a larger scale, in late medieval and
early modern civil and criminal courts throughout Europe.[13]

NOT LIABLE BY REASON OF INSANITY

Roman law supplied medieval Italian jurists with legal remedies for
addressing criminal insanity in court but only general principles for
tackling the problem of what to do with the criminally insane over
the long term. Though separated by almost fifteen hundred years,
Piera's case is a near perfect echo of a rescript issued by the Roman

emperor Marcus Aurelius late in the second century CE. When asked
whether one Aelius Priscus, a man who had killed his mother in a fit
of rage, should be held responsible for the crime, the emperor replied:
"If it is clearly determined that Aelius Priscus is in such a *furor* that,
due to continual alienation of mind (*mentis alienatio*), he lacks all
understanding (*intellectus*) and there is no suspicion that he killed
his mother under the guise of madness (*dementia*) then you can disregard the manner of his punishment since he is punished enough by
the *furor* itself."[14] Modestinus (d. 244 CE), a Roman jurist writing in
the fourth and fifth decades of the third century, also captured this
sentiment. His version runs: "if an infant or *furiosus* kills a man they
are not held liable by the *Lex Cornelia* since lack of understanding
protects the one and the unhappiness of his fate excuses the other."[15]

Roman jurists believed that, like children, the mad lacked judgment, depriving their actions of informed intent. As such, they could
not be held liable for damage to property or homicide.[16] In the case
of damage to property they likened the mad not only to children but
also to animals; in one colorful example, the second-century Roman
jurist Ulpian even said that a mad man had as much will as a roof tile
coming loose and causing damage as it fell to the ground.[17]

But the mentally disturbed had about them, too, an air of misfortune. They deserved pity not punishment. *Furiosi* and *mentecapti* of whatever variety stood on the periphery of legal personhood in a limbo peopled by minors, women, slaves, and, under
certain circumstances, the deaf, the mute, and the blind. Bereft of
self-consciousness, judgment, volition, or intent, as far as Roman
jurists were concerned, the life of the mad individual was no life
at all.

Roman jurists did not seek punishment for the criminally insane,
but they did mandate confinement. Marcus Aurelius's rescript
ordered that Aelius Priscus "be placed under careful restraint, and,
if . . . appropriate, he should even be put in chains, since this per-
tains not so much to his punishment as it does to his own safety
as well as the safety of his neighbors."[18] But who was to carry this
out? Ulpian claimed that if *furiosi* could not be controlled by their
relatives, responsibility for applying a remedy fell to civic officials.
The burden of confinement seems to have rested first with relatives
and, barring that, public institutions. So long as the person in question was no longer a public menace the nature of confinement was
immaterial.

FROM PRISON TO STREET IN REPUBLICAN FLORENCE

During Florence's republican period, judges applied Roman law principles to the problem of criminal insanity in the courts of the Capitano, a court of first instance and appeal, and the Podestà. Litigants,
in turn, used Roman law principles in these courts to have the sentences of their mentally disturbed kin mitigated or, if they could fashion strong enough arguments, completely forgiven. Occasionally the
Signoria, Florence's main executive council, intervened in these proceedings by *provvisione* (executive decree). In general, cases came
before these courts in one of three ways: by accusation of the injured
party, anonymous denunciation, or *ex officio*, that is, initiated by the
courts after a person had been apprehended *in flagrante delicto* or
on the basis of *fama* (rumor), the "unanimous clamor of unnamed
informants."[19]

Since cases involving criminal insanity tended also to involve violence or some kind of disruption of the peace they were typically prosecuted *ex officio*. As a result, they reveal little about how litigating
individuals or parties used the courts to settle disputes or, as some
historians have pointed out, pursue enmity.[20] They shed light rather
on how families and civic authorities interacted in court—sometimes
in collaboration, sometimes at odds—to address the problem of criminal insanity in their households and neighborhoods.

What we see in the pool of light that briefly illuminates mentally
incapacitated men and women as they passed through the courts of
late medieval and early modern Florence are the cracks in that structure. There simply were no public solutions to the problem of criminal
insanity. After offenders were apprehended and put in prison, family
members came forward to plead an exception, namely, that a relative
could not be held liable by reason of insanity. From that point on, the
problem of guardianship came to the fore. Here ambiguity reigned.
The question of what to do with mentally unstable and potentially
dangerous people plagued households, neighborhoods, courts, and
governing authorities for the entire period of this study.

Custodial institutions that look to modern eyes like obvious candidates for care or supervision of the mad, in general, and the criminally insane, in particular, were ill suited to the task in medieval and
early modern Florence. By and large, hospitals administered acute
care to the sick poor. Although severely mentally ill men and women
occasionally occupied their beds—or found themselves chained to

their walls—hospitals were neither prepared nor inclined to care for or house them long term.[21] Monasteries and convents were similarly reluctant to take on people who could not contribute materially or spiritually to their communities. They were not beyond refusing an unstable person admittance if they thought he or she posed a threat to their members.

Overall mad offenders ended up in prison with determinate—one or two years—or indeterminate (*per sempre*) sentences. Whatever the court's decision, they rarely remained there for long. Republican authorities temporarily incarcerated the violently insane to get them off the streets only to release them back into their communities, unloading the burden of their care and supervision back onto the shoulders of their relatives and, in particularly severe cases, their neighbors as well.

The problem was largely one of resources. Prison terms were meant to be temporary; prisons were not designed to house a large and permanent population nor could they materially support one.[22] The city of Florence had two main prisons: the Bargello and the Stinche. The Bargello, now a museum of the same name, was attached to the palace of the Podestà. It mainly housed political prisoners awaiting trial and fell under the control of whatever regime held sway in the Signoria.[23] Several streets away toward the eastern outskirts of the city loomed the Stinche prison, a massive stone edifice with three towers projecting above forty-four-foot walls. Although often referred to as a debtors' prison since debt was the most common offense among inmates, the Stinche incarcerated a variety of offenders.[24] Unlike the ambiguously state-run Bargello, by the mid-fourteenth century, a lay supervisory committee of four *buonuomini* operated it to profit the commune until the principate when it was controlled and financed directly by the ducal state.[25] In both republican and ducal Florence, costs of room and board fell to relatives of the person imprisoned. If those relatives were ill disposed to provide care or simply lacked resources to do so, prisoners languished unless charitable organizations stepped in to foot the bill.

Keeping the mentally disturbed in prison was an expensive proposition for state or privately operated prisons as well as families. The best financial solution for all involved once the threat of imminent danger had been at the very least mitigated was to entrust the criminally insane to his or her kin, those who by reason of blood or marriage presumably had the greatest incentive to care for them—a provisional, improvised arrangement at best. Thus even in cases where the civic authorities handed down what sounded like a life sentence, the criminally insane were habitually released back into their households and communities with little more than infamy preceding them.

We may observe this tendency at work in two early fifteenth-century cases, the first involving damage to property, the second homicide. In 1407, a certain Margarita of Prato was charged with arson—a very serious crime—before the Giudice degli Appelli, the Capitano's court of appeals. The case had been initiated *ex officio* by the Capitano and his officials since rumor of Margarita's illegal activities had repeatedly been brought to their attention.[26]

According to the case record, during the wee hours of one October morning in 1406, Margarita had gone to the house of her neighbors, Mea and Stefano, in search of a light for her lantern. Mea thought Margarita's presence at her door highly suspicious. She eventually gave Margarita her light, but not before telling her to go "'wisely and in health so that you don't damage anything. I heard that you set fire to the house and stables of Lionardo last December.'"[27]

Margarita went on her way that night only to set fire to the bakery of one Stefano Tomasini and two nearby houses.[28] Later that same month, Margarita appeared in Tizziano, a town in the Pistoian countryside. Her reputation preceded her. When she showed up at the house of one Andrea, seeking shelter for the night, his wife wanted none of it. According to her testimony before the Capitano, she told Margarita that she would not open her door to "the *pazza* of Florence who goes setting fire to straw." "'You are a mad woman,' she said, 'and I don't want mad women in [my] house.'"[29] The testimonies of Mea, Stefano, Andrea's wife, and others convinced the court that Margarita was widely held to be a public menace and one who cost her neighbors a good deal of money. The Capitano ordered his men to take her into custody where she confessed to several acts of arson.

Margarita had wreaked havoc on several communities; rumors of her alleged insanity had spread throughout Florence and beyond. But the court was sensitive to her circumstances. The Capitano's judge relaxed the sentence "on account of her confession and her insanity." Still he fined her 150 lire and required that she serve a one-year prison sentence to prevent her from harming others. If she did not pay the fine within ten days, the judge ordered that she was to be beaten through the piazzas of Pistoia and other public locations according to Pistoiese custom.[30] In other words, the court wished to show mercy while satisfying justice. Part of the satisfaction of justice involved providing some outlet to the rage her neighbors felt at the destruction she left in her wake. The damage that Margarita had caused, her *furor* and *dementia* notwithstanding, had destroyed the livelihood of several local families. Her offenses could not go unanswered.

There is no record that Margarita ever paid the fine. If she could not pay in lire she would pay publicly with her body. Either way, the court's solution to the problem of her pyromania was temporary at best. Having her flogged through the streets at the hands of her neighbors may have gone some way to appeasing public fury, but the negligible prison sentence demonstrates the lack of a long-term custodial solution. No arrangements were made for after her release. From this point on, Margarita's flame goes out; the case record ends. One can only guess at what became of her and the properties of her neighbors.

A case of 1415 similarly demonstrates the Florentine justice system's inclination to mitigate criminal sentences for the mentally disturbed as well as its tendency to pass responsibility for their care onto their families or neighbors. In February of that year, the Capitano's court initiated proceedings *ex officio* against one Anastasio of Florence for brutally murdering his mother. The court investigation found that Anastasio, armed with a wooden stick, attacked his mother while she was in her house, bludgeoning her to death. The notary remarked that property interests were a plausible motive for such behavior. At the same time, the record acknowledged that Anastasio and his brothers stood to inherit their mother's estate whether or not she died intestate. Since part of her property would devolve to him anyway, the court concluded that Anastasio really had no rational motive for striking her down.[31]

This case comes down to us in two forms: first, as a record of the investigation performed by the Capitano's court in 1415, and then four years later as an executive appeal urging his release from prison issued by the Signoria. The court of the Capitano initiated inquisition proceedings immediately after the homicide. They examined witnesses, evaluated evidence, decided upon and then executed a sentence. The judge formally announced the proceedings by means of a public citation in accord with statute. In response, Anastasio was to present himself at court, but neither he nor anyone else came forward on his behalf to defend or explain his actions. After the time allotted by law to answer the citation had passed, the court proclaimed Anastasio contumacious and a ban was invoked against him.

For reasons that are not clear, the Signoria issued a *bullectino*, an executive mandate to intervene in the Capitano's proceedings: "[I]t is clear, notorious, and manifest that at the time of the homicide as well as before and after, Anastasio was, had been, and is to this day *furiosus* and in the grips of the most powerful *furor* for which reason he should be released from penalty. Nevertheless, in order that no similar wrongdoing may occur let him pay his penalty with his body."[32] Civic authorities, and rather high-up ones at that, acknowledged that Anastasio had committed a terrible crime but decided that he had done it while mad. As the court concluded in Margarita's case, Anastasio deserved a mitigated sentence even if some kind of punishment had to be written into his flesh. He was accordingly condemned to prison for the term of his life by the authority of the Capitano.

In 1419, a petition was filed regarding Anastasio's case in the *Provvisioni*, the Signoria's day-to-day approval of petitions and promulgation of laws and decrees. The story went deeper than what the Capitano's proceedings of 1415 had revealed. The period leading up to the crime found Anastasio entangled in various legal battles with his brothers and suffering profound sadness. These entanglements drove him to such depths of despair that on one occasion he threw himself into the well of his house. In the words of the notary, he acted so strangely during this period that anyone of sound mind would have thought him beset by *dementia*. But Anastasio's behavior during his imprisonment in the Stinche had been unimpeachable from his entry in 1415 to the reopening of the case four years later. Based on his good behavior, civic authorities concluded he should be freed.[33]

Communal ritual marked the bestowal of that freedom. Anastasio was to present himself as an offering to God on the feast day of Saint John the Baptist (June 24): "at the accustomed time he should proceed to the church of San Giovanni Battista behind horn players with his head uncovered and a torch held in his hands as a public offering and especially on behalf of Benedetto de' Morelli," the man who had fought for Anastasio's release.[34]

The intervention of Morelli and the Signoria may seem strange, but this type of general amnesty, established by the 1322–25 redaction of the statutes of the Capitano, was common in Florence, Tuscany, and well beyond.[35] As an act of Christian mercy, the law allowed a certain number of prisoners liberation on three holy occasions during the year: Easter, Christmas, and the feast day of Saint John the Baptist. Technically not all prisoners were eligible. Only the poorest and most wretched were usually granted freedom and only fifty could be released at any one time. In order that no one abused the amnesty it could be granted to a person only once in the course of his or her lifetime. This practice of ritual purification had practical benefits. It offered criminals languishing in prison for the nonpayment of pecuniary penalties or with indeterminate sentences their freedom and it prevented the prison population from soaring to unmanageable numbers. It also allowed the Florentine community to play a role in the forgiveness of criminal offenses, particularly by those who had no family networks to look out for their interests.

MADNESS BEHIND CLOSED DOORS

What happened to the criminally insane after they dissolved once again into the fabric of Florentine society? Where did they go and in what company? Did Margarita set more fires? Did she get beaten through the streets of Prato? Did she end up in prison? And what of the matricide Anastasio? Did his brothers take on the burden of his care? Did they lock him up? Did they cast him out into the streets? Did he throw himself into a well, managing once and for all to kill himself? These are not questions court records answer in detail if they answer them at all. Once the courts closed the books on cases involving the mentally disturbed, historians tend to lose sight of them. For the most part, the experience of madness was lived behind closed doors.

A sensational mid-fourteenth century case of homicide captures something of the daily struggles families, friends, and magistrates faced to supervise the criminally insane. In January 1365, one Biagio of Prato found himself in the Stinche prison as a *furiosus* and *mentecaptus*.[36] He had killed a man named Santo without cause, which brought him to the attention of the Florentine authorities. Biagio's uncle, Filippo, pled an exception on behalf of his nephew. He presented to the court twenty-four articles, all of which claimed that the people of Prato, including Biagio's friends, relatives, and neighbors, considered him to be so mad that he could neither govern his behavior nor understand its consequences. These articles were read aloud in the vernacular to ten witnesses summoned to Florence, who were then asked to confirm or deny them and, where possible, to elaborate on them.

That Biagio had gone mad was not in dispute. Eighteen months before he killed Santo, he had led an unremarkable life. He went about his business; he had friends. And then something changed. There is no mention of a precipitating event or injury, but his family, friends, and neighbors universally agreed that madness swallowed him whole; he was continually beset by *furor* and bereft of memory.[37] To give some color to his behavior, two of his friends mentioned that they had both seem him on one occasion in one of Prato's piazzas, trudging through the mud in the pouring rain, tossing money into the air all the while yelling, "Who's up for a drink?"[38] Another of Biagio's neighbors noted that similar episodes drew the attention of the Podestà of Prato who demanded Biagio's confinement. He was duly shackled in iron and wooden fetters by his mother and unnamed others and remained like that except for the days that he broke his chains and escaped.[39] Witness testimony paints a pathetic picture of his time there. One witness claimed that he had seen Biagio chained in a ground-floor room in the manner of a dog.[40] Another noted that Biagio remained in that way *furiosus* and sunk in an "alienation of mind" for several months.[41]

It would be easy to level a charge of cruelty against Biagio's mother who had him bound, against his neighbors who bore witness or perhaps helped her do it, or against the magistrate who ordered such treatment in the first place. Such a judgment would be hasty and unfair. The highly constructed nature of court documents, from articles prepared by litigating parties to witness testimony, makes it very difficult to understand exactly what was going on in Biagio's household. We have only the consensus among witnesses as a guide for recreating the scene there. His friends, neighbors, and the friends of the man he killed unanimously agreed that he was out of control. As in Piera's case of two hundred years later, compassion played second fiddle to security.

There was good reason for caution. Despite his bonds, Biagio proved to be a constant menace to his own safety and that of others. At one point he managed to break free, flee the house, and dash through the streets with a crowd of people hard on his heels. The crowd finally caught him and dragged him back to his mother's house where he was fettered once more. On another occasion, Biagio wriggled out of his chains, ran to the window, and threw a lance through it, seriously wounding a man who happened to be walking by. Two of the witnesses noted that this man was none other than Piero Guelfi, one of Biagio's close friends before he had succumbed to *furor*. They also claimed to have been there to help Biagio's mother and other relatives drag Biagio from the window and chain him up again.[42] Those same witnesses assured the court that they used iron chains to restrain him and to prevent him from harming anyone else.[43]

Neighbors also testified that he continually tried to set fire to his bed. One Matteo remarked that Biagio would have burned the entire house down had a number of people, Matteo included, not secured him and dragged him to an adjoining room.[44] Another witness claimed that it was not merely a random number of people who had to rescue Biagio from the flames but men serving the Podestà of the city.[45]

Biagio's mother and sister, too, fell prey to his fury. A neighbor alleged that while Biagio simmered in continual *furor* he would strike his mother and tear the clothing from her back.[46] Even worse, Biagio would tell his mother and sister that he wanted to get underneath them and, while raising his own clothing, he showed them his "private parts."[47] Another witness claimed that in the company of others Biagio would say to his mother and sister that he wanted to know them carnally while acting as if he were conducting a business transaction (*si esset ad negotium*).[48] We are meant to understand here that he propositioned his mother and sister as if they were prostitutes.

The remaining six witnesses, all residents of the San Leonardo neighborhood in the district of Prato, were called to substantiate claims surrounding the murder of Santo, which occurred after Biagio escaped confinement for a second time. According to one of them, together with Santo, he and several others had come upon Biagio wandering naked somewhere between Prato and the streets of Pistoia presumably after he had escaped yet again. They covered him and with gentle words coaxed him to Santo's house where he was fed and warmed by the fire.[49]

Night brought trouble. Two of the witnesses testified that they awoke sometime after midnight. Independently they made their way to Santo's mill to find him lying dead on the floor. Biagio stood nearby armed with an unsheathed knife. Rather than engage Biagio, both men sought help from neighbors.[50] They returned with two men and eventually managed to corner Biagio. He stood in dumb silence while they bound him but began to chatter senselessly once he was in chains: "I was the son of Messer Pietro di Bardi!" "I am the companion of a priest!" "I am one of the Freschobaldi!"[51]

They brought Biagio to a nearby inn where, all through the night, as one witness put it, Biagio bellowed, bawled, and spewed forth complete nonsense. At some point Biagio's captors must have sent word to the Podestà for the following morning he dispatched men to take the madman into custody. At daybreak, the four men traveled with the nearly naked, raving Biagio to a bridge on the outskirts of Prato where they met the Podestà's officers. Biagio's uncle Filippo was also there. He hauled his unruly nephew up onto his horse, beginning an awkward march back into Prato.[52]

Nearly all of Prato gathered to see Biagio being led back into the city seated, with his uncle, uneasily atop a horse. One witness claimed that people along the way shouted, "Eccho Biagio paçço! [Look, it's Biagio the mad man!]"[53] Filippo held fast to his squirming nephew while another of his relatives skipped alongside to prevent Biagio from toppling to the ground. Witnesses claimed that over the heads of the heckling crowd Biagio made the sign of the cross in the manner of a bishop as he and this strange retinue advanced into Prato.[54] From there he was put in Florence's Stinche prison.

As long as Biagio's behavior remained safely in the realm of the bizarre and unruly the Pratese Podestà saw fit only to demand his incarceration and vigilant attendance by his mother and relatives in her house. The podesterial gaze stopped at the door of the household. It was only when Biagio committed homicide that he attracted the attention of the authorities again, going from private burden to public menace. By statute, cases of homicide in Florence's domains had to be turned over to the central authorities based in the city of Florence.[55] But even in the hands of the Florentine Podestà, after a brief thirteen-month stint in prison, Biagio was again released into the custody of his beleaguered mother and sister.[56]

Behind the episodes of Biagio's madness captured in court documents surely a longer drama played out across days and years. As his primary caretakers, his mother and sister may have been the main players, suffering the brunt of his *dementia*, but the effects of Biagio's madness rippled beyond the walls of his household. The drama spilled into the streets where he terrorized or, in the case of that strange procession, entertained his community. His neighbors, friends, and the municipal authorities of Prato were often called on to restrain him. The drama reached also into the district of Prato where he killed an innocent man. Once he committed homicide, Biagio of Prato temporarily became a Florentine problem. Without a legal or institutional strategy for long-term care and supervision, however, he was returned home. Had the court's sole interest been public safety, surely it would have kept Biagio imprisoned. After all, despite assurances given by his family and neighbors that Biagio had been bound in iron shackles, he had managed to escape twice, on the first occasion wreaking havoc on the streets of Prato and on the second killing a man in the district.

Short of tossing Biagio in the Stinche's *pazzeria* (the mad cell), as a for-profit institution that prison had little incentive to pay for his care. Biagio's upkeep there would have cost his family dearly day to day, month to month, and year to year. The best financial solution for court, prison, and family was to release Biagio into the custody of his kin with assurances that he would be locked up at home. There is no indication that the court troubled itself much over the nature of his confinement; the court made no threats to hold Biagio's relatives responsible for his behavior should he escape again. There is also no record of another escape or further misbehavior. Whatever disorder Biagio's madness caused it did not again attract the attention of magistrates or courts. We are left to wonder both what happened to Biagio when the walls of his home closed around him once more and what daily challenges his mother, sister, friends, and neighbors faced in caring for him.

The cases of Biagio, Anastasio, and Margarita are rare but representative. Whatever the crime, whatever a person's circumstances, whatever shocks they sent through households, neighborhoods, and cities, Florentine judges tended to forgive and release the criminally insane even if they had taken the life of another person. Families and neighbors had to assume their care or suffer whatever anarchy madness brought into household or street. That meant that the care of a mentally disturbed person was utterly contingent on the compassion or willingness of kin to assume that burden. No doubt some people fared well, living in relative comfort, while others suffered neglect and abuse. The court documents reveal something of these experiences, but in the end, walls and doors rise to block posterity's view.

CRIMINAL JUSTICE FROM REPUBLIC TO DUCHY

Like the reverberations of a distant bell, Biagio's case resounds nearly two hundred years later in that of Piera's, the bloody case that opened this chapter. Despite the two centuries and different institutional contexts that separate them, they are strikingly similar. Both Biagio and Piera were released from liability for their crimes by reason of insanity; both served more than a year in prison before being freed. The

Duke's initial reluctance to release Piera might suggest that he, in contrast to republican authorities, demanded greater assurances that she would not harm another person. Volubility in one documentary tradition against the relative silence of another does not necessarily reflect different realities. This is, of course, one of the drawbacks to using court documents as lenses onto the way things were in specific times and places. The important point is that, in the end, the result was the same. Without institutional resources, public or private, in republican or ducal Florence, Biagio and Piera returned home where their respective families assumed the burden of their care.

The similarity of the cases is especially important to bear in mind in light of recent scholarship, arguing that the transition from republic to duchy in the sixteenth century spelled disaster for the criminally insane. Dukes of Florence and their elite band of bureaucrats used criminal courts to exercise political power and social control. As a result, marginalized groups like the mad and, in particular, the mad poor increasingly ended up in prison or worse, as oarsmen in the ducal navy.[57] A number of thorny practical problems, however, compromised the strength of the Duke's grip on the system, not least of all the great expense that went into turning the wheels of justice.

Robust centralization efforts during the principate in the sixteenth century meant that significantly more instances of criminal insanity appeared in court and significantly more mentally disturbed people passed through Florentine prisons or found themselves pressed into galley service. But an increase in a particular type of caseload and more energetic intervention in the day-to-day business of the criminal courts from the top did not mean that civic authorities had gotten a handle on the problem or had changed their stance toward mad offenders. Taken together, the more than one hundred and fifty cases of criminal insanity prosecuted in the criminal courts of Florence between the mid-fourteenth and mid-seventeenth centuries show that the fate of the criminally insane changed but little from republic to duchy.

Some of the transformations in Florentine justice were long in the coming, their roots going back to changes in republican courts that evolved over the course of the fifteenth century; others accompanied the transition from republic to duchy. In a long series of executive reforms of Florentine justice beginning in the 1460s, the courts of the Podestà and Capitano, where cases involving criminal insanity typically ended up, became less and less relevant. In 1463 the Signoria

moved significantly to reduce the retinue of the Podestà followed in
1477 by the first abolition of the office of the Capitano. Both courts
were abolished once and for all in 1502.[58] Henceforth cases involving
criminal insanity fell by and large to the Otto di Guardia.

Like the Pupilli, the Otto did not begin its career as a court. It was
established in 1378 after a turbulent labor insurrection as an *ad hoc*
executive committee designed by the oligarchic regime to ferret out
conspiracies against the Florentine republic. Its eight officers were to
be elected from the seven major and the fourteen minor guilds of the
city. Unlike the judges who served the Podestà and Capitano, these
officers had no legal training. Initially they were tasked only with
conducting investigations into seditious behavior and reporting their
findings secretly to the Signoria. They could not try cases or issue
sentences.[59]

As the fifteenth century progressed, the Otto increasingly came
to enjoy powers of intervention in the decision-making processes of
the other criminal courts on the basis of state security.[60] In 1478, its
citizen-judges acquired the authority to act with *arbitrio*, that is, independently of executive authority and with exclusive reference to statutory law. By 1537 it had become the most important criminal court in
Florence. It took up residence in the Bargello, the former seat of the
Podestà, and assumed the management of the Bargello and Stinche
prisons.[61] There were other agencies with power to issue criminal condemnations, but the Otto exercised the broadest authority as a court
of first instance and appeal.

The rise of the Otto at the expense of courts like the Podestà and
the Capitano has pushed it to the center of scholarly debate addressing
the relationship between legal institutions and efforts at state building,
namely, how various regimes used criminal courts as tools for exercising political power or implementing programs of social control in late
medieval and early modern Florence. For some historians the creation
of the Otto and similar quasi-judicial offices in the late fourteenth century signaled the sophistication of Florentine justice and efforts by civic
authorities to maintain peace through public institutions rather than
private arrangements.[62] By contrast, other historians have interpreted
the evolution of the Otto into a full-scale criminal court as the unfolding of a series of seizures of criminal jurisdiction in service of an oligarchic elite, namely, the early Medici and their partisans.[63]

If criminal justice—the court of the Otto in particular—was a
tool in the hands of an oligarchic elite in the fifteenth century, it was

rough-hewn compared to the more finely wrought apparatus fashioned by Cosimo I and his administrators in the sixteenth century. They recognized the Otto's potential as an appurtenance of princely power and reformed it accordingly. The goal was twofold: first, to galvanize the authority of the Medici dukes as heads of the Tuscan state; second, to make criminal justice profitable. Cosimo's territorial and courtly ambitions required a good deal of money. He saw great potential for profitability in a criminal justice system unburdened by weighty overhead costs and capable of levying fines to line ducal coffers in lieu of meting out corporal or capital punishment. To this end he sought reforms that would replace the older republican juridical arrangements that seemed ungainly, expensive, and ripe for corruption with faster, leaner, more efficient practices, ensuring a speedy return of justice for everyone regardless of status.[64]

Centralization of criminal justice under the Medici dukes was achieved, in part, by changing the governing structures and procedures of courts like the Otto. Citizen-judges still staffed it and, at least in theory, maintained their *arbitrio*, but they lost a good deal of independent authority to the Duke and his operatives. Citizen-judges were usually patricians whose ability to use their office to advance personal agenda was limited by brief, nonconsecutive terms. By contrast, a team of career bureaucrats, who had legal training and advised the Otto's judges on points of law and procedure, held positions of much longer duration, serving at the pleasure of the Duke. The Otto's most important officer, the secretary, was among this corps of bureaucrats. He was the Duke's representative, reporting court business to him on a daily basis and, in turn, conveying the Duke's orders back to the court if he wished to intervene in a particular case or sentence.[65]

The Otto's citizen-judges continued to conduct investigations initiated by accusation, by denunciation, and *ex officio*. Once the information-gathering stage or stages were completed, they deliberated and made their decision. By virtue of their *arbitrio*, they could reduce or increase penalties, though the tendency was to negotiate settlements and soften punishments.[66] Cosimo made his influence felt by modifying the petition process. Beginning in his reign, sentences decreed by the Otto could be and often were adjusted through supplication. *Suppliche* were addressed directly to the Duke. Processed through the Otto's secretary, they often bypassed the Otto's citizen-judges so that the petition process amounted to a "kind of negotiation between violator and the grand dukes, in which the sentence was, in effect, a mutually agreed upon compromise."[67]

In theory at least, *suppliche* served to make criminal justice profitable by commuting corporal punishment, enforced labor, or confinement into cash for the ducal treasury. Profit motive was one of the factors driving Cosimo's decisions whether to intervene in certain cases.[68] The machine of criminal justice was expensive to operate. The Otto's administrative overhead was substantial, its profit margin narrow. In 1556, income from fines and penalties were 2,900 scudi. Expenditures cut that number by 2,605 scudi, leaving a paltry 295 scudi profit—a negligible amount considering the costs of war with Siena at that time rose to nearly 2 million scudi.[69] Moreover, Cosimo I and his administrators absorbed prisons like the Bargello and the Stinche into the ducal bureaucracy and supported them with funds from the ducal treasury. Because the maintenance of these prisons and their personnel was expensive, the Duke and his bureaucrats were more inclined to mete out monetary penalties, commute capital or corporal punishment to fines or forced labor, or simply to release nonviolent, onetime offenders.

To cut costs, they reduced the number of Otto personnel and resorted in large part to *suppliche*. The Otto lost yet more room to maneuver to the *auditore fiscale*, an office and financial organ of the ducal state that Cosimo established in 1543. The *auditore fiscale* reviewed decisions made by all courts and agencies with criminal jurisdiction, remaining on the lookout for crimes in which the duke might have had financial interest.[70] This was no toothless office; in 1558 the *auditore* removed all eight citizen-judges of the Otto at Cosimo's request for failing to impose penalties that would have fattened the public fisc.[71]

PRISONS OF MAD MEN AND SHIPS OF FOOLS?

In the new ducal system of justice, most of the criminally insane were shuttled through some kind of confinement; 75 percent ended up in the Stinche, 20 percent were pressed into galley service as oarsmen in the ducal navy. Even when taking into account some overlap in those numbers, they remain grim. If prison life was squalid, life on the galleys was nasty, brutish, and short. Once there the condemned joined the ranks of wretched oarsmen, what came to be a forced-labor group consisting of criminals, slaves, and impoverished volunteers hoping to make enough money to pay off debts. Oarsmen were chained to their posts by a fetter around an ankle. Their hair and beards, marks of distinction in society, were shorn. They lived in cramped quarters, packed with abject compatriots into a tiny space where they rowed, ate, and slept. Conditions were filthy, disease rampant. As one scholar has pointed out, "the galley became a hellish repository for rebels, misfits, and dissenters, common criminals, and captured bandits, rebellious monks, sexual deviants, unremorseful Protestants, and unrepentant Jews."[72]

The galleys and galley service reflect the new realities of geopolitics in the fifteenth- and sixteenth-century Mediterranean. The catastrophic fall of Constantinople to Ottoman Turks in 1453 followed in subsequent decades by increasingly aggressive expansion of the Ottoman seaborne empire into the western Mediterranean weighed on the minds of Christian rulers. Ottoman incursions into the Tyrrhenian Sea, which bathed the shores of Tuscany and Cosimo's new port at Livorno, induced him to build a robust navy. To lend prestige to the endeavor, to glorify and legitimate his reign, and to unite the well-heeled of Tuscany under a common banner, in 1561 and with papal support, he created the military order of Santo Stefano, whose mission was to protect Christian interests in the Mediterranean.[73]

An expedient way of powering this new fleet was with the bodies of criminals and, as some evidence suggests, mad men. Toward the end of 1565, the Otto di Guardia drafted a "List of Prisoners of the Stinche detained for criminal reasons."[74] The names of Paulo Franceschi, Baccio Masi, Piero Buonamici, Bartolomeo da Barga, and Bernardo Ulivi appeared on that list. The one characteristic they shared in common was that the court identified them as *pazzo*. Seven years later, three of these men, Baccio Masi, Bartolomeo da Barga, and Bernardo Ulivi, appeared on another list, titled "List of Crazy Men in the Stinche to be sent to the Galleys."

Little ink was spilled over Paulo Franceschi. We know that he was imprisoned in June 1546, nearly twenty years before *per pazzo* (for being mad). In 1549, he was one of forty men and four women who were released from prison by special amnesty on the feast day of St. John the Baptist.[75] How he came to be in prison once more the record does not say. Court records are a shade more revealing about Baccio Masi. For one, he was identified as a poor *mendico* (beggar) from the Mugello. In 1561, he was sentenced to imprisonment, a fine, and corporal punishment in the form of two *tratti di fune*, or drops of the rope,

for having assaulted someone and cut a vine in someone else's gar-
den.[76] In the *tratti di fune* the hands of the offender were tied behind
his or her back with a cord (*fune* or *corda*) that was then pulled.
The victim was lifted off the ground and then dropped just enough
to cause serious and potentially permanent damage to the arms and
shoulders.[77]

Baccio's support in prison came not from relatives, of which he
seemed to have few, but from *limosine* (charity). In 1566, Baccio petitioned the Otto for release. He claimed that though he might have
been *pazzo* before, he had made a full recovery. Together with the
guards of the Stinche, a relative from his mother's side confirmed that
"he had become sane."[78] There was a complication, however. The
court noted that Baccio's name had already appeared on the list of
offerta (offerings), that one-time gift of charitable amnesty. Baccio
had been in trouble before and not for an insignificant infraction. The
record does not state whether he had actually received this amnesty,
but it does claim that he had killed his mother and burned down
an unnamed person's house.[79] The Duke rejected the petition. The
Duke's response in no way discouraged Baccio from trying again. In
1566, he asked the Otto to forgive the fine; in 1567 and 1569 he asked
for liberation as an offering to St. John.[80] All three of these petitions
fell on deaf ears.

The petition of 1569 sheds further light on the Duke's reluctance
to grant Baccio special amnesty. In 1561, so the record goes, the Otto
had judged Baccio to be so mad that he had to be bound for several
months while in prison. His bonds were practical rather than punitive: "while he was in prison he did various and diverse crazy things.
In particular, he threw himself in the well of the prison."[81] Baccio
was over sixty years old at that point and had spent the previous eight
years in prison. What family he had insisted he was sane and had
been for a good five years at least. Moreover, his charitable support
was drying up. If he remained there surely he would die of starvation. A cognate relative and several nephews claimed that they would
assume his care. Despite testimony corroborating his sanity, the final
response given on September 26, 1569, was negative for nonpayment
of his fine. Baccio remained there until 1572 when he was selected for
galley service.

The stories of two other men on the list, Piero Buonamici of Florence and Bartolomeo of Barga, resemble that of Baccio. In 1564,
Piero was put in the Stinche in 1564 for having killed a servant in his

friend's household. Various of his relatives petitioned on his behalf three times, claiming that Piero's sanity had returned and that he had made peace with the dead man's family.[82] The Duke rejected all of these petitions without explanation. Similarly, Bartolomeo was put in the Stinche in 1565 for killing a friend of his, injuring two others, and running *furiosamente* through the town of Barga armed. Petitions were made on his behalf claiming that he had returned to his right mind and should be released. Again the Duke refused the petitions and demanded that Bartolomeo remain in prison.[83]

The Duke's decision not to free these men should not be interpreted as unjust or punitive. Nor should it necessarily conjure up the specter of Foucault and his evocation of ships of fools. The calculations that the ducal justice system made when faced with violent offenders were pragmatic rather than punitive. Three of the five men had committed homicide and at least two of them continued to be violent or unruly. The mental condition of these prisoners seemed to improve—rather conveniently—when the cost of their upkeep became too burdensome to their kin. The Otto and the Duke may have worried about financing the prison, but not at the cost of public safety. Repeat offenders like Baccio Masi and Bartolomeo Barga were too risky to release onto the streets unless families could give concrete assurances that they would be properly and securely supervised—something Paolo da Falla only managed after three years of negotiation with the court.

Bernardo Ulivi had not killed anyone, but his aggressive behavior on the streets of Florence had landed him in the Stinche several times between July 1566 and December 1568 *per pazzo pericoloso* (for being a dangerous mad man).[84] He seems to have ended up there after the guards of the Bargello found him one night, brandishing a pitchfork and threatening his friends.[85] They brought him to the Stinche. Officers of the Otto thought his behavior and bearing strange enough to warrant being called *pazzo*. The authorities released him after Stinche personnel testified that he had recovered his senses though on the condition that he "be sent away on a ship," that is, consigned to a galley. The secretary of the Otto believed that "if [Bernardo] went on a ship he would no longer end up in the Stinche," certainly an outcome the Duke preferred with an eye to his treasury.[86]

A few months after the first petition Bernardo wrote to the Otto asking them to release him as they said they would: "he intended to go on the ship, but it wasn't in the region so that he could immediately

go aboard." He did not wish "to falsify their order; he wanted to be
a good, obedient son" but hoped they would grant him freedom until
the ship arrived and he could join its crew.[87] He was duly released.

A few days later, Florentine guards found him prowling at night
armed. They brought him before the Otto, who claimed that he
was out of sorts. Bernardo petitioned the Otto again seeking release
because he had returned to his senses. The Otto was dubious. "This
was his second stint in prison *per pazzo*," they noted. Witnesses had
come forward the first time, too, to say that "he was *risanato* (cured)."
With his brother's consent he was freed. But he fell afoul of the law
in a matter of days. Again witnesses came forward to say that he had
gotten better. Seventeen witnesses, including prison personnel, came
forward to testify that Bernardo's soundness of mind had returned.[88]
This time, however, neither the Otto nor the Duke's secretary could
be swayed. Bernardo was still in prison in 1572 when he appeared on
the "List of Crazy Men in the Stinche to be sent to the Galleys."

When trying to make sense of these lists it is important to keep in
mind that these men were repeat offenders with little to no family support. Why their families abandoned them remains unclear. But since the
family was the primary custodial institution, without the willingness of
kin to take on their care, the Duke's solution was either to keep them in
prison—an expensive proposition for the state if their families refused to
pay their expenses—or to send them to the galleys where they would at
the very least serve the Tuscan state and Christianity at large. In these
cases, Florentine dukes tended to choose the interests of the state.

Horrific though life on the galleys might have been, some inmates of
the Stinche actually preferred to have their prison sentences commuted
to this service since it excused their fines. A few pages after the "List
of Crazy Men in the Stinche to be sent to the Galleys," a "List of Prisoners in the Stinche to be sent to the Galleys in substitution for their
condemnations" followed.[89] By way of example, one Francesco "[is sent
to] the galleys for two years to replace his condemnation of 50 scudi
and two years' confinement in the Stinche plus 300 lire in expenses."[90]
Here some ten or so men exchanged large fines and imprisonment in
the Stinche plus their expenses there for galley service.

MADNESS BEHIND CLOSED DOORS REVISITED

It is unlikely that a well-connected—or perhaps well-familied—man
of means would have ended up on that list of men destined for the

galleys either for repeat offenses or to pay off a debt. In the medieval and early modern criminal justice systems of Florence and Europe more broadly, those who could not pay fines with money paid with their bodies. Then as now, poor families had fewer options than the wealthy when it came to dealing with their mentally disturbed relatives.

In the most violent cases, dukes demanded assurances that offenders would not harm others before they were released. If families could meet such requirements, their kin were often entrusted to their care. Paolo da Falla's preparations for his wife Piera's supervision provide a good example; he had a special room built and hired a guardian to watch her. The family of a man named Barone Cappelli made similar arrangements after he had stabbed one of his brothers to death. In September 1562, Barone's sister Francesca petitioned the Otto for his release from prison into her custody at home. She claimed to have "built a better and stronger room where she would supervise him." He would be secured there with a chain around his ankles. The Duke's secretary, Lorenzo Corbolo, went himself to examine this room. He reported back that Francesca had indeed prepared a ground-floor space that measured about 9.6 by 12.5 feet (5 by 6½ *braccia*). Its walls were sound. One entered and exited through a "strong, low door." There was also a "high, reinforced window with a hole to pass food through.["91] All things considered, it seemed to Corbolo that "one could stay there in greater comfort than in that other place," and here he meant Barone's cell in the Stinche prison. The Duke seemed satisfied. He replied, "if the place is secure, send him there."[92]

Surely such renovations to a house cost a good deal of money. It is likely, then, that the poor remained in prison longer than those whose families had capital or connections. This tendency need not have arisen because the governing elites of Florence targeted the poor as deviants but because well-to-do families had resources available to make the kind of arrangements the courts and the Duke could support.

Those who could not pay to have special rooms built in their homes faced greater challenges when their mentally disturbed relatives fell afoul of the law. In June 1561 Spinetta, whom the record calls *povera donna* (poor woman), begged the Otto to help her pay for the care of her husband, Domenico. He had been in prison for three months and the costs of his care had so "reduced her [resources] that she could no longer support him without help." It was actually goodwill that put her in this predicament in the first place. Spinetta's father worried about his daughter's safety at the hands of her mad husband. Together with other relatives, Spinetta's father petitioned the Otto to have his wild son-in-law imprisoned. They maintained that "[Domenico], vexed by melancholy humors, had lost his senses, doing things that endangered his life and the life of his family." According to the record, the Otto "wanted to consider having him chained up at home," though he would remain in the Stinche during their deliberations.[93]

Neither solution suited Spinetta. She claimed that she and her family "had no way of supporting [Domenico] whether it be in the Stinche or at home." She wondered if perhaps the hospital Santa Maria Nuova might accept him where they could offer the food and care appropriate to a person with Domenico's condition. Perhaps they could even cure him. The Duke was not totally opposed to the idea but left the final decision up to the director of the hospital: "Let the director of the hospital cure him if he can. If not, he should act in accord with the rules of the hospital."[94] This outcome did not bode well for Spinetta. Like other hospitals in Florence through the sixteenth century, Santa Maria Nuova ministered acute care mainly to the sick poor or at least those deserving of charity. It was not in the habit of housing the mentally ill.[95] Domenico may have won a bed for a few days, but a stay longer than a week was unlikely.

A case of 1570 presents a similar conundrum. Like Spinetta, Alessandra degli Albizi found herself married to a man who fell into a "madness that endangered his whole family and was an intolerable nuisance to his neighbors."[96] His behavior so irritated them that they wrote to the Otto in support of Alessandra's petition. One among them had rather a lot to say:

> I Zanobi di Mattheo . . . attest that Giovanni da Mare is seen to make many astonishing gestures and day and night to yell and say many inappropriate things so that one can certainly believe that this poor man has gone crazy and, to us, his neighbors, it is no small labor to have him for a neighbor; he is dangerous not for doing something scandalous and bad [but] seeing him throw bricks out the window and anything that comes into his hands.[97]

Something had to be done about Giovanni; the question was what. Alessandra had to support their two young children; she could not also take care of her husband nor did she want him living with them. She asked that the Duke grant Giovanni a place in Santa Maria

Nuova where "he would be watched in the same way that others had been admitted to that hospital." She added, "the great necessity of the sick man and the satisfaction of all of her neighbors" warranted it. But Alessandra was mistaken. The Duke's response made that clear: "Santa Maria Nuova does not admit *pazzi* unless they are *miserabili* (paupers); if she wants to put him in the Stinche it can be done, but she must consider that she has to pay his expenses."[98]

Domenico's behavior may have been strange, irritating, even potentially dangerous. Alessandra had to weigh the inconvenience of having him at home—the time and resources it took to supervise his behavior and the shame she and her children endured in the eyes of their neighbors—against the expenditures she would have to make to support him in prison. She would pay the price in cash or honor either way; neither the Duke, the courts, nor the hospitals of Florence were equipped to help her.

BARGAINING WITH THE MAGISTRATE

Cosimo I took control of criminal justice to use it as a tool of executive power. He and his administrators sat at the top of an arbitrary system they in large part controlled even if their control was not absolute. Still financial strains on the system coupled with procedural changes, the streamlining of the appeals process through supplication, and the move from Latin to the vernacular often ended up serving interests of litigants by giving them space to negotiate the terms of sentences. More often than not, the Otto and the Duke showed themselves willing to accommodate petitioners to deliver justice swiftly and, if possible, cheaply.[99]

But profit motives were not the only concern. Desire for order also fueled the engine of justice and this was often determined on a case-by-case or household-by-household basis. Bringing order and discipline to households and communities was not accomplished unidirectionally from the top down or the bottom up. Litigants and civic authorities met in the arena of the courts to participate in this process of social ordering together. Some cases found petitioners asking that the courts mitigate sentences after their relatives had been proved guilty; others show petitioners calling on the courts to help them bring order to the anarchy madness introduced into their households and communities. Otto personnel, from citizen-judges who conducted investigations to the Duke's liaisons to the Duke himself, were

often—though certainly not always—willing collaborators in the
process of trying to figure out what to do with the criminally insane.

Of the over one hundred and fifty cases of madness prosecuted
in the criminal courts of Florence between the mid-fourteenth and
mid-seventeenth centuries, 11 percent involved homicide, 20 percent
assault, 7 percent illegal possession of weapons, 2 percent damage to
property, and the remaining 60 or so percent drunk and disorderly
behavior, imprisonment for debt, fraud, theft, and crimes against
honor. None of these offenders received capital punishment. Most
were instead ordered to serve prison terms or stints in the galleys, pay
fines, and/or or receive corporal punishment. Only about half of these
sentences were carried out in full. In 70 percent of those cases, the
court further mitigated sentences by reducing, commuting, or revok-
ing prison terms, corporal punishment, or fines. These numbers illustrate the flexibility of the Florentine justice system. They also reveal
the role both litigants as well as civic authorities played in ordering
their social spaces by setting the bounds of rational or acceptable conduct from household to street.

Since petitioners could argue their cases in Italian, they were able
to paint the spectrum of madness in subtle hues, distinguishing one
form from another through semantic shading. In this way, Tuscans
could use the universal concept of madness as a legal category, without resorting to its most extreme forms thereby depriving a relative
of his or her legal capacity once and for all. One of the areas open
for negotiation falls under the category of youthful indiscretion. In
civil courts, the idea of youthful indiscretion tended to cluster around
spending habits. In criminal courts, they rather clustered around cases
of hot-headed young men committing acts of violence. The stakes
were all the higher if they were armed.

Part of Cosimo I's bid for power and the establishment of public order, particularly in the city of Florence, involved the control of
arms. In February 1537, all noncitizens were barred from having and
using crossbows. The fine for breaking this law was twenty lire and
two *tratti de fune* (drops on the rope). In July of that year and in May
1539, Cosimo I ordered a general ban on all offensive weapons. The
Otto fined those who used rocks or carried knives, clubs, and small
swords ten scudi and two *tratti di fune*, while those carrying daggers
were to receive a fine of twenty scudi and three *tratti di fune*. The
regulation of arms intensified after 1547. Fines of twenty-five scudi
and two *tratti di fune* were levied for possession and use of firearms.

The police were even permitted to enter into homes suspected of possessing them.[100]

Despite these efforts, weapons were ubiquitous. Late medieval and early modern cities were violent places. The records of the Otto are rife with accounts of beatings, stabbings, and shootings. But weapons were also the trappings of gentlemen. As one scholar has noted, Tuscans believed that if a man wasn't armed, he must be a priest.[101] The need to display and protect one's honor combined with the possession of arms only increased the lethality of violence.

Some arms carried more honor than others, but just about anything could be used as a weapon. Rocks, for example, were the perfect weapon of opportunity and were often used as missiles to be lodged at houses or heads. In eleven cases prosecuted between 1540 and 1600 that explicitly involved the illegal possession or use of weapons, parents and relatives turned youthful imprudence into an insanity plea. In more than half of them, this strategy won either a full pardon or a relaxed sentence.

Petitioners in these cases used a range of terms to capture the excusable lack of judgment that sometimes attached to young men. In February 1543, for example, one Agnolo of Camprena described his seventeen-year-old nephew who had been caught with a dagger as "scemo di cervello" (foolish). He was carrying the dagger not out of malice but rather "leggerezza" (carelessness) and "dapocaggine" (stupidity). The Otto had sentenced the boy to three *tratti di corda* and a fine of twenty scudi that would increase to thirty-five if he did not pay. Agnolo asked that the Duke forgive his nephew the fine for being a youth "of little thought and intellect." The *corda*, however, could stand; Agnolo thought it would be insurance against making a similar mistake in the future.[102]

There is no record of the Duke's response. As an easily concealed lethal weapon, a dagger posed a real danger; possessing one was considered one of the more serious arms offenses. Nevertheless the Duke tended toward leniency in these cases. In a case of 1557, for example, one Lorenzo Giacomini petitioned the Otto on behalf of his twenty-one-year-old son, Giovanni, who had thrown a rock at the head of a certain Francesco one night when he was out carousing with friends. Francesco sustained injury but seems to have survived. The Otto fined Giovanni one hundred and fifty lire for the crime as well as ten scudi plus one *tratto di fune* for using the rock as a weapon. Lorenzo asked the Otto to excuse his son's "disobedience" because he was of little mind (*poco cervello*). Lorenzo added that as a poor man caring for a wife and three children, he could not pay the fine. The Duke ordered that Giovanni receive the *tratti di fune* but excused the fine.[103]

Matteo Passani used even more subtle terms to capture his son's youthful imprudence. The night guard had tossed young Giuliano into the Bargello after they found him carrying a sword. In keeping with their usual practice, the Otto sentenced him to two *tratti di fune* and a ten scudi fine. As Lorenzo and Agnolo had done before him, Matteo argued that his son was like a "sciocho" (fool) and even a "fanciullaccio" (naughty child). Like the other boys, he acted not out of "nimicitie" (enmity) but "mera pazzia" (sheer madness). Witnesses agreed that Giuliano was a bit daft. His employer remarked that he was the workshop "uccello" (idiot).[104] Unlike the other petitioners, Matteo worried that the *fune* would unduly harm his son; it would certainly bruise family honor. He asked the Duke, then, to release Giuliano from corporal punishment. Here the Duke refused; he insisted on the *fune* but forgave the fine.

The goal in these cases was to persuade the Duke that these young men, usually under the age of twenty-five, were not so much crazy as imprudent. Their foolishness like their youth would presumably pass with time. For the most part, the Duke agreed. The crime could not go unanswered, but sentences were not written in stone. On the books, the illegal possession of weapons received some combination of corporal punishment and a fine. The Duke may have wanted to profit from criminal justice, but it was not his or the Otto's practice to squeeze funds from those who could not pay. They were often willing to let the fine go so that an entire family was not punished along with the offender.

The Otto and the Duke were less amenable to forgiving corporal punishment, however, because of its role as a deterrent. The meting out of justice in medieval and early modern Europe was a public affair. In Florence, offenders received their blows or lashes at columns in the old market. The publicity of justice was intentional; such displays were meant to shame, humiliate, and dishonor wrongdoers while discouraging others from similar behavior.[105] It was one thing to agree that boys will be boys, quite another to let them get away with it.

Public order was not imposed solely from the top by civic authorities and achieved only through coercion. In cases of criminal insanity, individuals, households, and neighbors worked together with courts and the Duke to find some way of maintaining peace that served both private and public interest. September 1588, for example, found one Guglielmo from around Prato petitioning the Otto to commute his son Taddeo's sentence from three years' service in the galleys to incarceration in the Stinche. This was a remarkable request since that Easter Taddeo shot at his father with an *arquebus* (firearm). He missed and went on the lam. Had Taddeo answered the court summons that followed, his sentence would not have been so harsh. He chose rather to flee, forcing the court to declare him contumacious.

Still, Guglielmo begged the court for mercy. He insisted that Taddeo acted "per mancamento di cervello" (on account of a lack of mind). "Pazzia" and "furore" had been steadily growing in him since he was a boy. By the time he was twenty-six, he had repeatedly terrorized his family and community with "many acts of brutishness and insanity." The record noted that Taddeo's "poor father" recognized the "grave danger" Taddeo posed but argued that "he had not killed anyone." He held out some hope that Taddeo might get better. If he were put in the Stinche "it might please God to restore his mind to him." For all its squalor, the Stinche had an infirmary and attending medical practitioners as well as priests who saw to the spiritual needs of the inmates. The galleys offered no such support. All the Duke required was surety that Taddeo's expenses in the Stinche would be paid.[106]

By April, Guglielmo had sent the collective testimony of his town councillors, who could represent the general views of the people living there. It was their impression that Taddeo was often "out of his senses" (*spessisime volta fuora di suoi sensi*) and that "it would be dangerous to let him remain free." They drew their evidence from public voice and fame. It was hard to avoid Taddeo's raucous behavior, "when every hour he yells at the top of his voice at this or that person." Those who had the misfortune of getting too close to him said that "underneath his natural madness (*pazzia naturale*) was the odor of wine." He was publicly considered a mad man and a drunkard ("pazzo" and "ubriaco"). The last testimony was from the Stinche's notary, confirming that Taddeo had a "mallevadore" (guarantor) who said that arrangements had been made to cover the costs of his "vitto et vestito" (food and clothing) in the Stinche.[107]

Both Guglielmo and his town's councillors described Taddeo as an angry, violent drunk. He had menaced their community for the entirety of his life and almost killed his father. They all shared the view that confinement was probably the best solution. Taddeo may not have ranked high on the list of preferred dinner invitees in his small parish community, but no one—not his father who had been shot at, not his neighbors who had suffered his drunken outbursts, or the town authorities—seemed to wish on him or his household the dishonor and barbarity of the galleys.

Cases like Taddeo's are unique, but they do have something to say about the way families, communities, and courts collaborated to deal with the criminally insane. Even in situations where the mentally disturbed were chronically disruptive, the first impulse of households, neighbors, and civic authorities was not necessarily to exclude them from the community by exiling them, throwing them in prison, or consigning them to a galley.

Families and communities were willing to suffer a certain amount of troublesome behavior in their public squares. Whether it was out of deference to his father or pity for the crazy, drunken young man, Taddeo's neighbors put up with his abuse for almost a quarter century. It was only when he tried to shoot his father—whether to kill or to injure we can only guess—that Taddeo drew the attention of the central court in Florence. That was the last straw. Taddeo was no longer a nuisance, he was a potential homicide. The court had to intervene, but again, it was willing to adjust the sentence to satisfy Guglielmo so long as Taddeo's costs were covered.

The Duke's mercy, however, went only so far. Despite what would seem like extenuating circumstances, these cases did not always succeed. We have already seen that cases involving criminal insanity often hinged on the costs a family had to bear to support a mad man or woman in prison. Those costs were compounded if the person in prison had also been a family's main breadwinner. This was the problem a weaver of Florence named Maria faced when her son Bernardo was put in the Stinche in 1568 "under the pretext (*pretexto*) that he had become *pazzo*." Maria insisted to the court that this was not at all the case. Bernardo's behavior was certainly odd, but not mad. "Every month or every six weeks," she explained, "[Bernardo] entered into certain haughty diatribes about things of no consequence. He injured not a soul during these strange rants, which only lasted at most three days, after which time he returned to his wood shop and worked as if nothing out of the ordinary had happened." As evidence, Maria claimed that her neighbors had witnessed this strange behavior. She asked that the Otto free Bernardo and restore him to his family so that—and this is the crux of the matter—she and her family would not die of hunger from the petty offenses he caused during his bombastic episodes. She promised that he would be shut up in their house or, if the Duke preferred, that he would leave the city of Florence.[108]

Maria's plea did not succeed, but neither did it totally fail. The Duke's office responded with the phrase, "Non accade altro." This answer was equivocal; it did not mean that he had rejected the petition once and for all but that, for the time being, nothing was to be done. Her circumstances and the tendency of the court to negotiate with petitioners required that she at least try to make her case. According to her petition, Maria was a widow of modest means with three children in her care. She had a daughter of marriageable age who was, as she put it, "without any help," which might indicate that she had no dowry. Maria also had a young son under the age of eighteen who earned little to nothing. Thus Bernardo was the breadwinner of the family, earning the family's keep through his skill as a "legnaiuolo" (carpenter). Without his income and forced to pay his prison expenses, Maria feared that the family would fall into destitution and ruin.

It is relatively easy to account for why Guglielmo's petition succeeded but harder to understand why Maria's did not. There was general agreement that Taddeo was a menace and should be confined. Furthermore, Guglielmo was willing to cover his prison costs if the Duke commuted his sentence. This was a win-win situation. Guglielmo had to pay, but his troublesome son might be cured in the Stinche. In the galleys he was more likely to suffer and die. Here household, community, and state were able to work together to find a feasible solution to the problem of Taddeo's care.

Maria's case is harder to square. She portrayed her son as being relatively harmless in her petition to the Otto. Was he? Is it perhaps what the record does not divulge that determined Bernardo's fate? What exactly was it that he said when he launched into his strange rants? Were they too offensive to his neighbors? Subversive? Whatever the case, Maria was willing to move her son out of the city to avoid prison costs and perhaps to install him in another job. The fact remains, it was worth the effort to take her chances with the courts. Her case notwithstanding, the tide was usually with rather than against petitioners.

Sometimes the drama played out not in the streets but within households where the nature of family relations conspired against finding an easy solution to the problem of criminal insanity. In such cases, members of a household might call on the Duke via the Otto to help them navigate the perilous waters of family politics. In 1573, one Ginevra found herself in just such a situation when she asked the Otto to intervene in a delicate case involving her violent brother-in-law, Piero.

In July of that year, Piero petitioned the Otto from the Stinche. He had been there for about six months "for a little fight he had with his sister-in-law Ginevra." His sentence called for a year, but Piero had fallen ill and thought the Otto might consider forgiving him the rest of the confinement. The secretary of the Otto noted that Piero had injured Ginevra quite badly but had avoided the ordinary penalty for assault because he was "mezzo pazzo" and "furioso." The Duke did not grant the petition.[109]

Piero was released sometime in December when his full sentence finally elapsed. The terms of his release required that a guarantor come forward on his behalf to swear that he would not attack Ginevra again on penalty of two hundred scudi.[110] A month later, however, after Piero had secured a guarantor who duly assured the Otto that he would not harm his sister-in-law, Ginevra petitioned the Otto in desperation. What Piero had referred to as a "little fight" in his petition had been, in her telling, much more. In her version of that incident, Piero "innocently delivered two deadly blows to her head for no other reason than his *mattia* (insanity) and *poca religione* (lack of religion)." A "medico" attended to her wounds. The Otto initiated a case *ex officio* against Piero. They determined through investigation that he was "mentecapto" and issued a mitigated sentence accordingly.[111]

Ginevra bristled at the outcome. She secured a lawyer who argued on her behalf that the Otto attached a "light punishment to a grave offense."[112] In her mind, the court had failed to find a person who would speak in support of her side of the story. Ginevra also had little regard for the idea that her safety could be assured by threat of a two hundred scudi fine. That Christmas, in fact, she claimed that Piero "insolently showed up at her house to bang on her door not once but twice." She refused him entry, saying that her husband, his brother, was not at home. It was clear to her that Piero was still "mentecapto." To convince the Otto, she enclosed witness statements by "gentil homini" who confirmed that Piero "did not cease to pass through her neighborhood, threatening to kill her."[113]

Ginevra was a prisoner in her own house: "out of fear and a great suspicion of [Piero] she could not go to mass or to confession, always fearing that he might be behind her." The Otto's paltry threat of a two hundred scudi fine meant nothing. They could have set the penalty at two thousand scudi and "she still would not be safe [since] she was dealing with a *matto*." In other words, what good would a reasonable settlement do for a man who was not reasonable? Ginevra pointed out that Piero had already proved that "he took no account of the magistracy." No sooner was he freed from prison than he was banging down her door, threatening her life. The Duke responded that the "Otto should ensure that this poor woman be able to live safely."[114]

But the story was more complicated still. Ginevra followed her lawyer's petition with one of her own, addressed directly to the Duke and written in her own hand. "I say to Your Eccellency," she wrote, "how happy I am that Messer Francesco Lapini as my lawyer presents to you the supplication concerning that matter of the confinement of Piero Chelli, my [brother-in-law] since it is not safe for me to venture out and especially since I do not wish that my husband know about it . . . since it involves his brother." Ginevra suspected that, given the choice between her and Piero, her husband would side with Piero. "If Francesco [her husband] were to find out about it," she claimed, "he would want more for his brother than for his wife." It was her husband, after all, who begged pardon for his brother when he assaulted Ginevra the first time without her knowledge so that she could not relate her side of the story. In Ginevra's words: "when my husband found me wounded in bed he went to the Otto in my name without my knowing about it so that his brother would receive a lesser penalty." In the end Ginevra wanted only that Piero remain in some kind of confinement so that she could go about her business without fear of attack. In February, the Duke gave the Otto the authority to ensure her safety so long as their decision was in accord with statute.[115] What form that assurance took was not spelled out.

This case raises more questions than it answers. If we take Ginevra at her word, it would seem that she was repeatedly terrorized by her brother-in-law. Her husband knew about it but defended his brother's interests against those of his wife. That may very well have been the case; witnesses came forward to corroborate her story and the Otto and the Duke seem to have been swayed by it. Without her husband's account or Piero's for that matter, there is no way of knowing what was actually going on in that household and what alignment of interests there were. A brief line in the petition Ginevra's lawyer sent to the Otto suggests that, as usual, the case was about patrimony. Ginevra's petition claimed that Piero "was a bachelor . . . who had made a gift of his estate to his brother [her husband] which came to 50 scudi a year."[116] As far as she was concerned, her husband did not want to turn off the cash flow even if it meant tolerating her abuse. Again, without any way of filling in the back story, the details of the case remain mysterious. Be that as it may, Ginevra's secret dealings with the Otto and the Duke illustrate again collaborations between individuals and the court to address the challenges mental disturbance might visit on a household.

Modern sensibilities may look with approval on the practice of not holding the criminally insane responsible for their crimes and with horror on the lack of long-term custodial solutions for them. Between the fourteenth and seventeenth centuries, the city of Florence and her subject Tuscan domains lacked public or private institutions that could take them in. Prisons were not financially equipped to house permanent populations; until the mid-seventeenth century hospitals did not treat or specialize in the care of the mentally ill, administering acute care only to the sick poor. Furthermore, unless families could make a monastery or convent a financial offer it could not refuse, as happened with Piera, they were reluctant to accept violent mad offenders into their communities. For the entire period spanning the fourteenth through mid-seventeenth centuries, families and civic authorities confronted the same challenges and, on the whole, applied the same solutions to the problem of criminal insanity.

These cases do not signal the failure of republican or ducal justice or the barbarity of Florentine society as modern textbooks in abnormal psychology claim for this period in European history.[117] They illustrate, rather, the practical and material challenges facing families and civic authorities as they confronted the problem of what to do with the type of person who could not be held liable for breaking the law by reason of insanity. More revealing for historians, they demonstrate how a later medieval and early modern European criminal justice system worked in practice.

Between the fourteenth and seventeenth centuries, political and legal power increasingly revolved around first a republican then ducal center. Like the early Medici and their partisans who came to exercise extraordinary executive power beginning in 1434, Cosimo I and his administrators saw legal institutions, particularly those with criminal jurisdiction, as important mechanisms for legitimating, maintaining, and exercising political power.

Particularly with the arrival on the scene of the Medici dukes in the 1530s, the Florentine system of justice changed from one of Romano-canonical procedure conducted in Latin to one of summary justice conducted in Italian and centered on appeals to the Duke. This new procedural and linguistic context actually served petitioners by allowing them a modicum of latitude in arguing their cases. Petitioners used a vibrant semantic palette to depict their mentally troubled or perhaps mentally deficient relatives to negotiate the terms of their sentences and mitigate or commute punishments. As we shall see in subsequent chapters, the richness and malleability of language of madness gave it strength and precision as a disputing strategy.

Arbitrary though this system was, it allowed petitioners to justify or excuse strange, eccentric, and even violent or homicidal behavior without depriving someone of his or her life or legal rights. Civic authorities were willing collaborators in this process. The goals of families were sometimes at odds with those of the state, but for the most part they worked together to order households, streets, and communities in ways that served public and private interests.

CHAPTER 3

Spending Without Measure

Madness, Money, and the Marketplace

Whoever comes to me and does not hate father and mother,
wife and children, brothers and sisters, yes, and even life itself, cannot be my disciple. . . . So therefore, none of you can become my disciple if you do not give up all your possessions.

—LUKE 14:26, 33, NRSV

I know that it is madness to throw away what you possess. The man
who has never experienced the sorrow and frustration of going to ask
others for help in his need has no idea of the usefulness of money.

—LEON BATTISTA ALBERTI, *The Family in Renaissance Florence*

In the winter of 1206, an enraged father brought his prodigal son
before the bishop of Assisi, demanding that he renounce his rights
of inheritance. The father was a merchant of means, the son, good-
natured but prone to wasting money and carousing with friends.
A few months earlier, he had sold his father's stock of scarlet cloth
in the nearby town of Foligno. On his way home he stopped at the
ramshackle church of St. Damian. Instead of bringing the money
he had earned to his father, he offered it to a poor priest to repair
the church. Aware of his reputation and fearing retaliation from
his family, the priest allowed him to stay but refused the money.
What the priest did not know was that the young man was in the
midst of a spiritual transformation. The frivolities he relished in
the past had lost their appeal. He preferred poverty to extrava-
gance and humility to vanity. He left the money on a windowsill in
the church and, after hiding for some time, eventually returned to
Assisi empty-handed.

Spiritual struggles had given the young man a newfound sense of
joy, but they had taken a terrible toll on his body. When the people of
Assisi saw his wretchedness they believed that he had gone mad. They

pelted him with mud and stones from the streets, shouting insults at him as if he were insane. His irate father beat him and dragged him home where he bound him in chains. But his mother took pity on him. When his father left town on business, she set her changeling son free. He went into hiding, where he remained until the wrath of his father called him back to Assisi once more. In a final effort to bring his son to heel, the father sought out the help of the bishop, hoping that a public solution would succeed where private strategies for curbing his son's behavior had failed.

Resigned to his new path, the young man appeared before the bishop. With no word of explanation, he stripped himself of his clothes and handed them back to his father. Standing naked before those present, he renounced his birthright and pledged his life to the service of his true father, God. In tears, the bishop covered the young man's nakedness with his lavish cope.

This once prodigal youth would go on to lead an immensely popular spiritual movement, drawing to him and his cause disciples from all over Europe in a matter of years. Those who followed him were known as Franciscans after their eponymous founder, Francis of Assisi. He was canonized on July 16, 1228, a mere two years after he died.[1]

Nearly four centuries later in the city of Florence, another young man also stripped naked in a piazza. He gave his clothing and all that he had with him away to the people around him. Instead of winning the praise of a bishop, the support of devoted followers, and eventual canonization, the "crazy things" that he, Zanobi Niccolini, did in public brought "shame to him and his relatives." The authorities captured him and threw him in prison. His brother, in turn, brought the case to the Pupilli. Zanobi, he argued, had "taken leave of his senses." The Pupilli should assume his care as a *mentecatto*. The Duke's office granted the petition and Zanobi passed from prison into the hands of his family under the supervision of the court.[2]

Both Francis and Zanobi publicly renounced their worldly goods; both men were deemed mad by those around them. And yet where Francis became one of the most famous and well-known of Christian saints, whose life generated a rich hagiographical, visual, and institutional tradition, were it not for the brief account of his alleged mental incapacity in the records of the Pupilli, Zanobi would have been consigned to obscurity.

The stories of these two men, thirteenth-century saint and sixteenth-century mad man, evoke the range of attitudes to wealth that existed in medieval and early modern Italy. Francis's tale evinces the long tradition of Christian contempt for the material world, particularly its tendency to lure men and women away from God. Zanobi's case, by contrast, shows not only that Italians worried a great deal about how their relatives managed or mismanaged money, property, and patrimony but that they based their judgments about a person's mental capacity in no small part on economic behavior.

These stories map onto a broader European narrative. From the twelfth through the sixteenth centuries, a set of interrelated though often conflicting religious, intellectual, and sociopolitical ideas about wealth and its uses governed economic behavior and shaped judgments about spending.[3] The unprecedented influx of money into regional economies made large-scale accumulation and expenditure of wealth not based solely in land possible for a growing commercial class. It simultaneously generated debates about what the acquisition and use of money meant for a person's immortal soul. Dissenting voices never disappeared from the scene, but, in general, a more tolerant attitude to wealth and its uses developed in Italy between the twelfth and seventeenth centuries as credit and consumption were normalized throughout Europe.

The stories of Francis and Zanobi also provide a key to understanding changes in Florentine law that increasingly came to associate certain types of spending habits with madness. Florentine statutes from the fourteenth through the sixteenth century express a deep and abiding concern about the integrity of property and patrimony. At their core, guardianship laws instituted in the 1320s protected patrimony by giving families access to legal remedies against the misguided, irresponsible, or reckless financial behavior of their relatives. These laws targeted two types of people: those who lacked the mental capacity to make sound financial judgments—*mentecapti* and *furiosi*—and those who willfully squandered their patrimony—spendthrifts (*prodighi*). Where the mentally impaired *could not* manage their property well, spendthrifts *would not* manage their property well. In Roman law, both types of person warranted a guardian: in the case of the *furiosus*, to care for person and property, in the case of the *prodigus*, solely to manage property.

After 1540, when stability returned to a juridical system that had undergone more than half a century of reform, the Pupilli became the catchment area for cases of financial incompetence and recklessness.

In this more centralized context, Tuscans came more and more to conflate the Roman concept of the spendthrift and forms of mental incapacity, traditionally categorically distinct states. Only a truly mad person would throw money away to the detriment of his lineage. Where in the thirteenth century Francis's renunciation marked him as saint, in the sixteenth century, Zanobi's renunciation branded him a patrimonial saboteur and traitor to his kin.

This chapter turns from strategies employed by families and the Florentine state to provide long-term care for severely mentally disturbed or criminally insane kin to aspects of guardianship that sought to regulate economic behavior within a household, in particular, to check problematic spending habits. Like the guardianship cases of the previous chapters, cases involving economic incompetence demonstrate the pragmatic and instrumental use of legal institutions as well as the limits of their intervention. Male and female litigants leveraged the economic definition of madness to regulate economic behavior in their households and to invalidate contracts made by reckless relatives—a tactic that was used by individuals to protect family patrimony, by republican legislators and judges, and especially by ducal administrators to police transactions in the marketplace.

By linking the categories of prodigality and mental incapacity—implicitly during the republican period, explicitly in ducal Florence—Tuscans built a powerful legal weapon against behavior that imperiled the property, reputation, and future of a patriline. When it succeeded, this strategy could both prevent future acts of financial imprudence and reach into the past to overturn ill-advised or illegal contracts. Important changes taking place in the Florentine economy and credit market may have shaped this legal strategy. As Richard Goldthwaite has argued, Florentines had to adjust to the continual increase in the quantity and distribution of liquid capital and the drop in the cost of money. Simply put, in the sixteenth and seventeenth centuries, the rich and middling classes had more disposable wealth relative to their fifteenth-century counterparts.[4] More disposable wealth meant that unchecked spendthrifts had more money to burn. Since a systematic study of prodigality in late medieval and early modern Florence has yet to be done, making a connection between the availability of liquid capital in the Florentine market and the rise in cases of prodigality must remain impressionistic. But cases that conflate madness and prodigality capture something of the anxiety families and civil authorities felt about the proper use and abuse of wealth. They also capture the strategies families and legislators deployed to soften the impact a spendthrift might have on his household and, more broadly, his community.

Tuscans used the courts to mitigate the consequences of bad spending habits, but they could not save the spendthrift from the grim fate that awaited him after death. Dante consigned these condemned souls, who "'were so squint-eyed of mind in the first life—no spending that they did was done with measure,'" to the fourth circle of hell. There they rolled great weights with their chests in a circle only to clash them against weights rolled by hoarders. For "ill giving and ill keeping" in the brief span of life, they would spend eternity in this vain and farcical battle.[5] If the horror of the afterlife were not enough to make spendthrifts reconsider their actions, perhaps at least laws that defended patrimonial rationality could render them powerless to destroy their families.

EUROPE'S TWO ECONOMIES

Medieval and early modern men and women making decisions about how to spend their money were faced with a series of competing moral, social, and philosophical choices. Should they renounce their goods out of veneration for Christian poverty or use them to advance family interests? Should they employ their wealth to repair or construct churches, chapels, and shrines or build large and lavish palaces to house and honor their relatives? Should they commission religious objects destined for display in holy places or furnish domestic halls and rooms with *objets d'art* to display their power and prestige? The complex interplay of these ideas—often in conflict though not mutually exclusive—animated the choices people made in the marketplace.[6]

Francis embodied a Christian attitude to economic morality, which championed contempt for the world and worldly things. His renunciation recalled Jesus' command to the rich young man in the gospel of Matthew: "'If you would be perfect, go, sell what you possess and give to the poor, and you will have treasure in heaven.'" It recalled, too, the words that Jesus spoke to his disciples after the rich young man went away in despair: "'Truly, I say to you, it will be hard for a rich man to enter the kingdom of heaven. Again, I tell you, it is easier for a camel to go through the eye of a needle than for a rich man to enter the kingdom of God.'"[7] One of Christianity's core beliefs was that wealth bore the odor of sin and one sought it to the detriment of his or her soul.

Jesus' most ardent supporters recognized how difficult it would be for Christians to forsake their families and material comfort. Those who performed such extreme acts of devotion might even appear crazy. There is in the Christian tradition a play on the wisdom of the supposed fool against the folly of the allegedly wise. Francis was what St. Paul would have called a "fool for Christ," a person who rejected terrestrial vanities in favor of godly knowledge.[8] "Fools" like Francis were, as St. Paul said, truly "wise in Christ" because they understood that it was only by forsaking earthly life—the attachment to both material things and human relationships—that one could hope to approximate holiness.

These values conflicted with the realities of the new market economy. By the time Francis experienced his spiritual awakening around 1200, Italian merchants like his father had been engaged in commercial activity in an urban, monetized economy that had existed throughout the Mediterranean and western Europe for over a century. From the eleventh century onward Italian merchants had ventured far and wide to discover and develop new markets; over time they invented interest-bearing credit instruments that freed capital for business enterprises and built trading networks that helped reduce risks and improve the efficiency of their transactions.[9] Usurious contracts greased the wheels of this machine.

Usury was problematic because it offended both Christian theology and Aristotelian philosophy. Scripture said that gifts of money should be freely given with no expectation of profit. Any amount returned beyond the initial value of a "gift" was considered usurious and usury was a sin.[10] Aristotle was troubled by the unnaturalness of money, a dead thing that managed to reproduce itself. For him, money was a medium of exchange rather than a source of value in itself.[11]

A number of medieval thinkers, including the famous Dominican theologian Thomas Aquinas, adopted this position, railing against the immorality of usury. Aquinas's younger contemporary, Dante, left little doubt that the practice imperiled the soul. Like Aristotle he believed usury was an assault against nature. As such, he plunged usurers deep into the seventh circle of hell, where they sat under a rain of fire, each wearing a money purse emblazoned with their family crest around their necks.[12] This was a cruel fate indeed for people like Francis's father who had struggled to build patrimonies that they could pass on to their progeny. The material wealth that brought honor to their names and transported them across generations encumbered and imprisoned their souls.

But late medieval and early modern Italians excelled at reconciling the cosmic demands made by God and the earthly demands made by their families. As Peter Brown has shown for a much earlier period, it was often men of the church who provided the ideological justification for practices like usury. The medieval canonist Henry of Susa (ca. 1200–1271) and the Augustinian friar and theologian Gerard of Siena (d. ca. 1336), for example, privileged the Roman law attitude that usury was tolerable within certain parameters.[13] This more permissive thinking coupled with the power of merchants and investors on the local scene fostered a political environment favorable to a market economy.[14]

Despite the growing popularity of Franciscan calls to poverty, the thirteenth and fourteenth centuries saw the emergence of legal and political institutions designed to protect private property, uphold the sanctity of contracts, and enforce rules governing creditor-debtor relations. The best example of this development was the creation of the Florentine Mercanzia in 1308. In general, this court settled debt disputes. Perhaps its most important function was to recognize civil actions by foreign creditors against Florentine debtors in order to protect the creditworthiness and reputation of Florentine merchants and bankers abroad.[15]

Money and politics were inextricably connected in the Italian commercial republics. This was nowhere more true than in the realm of public finance.[16] The creation of the Florentine public debt in 1343–45 may have generated a "storm" over the morality of communal loans between 1353 and 1354, but the debate turned less around the fact that the Monte comune was usurious than that it generated an exploitative and speculative secondary market.[17] By the fifteenth century, public debt and traffic in its credits were routine parts of the Florentine economy.[18]

The creation of other state-run credit institutions followed suit. The Pupilli was one such institution, though the Florentine Dowry Fund (Monte delle Doti), established in 1425, is certainly the more famous. Families could deposit money into this fund on behalf of their unmarried daughters for terms of seven and a half to fifteen years. If the girl was married by the end of the term, her husband collected a cash dowry made up of principal plus compound interest.[19] By the late fourteenth and fifteenth centuries, the Florentine commune, like many other Italian cities, financed its enterprises through usurious practices.

If Florentines were conflicted about the metaphysical consequences of making, renting, and using money they could not deny that credit had an important role to play in all of their lives. Liquidity alleviated moments of crisis, but it also allowed people to make capital investments for their professions and to meet daily household needs.[20] When the banker's guild imposed a hefty fine on the usurious practices of its members in 1367, such transactions simply moved outside of the guild to serve a ready market.[21] The Florentine government began its first systematic attempts at regulating rather than extirpating the low end of the credit market in 1437 when it allowed a certain number of Jewish moneylenders to conduct their business under the condition that they not charge excessive interest.[22] This legislation recognized the need for credit while attempting to transfer the stain of usury from Christian to Jewish hands.

By the end of the fifteenth century, certain of the mendicants themselves had recognized the common need for credit. Franciscans, in fact, were the driving force behind the creation of *monti di pietà*, charitable civic pawnshops that provided inexpensive loans to people who otherwise had no access to credit. In practice, a poor person could pawn an item of little value to secure a small, low-interest loan. The owner of the loan could redeem it at any time within a year simply by paying it back for either a small fee or at around 5 percent interest. The *monti* could sell or auction unredeemed loans at the end of a year.[23] Franciscans established the first *monte di pietà* in Perugia, the model for subsequent *monti*, which quickly spread north through Lombardy, Emilia, and the Veneto and as far south as Sicily.[24] Papal approval came first on a case-by-case basis, beginning with the *monte di pietà* at Orvieto in 1464 and then universally by a bull of Leo X in 1515.[25]

Beginning in the 1470s, the Franciscan rector of San Miniato used his pulpit to promote the creation of a Monte di Pietà in Florence. As in other cities, the Florentine Monte was intended to serve moral ends. There was some initial opposition, but by the 1490s no less than the fiery Dominican Girolamo Savonarola tempered his moral objection to usury on the grounds that this publicly funded debt protected vulnerable Christians from rapacious Jewish moneylenders. After several decades of lackluster performance, by the 1540s its coffers had swelled thanks in large part to its principal clientele, the middling classes. Its success attracted the attention of the Medici dukes, who used it as a source of liquidity and an instrument of statecraft.[26]

At the close of the fifteenth century and over the course of the six-teenth, Florence established other credit institutions, most of which were closely connected to the ecclesiastical establishment.[27] Florence's leading welfare institutions, Santa Maria Nuova, its largest hospital, and the Innocenti, its largest foundling home, opened depositories where people could receive a modest 5 percent interest on deposits. In theory, these institutions could use such deposits to fund their activities while offering those of the middling class access to savings and investment.[28]

At the same time that Italians were carving out a space for per-missible types of interest-bearing transactions, they found ways to justify the consumption and expenditure of wealth by distinguishing between moral and immoral uses of it. Mendicant friars and theologians were again often the loudest voices on either side of the chorus. Francis was one among a sea of thirteenth-century reformers who reacted to the profit economy by fashioning a new kind of lay spirituality built on voluntary poverty.[29] If wealthy merchants and bankers would not renounce their riches, mendicant friars vigorously urged them, at the very least, to put their gains to moral use through charity. In response, urban elites began to assume a leading role in the support of welfare institutions like orphanages, hospitals, and confraternities. This new "ethic of philanthropy" took some of the stink off wealth and turned the urban elite from usurers into philanthropists and patrons of the Church.[30]

Where Franciscans led the charge to create morally acceptable credit institutions like the *monti di pietà*, it was Dominicans who first put a more positive spin on large-scale expenditure. In the thirteenth century, Thomas Aquinas adopted Aristotle's more sanguine view of what ancients and moderns alike referred to as magnificence, a form of lavish public spending. The outlay of even enormous amounts of money could be considered a moral virtue provided it was appropriate to the means of the spender and served honorable ends, the building or repairing of churches, for example.[31]

In the 1330s, the Dominican Galvano Fiamma developed this idea to provide the Visconti of Milan with the ideological justification for large and extravagant building programs that expressed princely greatness in the hopes of providing unity to a region plagued by political discord.[32] A little less than a century later, Florence produced her own chorus of humanist and Dominican voices who sang the praises of magnificence in republican rather than seigniorial tones. Leonardo

Bruni said around 1419 in defense of displays of wealth, "[a]s health is the goal of medicine, so riches are the goal of the household. For riches are useful both for ornamenting their owners as well as for helping nature in the struggle for virtue. These riches also benefit our children who are raised more easily by riches to honor and dignities." The fifteenth-century humanist Poggio Bracciolini similarly saw magnificence as the soil in which great cities and cultures thrived.[33] Dominican friars followed suit, promoting what one scholar has called a "theology of magnificence."[34] From their pulpits they called on great Florentine families like the Medici to put their fortunes in the service of Florence and the Florentine people through large building projects. Over the course of the fifteenth century, Florentines were coming more and more to regard magnificence as both a civic virtue and an effective tool for self-fashioning. Lay and clerical urbanites who simultaneously lived amid and created an "empire of things" increasingly recognized the utility of wealth as a device that could be employed for strategic social and political purposes.[35]

In the long run, the need for credit at the low and high ends of the marketplace coupled with a more positive regard for grand displays of wealth in the public sphere mitigated even if it did not extinguish traditional religious hostility to wealth.[36] Opposition to usury and uneasiness about expenditure continued to flare up periodically in Florence in the sixteenth and seventeenth centuries.[37] The great bonfires of the vanities, orchestrated by Bernardino of Siena in the 1420s and, more famously, by Savonarola in the 1490s, invited good Christians to cast into flames the material things that bound them to sin. Many of them eagerly heeded the call. Nonetheless, by Zanobi's day, concerns about money had shifted from worrying about the sinfulness associated with consumption to concerns about on what and to what end money was spent.

If the Christian moral economy had among its principal values poverty, humility, and renunciation, the market economy valued "credit relations, trust, obligation, and contracts," fueled in part by what I call patrimonial rationality.[38] Economic theory that sees individuals in the marketplace as rational, self-interested actors seeking to maximize their profits does not capture the nature of human relations in this economy nor does the term "economic rationality."[39] The more fitting term is "patrimonial rationality."

Patrimonial rationality describes the belief held by families and governments that the prudent preservation, management, and devolution of patrimony were of supreme importance. It suggests that economic decisions could not be made outside the context of the family or independent of social concerns. Patrimonial rationality was an "ethical habit," to borrow a phrase from Francis Fukuyama, implying the subordination of individual interest to that of one's lineage.[40] But it was also a practical strategy for protecting the material interests of a lineage by using the courts to deactivate spendthrifts in the marketplace.

The appearance and diffusion of a large body of literature dedicated to household management amplified the principles of patrimonial rationality in the fifteenth and sixteenth centuries. The discovery of Xenophon's *Oeconomicus* in 1427 was the model for the polymath Leon Battista Alberti's *Libri della famiglia* written between 1433 and 1441. Here Alberti instructs Florentines on how to use their wealth to advance family honor and interest while providing a justification for the intensifying consumer habits of the fifteenth century.[41]

By the sixteenth century, these treatises were the mainstays of an economic disposition that saw the world of goods as an instrument for cultural, social, and political hegemony.[42] In this thinking, the wise paterfamilias who made sound economic decisions and so passed on intact to his heirs a respectable estate, despite the countervailing forces of partible inheritance, was the honorable and rational man. His moral dilemma was not so much that he had accumulated wealth as it was how he should spend it to his family's best advantage. The mad man, by contrast, mismanaged or squandered patrimony to the shame and detriment of himself and his heirs. Patrimonial rationality did not contradict the principles underlying Christian morality. Honoring God the Father and honoring one's earthly father could be mutually reinforcing ideas. As Italians grew more accustomed to life in the market economy, they domesticated the champions of voluntary poverty like Francis. An ethic of philanthropy replaced an ethic of renunciation. By as early as the fourteenth century, St. Francis had become the "patron and protector of merchants."[43]

PATRIMONIAL RATIONALITY AND THE WRATH OF PIETRO

The complexity of Italian attitudes to wealth is perhaps nowhere more powerfully captured than in paintings of Francis's renunciation of worldly goods between the fourteenth and sixteenth centuries.

These images lay bare the contradictions that nourished attitudes to spending. St. Francis's disavowal of wealth and the rejection of his patrimony might have signaled sanctity, but it also denied the importance of familial relationships and the property and patrimony that materially and generationally bound them together. He renounced not merely worldly goods but everything that his father had worked to build and pass on to him, honor, reputation, and status as well as the material appurtenances of a cloth business. Francis was at odds with the spirit of patrimonial rationality.

Early accounts of Francis's life, particularly those of Thomas of Celano and the *Legend of the Three Companions*, emphasize Francis's prodigality as a young man. This characterization did not sit well with later hagiographers who whitewashed his alleged youthful indiscretions. Bonaventure of Bagnoregio's (1221–1274) *Legenda Maior*, the official version of Francis's life completed in 1263, tends to play his prodigality down. Although Francis enjoyed merrymaking he did not egregiously abuse money despite living among greedy merchants like his father, Pietro di Bernardone. Bonaventure, in fact, casts Pietro as the arch villain in the story. He is overly concerned with the worldly at the expense of the celestial. He is covetous, cruel, and, when confronted by his son's disobedience, violent and without mercy.

Artists who depicted Francis's life after the 1260s based their representations largely on Bonaventure's official account, while simultaneously enriching and complicating it.[44] When Bonaventure narrated Francis's renunciation he left out how those witnessing the scene, particularly Pietro, responded to the young man's extraordinary behavior. Artists commissioned to paint this moment had to imagine it. That said, they did not have to conjure it ex nihilo. Bonaventure provided somewhat of a blueprint by describing Pietro's earlier responses to Francis's conduct, much of which consisted of him beating his son, but representations of Pietro in painting in and around Florence are not all negative. Rather, depictions of the renunciation exploit the tensions that characterized the economic culture of the time.

No discussion of Francis's renunciation in painting is complete without a passing glance at the St. Francis Cycle in the upper church of the basilica of San Francesco in Assisi. [Fig. 4] Painted sometime between 1288 and 1297, it became a model for later renderings of the scene.[45] Here Francis's renunciation of his terrestrial father in favor of his heavenly Father is clear. Francis pays no attention to Pietro, fixing his gaze on the heavens. A divine hand pokes

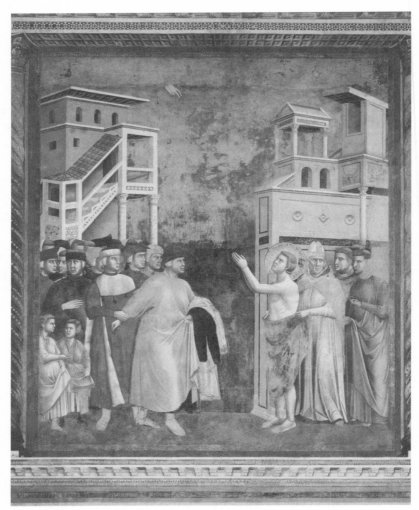

Figure 4.   Attributed to Giotto di Bondone (1266–1336). *Saint Francis Renounces his (Earthly) Father.* Upper Church, S. Francesco, Assisi, Italy. Reproduced with permission from Alfredo dagli Orti/The Art Archive at Art Resource, N.Y.

out from the clouds to bless Francis and sanction his abandonment of earthly things. Francis's serenity stands in stark contrast to the rage of his father, who is placed a few paces from his son. Onlookers must restrain Pietro in midstride as he makes for Francis. They hold back a fist poised to strike. In the 1320s Giotto (1266–1336) and in 1452 Benozzo Gozzoli (ca. 1420–1497) reproduced the raw

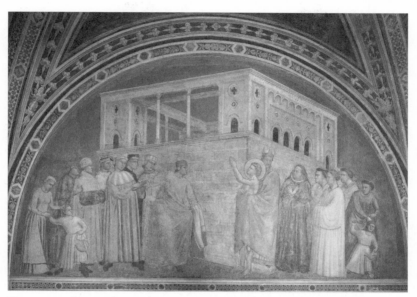

Figure 5.   Giotto di Bondone (1266–1336). *Saint Francis Renounces his (Earthly) Father.* From the Life of Saint Francis. Cappella Bardi, S. Croce, Florence, Italy. Reproduced with permission from Scala/Art Resource, N.Y.

anger and barely contained violence suggested by the portrayal of Pietro at Assisi.[46] [Figs. 5 and 6]

Other artists gave Pietro a more complex blend of emotional hues. In his depiction of the renunciation for the Borgo San Sepolcro altarpiece painted between 1437 and 1444, Sassetta (ca. 1392–1450) softens Pietro's reaction. [Fig. 7] His demeanor is less suggestive of cruelty than it is of desperation and anxiety. He is checked by those around him, but the hand he extends to his son is not balled into a fist; it is splayed open in a gesture of entreaty. He seems to implore his son to stop and reconsider the gravity of his actions. In comparison to the renderings from the St. Francis Cycle and Giotto, Pietro's face does not so much betray anger as alarm, distress, and grief. In the renunciation scene that Ghirlandaio (1448–1494) painted for the Sassetti Chapel of the Vallombrosan church Santa Trinita between 1482 and 1485, Pietro, grim and determined, makes toward Francis menacingly, but exactly what he is about to do is unclear. [Fig. 8]

As in the earlier paintings, spectators hold him back, suggestive of violence. Pietro carries the clothing Francis cast off but also holds

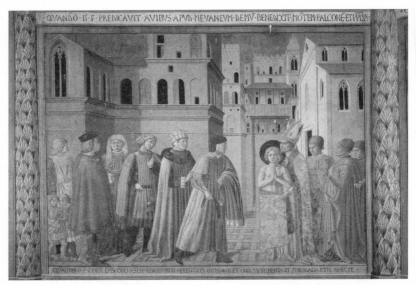

Figure 6. Benozzo Gozzoli (1420–1497). *Stories of the life of St. Francis: Saint Francis Renounces his (Earthly) Father.* S. Francesco, Montefalco, Italy. Reproduced with permission from Scala/Art Resource, N.Y.

in one hand Francis's belt, perhaps an allusion to the chains he used earlier to detain Francis at home as well as to the rope cord Francis would later adopt as a symbol of his poverty.

All of these artists, from the Master(s) of the St. Francis Cycle to Ghirlandaio, heighten the drama of the scene by putting a space between Pietro and Francis.[47] This division cuts the painting in two, splitting the figures into two camps, those with Francis and those with Pietro. It sets up a dichotomy between sacred and profane, spiritual and secular. Even so, the pregnant space accentuates the contradictions that separated Francis and Pietro's worlds by driving a visible wedge between two value systems, on the one hand, renunciation, poverty, and humility, on the other hand, materialism, avarice, and conceit.

Through the device of this space, the artists have invited beholders to meditate on their attitudes to worldly things, knowing perhaps that although viewers might admire Francis, they were certainly not without sympathy for Pietro. Sassetta and Gozzoli stress the distance by using architectural elements physically to partition the heavenly world of Francis from the terrestrial world of Pietro. Ghirlandaio intensifies

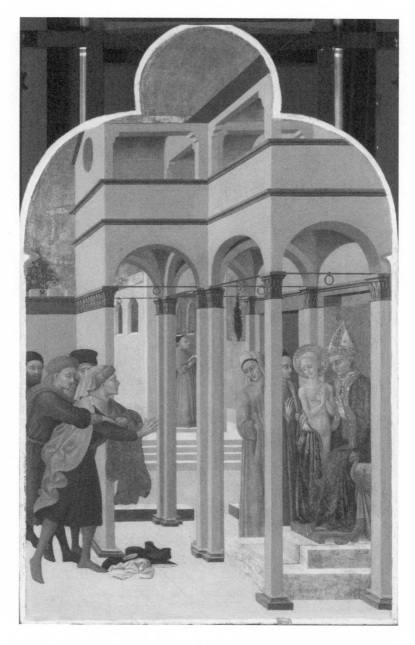

Figure 7.   Sassetta (d. 1450). *Saint Francis Renounces his (Earthly) Father.* From the "San Sepolcro Altarpiece." Reproduced with permission from the National Gallery, London.

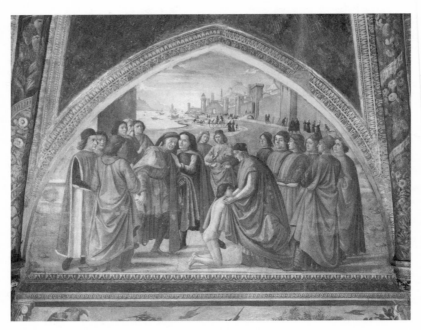

Figure 8.   Domenico Ghirlandaio (1448–1494). *Saint Francis Renounces his (Earthly) Father*, S. Trinita, Florence, Italy. Reproduced with permission from Scala/Art Resource, N.Y.

the distance between father and son by positioning Francis with his back to Pietro on his knees before the bishop as if he were making a formal profession of faith. Ghirlandaio evokes also the sanctioning of the Rule by the pope, narrated by Bonaventure in the *Major Legend* and depicted by the Master(s) of the St. Francis Cycle.[48] In this way, Ghirlandaio sets the wrath of Pietro against the ecclesiastical hierarchy's approval of Francis's renunciation.

The juxtaposition of worldviews, that of the merchant represented by Pietro and that of the saint represented by Francis, would have resonated with a large portion of Florentine society from the merchant elite like the Bardi and Sassetti who commissioned chapels that included the renunciation scene to those who participated in the low end of the market economy.[49]

In maintaining this space between father and son and capturing the complexity of Pietro's response to Francis's renunciation, these artists led their viewers to feel a range of emotions—simultaneously wonder at Francis's extraordinary sacrifice and disapproval of his father's inability to see sanctity in his conduct; by the same token, indignation at Francis's disregard for his patrimony and compassion for Pietro, who watched his son throw away all he had painstakingly built for him and their lineage. In these paintings Francis is recognizably holy, but he is also recognizably a patrimonial saboteur. In the market economy such behavior was not only imprudent, but from the fourteenth through the sixteenth century in Florence it was increasingly considered mad by magistrates and litigants in courts of law.

PROTECTING PATRIMONY IN FLORENTINE COURTS

Ancient Roman, medieval, and early modern Italian jurists saw something inherently unreasonable in the mismanagement of wealth. The famous jurist Bartolus da Sassoferrato (1313–1357) claimed that, without any specialized training, the average head of household should have the capacity to manage and transmit a patrimony as well as the ability to foresee the risks and benefits of his administration. These activities implied a basic grasp of the legal mechanisms for bringing them about. Borrowing from Aristotle, Bartolus called this type of know-how economic prudence (*economica prudentia*), a fundamental characteristic of the rational person.[50]

In Florence as in other Italian cities, failure to make sound financial decisions could be associated with mental incompetence in court. In the 1348 case of Tessa from Chapter 1, Tessa's brother Giovanni made such a connection. The poor care that she took of herself and her property was proof of mental incapacity.[51] Almost exactly a century later, another Giovanni petitioned the Podestà on behalf of his sister Niccolosa. Cola, as she was called, "was and had been for several years *mentecapta* and lacking in all access to her rational faculties (*omni prorsus usu ratione carens*)." On account of this "*imbecillitas* of mind, sense, and intellect she [could not] manage her affairs or see to any of her business . . . so that her goods and rights were falling to waste."[52] The year 1548 found yet another Giovanni in court, this time claiming that his mother, Costanza, "not being of sound mind [required] intervention in certain acts and instruments." One of the ministers of the Bigallo confirmed that Costanza had been in such a state "for many years" and that "she needed supervision and to be governed by others since she could not govern herself with her own judgment."[53]

In these cases, inability to manage property and patrimony signaled mental incapacity, justifying the loss of legal personhood. There were other ways of getting the same result in court. The Pupilli's founding purpose was to protect the interests of society's vulnerable property holders—minors and widows. It later added the severely mentally and physically impaired. The Giovannis could have successfully sought guardians for Cola and Costanza based on the fact that they were widows. Why claim mental incapacity, too?

With no more information than that two of the widows were old enough to have sons who had reached the age of majority, we cannot know how benign the intentions of the Giovannis were when they used the courts to remove the women from control of their estates. Whatever circumstances sent these men to court, it is clear that they had previously met with relatives to discuss the women's fate. They had already made and agreed on arrangements for the management of their estates once the court accepted the petitions. What we do not hear is the voice of the women themselves. We do not know if they objected to these arrangements or if they were even capable of objecting to them. The language of the cases suggests that all of these women were actively conducting their affairs against the wishes of their male relatives. Exactly what they were doing remains unknown.

In the case of Tessa, Giovanni threw the full arsenal of the language of mental incapacity at her, perhaps as a way of preventing any and all participation in the marketplace. In the cases of Cola and Costanza, their alleged mental incapacity strengthened the claim that as widows they required guardians to supervise their affairs. It is possible that the Giovannis added mental incapacity to other arguments to remove any doubts or objections the court may have entertained in reaching a final judgment. The connection between mental and economic incapacity was plausible enough for the court, which granted two of the petitions. For lack of evidence, the third outcome remains a mystery.

This selection of early cases might suggest that vulnerable women were targeted by grasping male relatives. Surely that was true in some instances. But women availed themselves of the courts, too, as a case from 1577 demonstrates. In December of that year, one Lessandra sent a petition from Empoli to the Pupilli in Florence, claiming that her husband, Piero the jug maker, had suffered a sickness that had robbed him of his judgment. From the time of the sickness, she argued, he showed signs of *dementia*: "He contracted poorly, selling properties at a very low price and did others things in grave prejudice to his wife and his [four] children." Lessandra enlisted the help of the Pupilli to find a remedy for the mess (*disordine*) Piero had made of their finances. She asked that they assume his care as a *pazzo* and a "person incapable of managing himself or his family." Four witnesses corroborated Lessandra's claims, confirming that he was "*mentecatto, pazzo* and poorly administering his affairs."[54] The Duke's office instructed the Pupilli to send the case on to the Magistrato Supremo for review. Thereafter, the trail is lost. Like the case of the three Giovannis and the three widows, Lessandra explicitly associated irregular or imprudent economic behavior with mental incompetence in the hopes of bringing order to the household her husband could no longer run.

RESTRAINING THE PRODIGAL SON

The spendthrift did not join the ranks of the mentally and physically incompetent as a legal category until 1565 in the statutes of the Pupilli, but his unwelcome presence in households had been the subject of Florentine court cases as early as the fourteenth century. Leon Battista Alberti had nothing but contempt for these patrimonial saboteurs who threatened to destroy their families, not because of their inability to make sound financial decisions but because of their refusal to do so.

In book 3 of his dialogue *On the Family*, Alberti's model paterfamilias, Giannozzo, says to his friend Lionardo, "Consider whether there is anything more apt to cause the ruin not only of a family but of a village or a whole community than those—what do they call them in those books of yours, those persons who spend money without reason?" Lionardo replies laconically, "Prodigals." Giannozzo shrugs off the technical term and adds, "Call them what you like. If I had to give them a name, what could I find to call them but 'a damned pestilence?'"[55]

Florentines saw prodigality as a grave threat to their households. According to Alberti's Giannozzo, spendthrifts used their resources to satisfy materialistic whims, from gambling to the excessive purchase of high-cost items like clothing, horses, jewelry, and hunting animals. These activities attracted the worst society had to offer. Spendthrifts, Giannozzo observed, tended to keep company with "vile and dishonest men, musicians, players, dancers, buffoons, pimps, [and] rubbish dressed in livery and frills."[56] Their behavior offended family, honor, decency, and reason, bringing shame and ruin in its wake. More than that, their destructive self-interest undermined the corporate, familial spirit of patrimonial rationality.

During the 1320s, a century after St. Francis's death and around the same time that Giotto was painting the Bardi Chapel, Florentine legislators were busy writing laws that gave families a measure of control over the problematic economic behavior of their relatives. Statutes gave heads of household broad rights of action against dependents who operated imprudently, recklessly, or illegally in the marketplace. If, for example, an uncle informed the court through formal petition that his nephew was mismanaging his affairs to the detriment of his family and other interested parties, the Podestà and his judges were required to ban citizens from lending to or contracting with that wayward nephew.[57] The 1415 redaction of these statutes added that a person poorly or wickedly conducting business could be legally banned for one year from making any (and all) legal contracts.[58]

Furthermore, if a male descendant chose to "lead a disgraceful life by gambling and frequenting taverns with people of ill repute in defiance of his relatives . . . upon the petition of the father or grandfather, the Podestà and his judges [were] required . . . to capture, incarcerate, and detain him either in prison or wherever the father or grandfather wished until he regained the upright path."[59] These laws gave families, in concert with the court, the power to deactivate a relative in the marketplace if they thought he was making illegal contracts, gambling, or keeping company with the wrong element.

The laws did not explicitly name spendthrifts as a category of person but drew inspiration from the Roman law concept of the *prodigus*, a person who imperiled his or her patrimony by squandering material resources in any way.[60] In Roman law, this category of person appeared alongside the severely mentally or physically impaired as in need of a guardian because, like them, he was considered unfit to manage his financial affairs. If he wanted to exercise rights or obligations or make a contract he could only do so through a *curator*. This rule applied to extravagant women as well, though in the Florentine courts women rarely if ever appeared as spendthrifts.[61]

Although jurists tended to address the mentally impaired and spendthrifts in the same laws, ancient Roman jurists had drawn subtle but clear distinctions between the two categories. However unreasonable the behavior of the *prodigus* might seem, his incapacity was thought to extend only to the management of property and the ability to enter into contracts. To be sure, *prodighi* were known to act like the insane, but the misuse of their rational faculty was not considered involuntary, nor was it seen to extend to all facets of thought and behavior as in the case of *furiosi* and *mentecapti*. Thus Roman magistrates assigned a *curator* for the *prodigus* only to manage his property and supervise his affairs.[62] *Prodighi* remained, however, masters of their own persons.[63] By contrast, a *curator* assumed the care of both person and property in the case of the *furiosus*.[64]

In May 1375 one Lapaccio petitioned the Capitano to have his brother Guido put in Florence's Stinche prison. Lapaccio claimed that Guido for quite a few months had led, and continued to lead, a shameful and indecent life. He gambled, went to taverns, associated with unsavory characters, and was himself of questionable repute. In general, Guido squandered his wealth with no regard for economy.[65]

This behavior was only one manifestation of a deeper problem. According to Lapaccio, Guido suffered from *furor*. He was *fatuus* and out of his mind (*vagans extra mentem*). More to the point, Lapaccio argued that his brother's immoderate lifestyle threatened to bring shame and impoverishment to them both. As Guido's closest living relative, Lapaccio petitioned the Capitano's court to have him captured, bound, and incarcerated until such time as Guido reverted to honest living and good judgment. In keeping with statute, he was not to be released without the express consent of the Capitano, his successors, or Lapaccio. Witnesses supported Lapaccio's account, adding that Guido was so *fatuus* and *delirans* that they often saw him yelling and running through the streets of Florence hitting men and boys as he went. His habits, they maintained, were like those of foolish (*fatui*) men. The Capitano ordered his police force to go out and take Guido into custody. Once apprehended, the court interviewed Guido and found him to be "a man who poorly managed his affairs, ill used his property, led a wicked life, spoke poorly and, finally, was mad, raving, and out of his mind."[66]

Prior to legal intervention Guido was a full legal agent; he was not in the power of a father, grandfather, or uncle. He could dispose of his property on his own terms even if that meant utterly wasting it. Roman law and Florentine statute and culture—defenders of the sanctity of patrimony—took a decidedly negative view of such behavior. Already in the fourteenth century, Florentines could represent the misuse of money as a failure of reason. Lapaccio did not use the term *prodigus* in his case against his brother, but he described Guido's abuse of his patrimony coupled with immoral behavior as evidence of his insanity. The strategy was effective; for how long, the record does not say.

OTHER PEOPLE'S MONEY: DEFRAUDING
YOUR CREDITORS AND KIN

During the republican period, the courts of the Capitano and Podestà handled cases involving economic imprudence or recklessness. By contrast, the Pupilli came late to the game; its court did not begin to take on such cases until after 1540, and its statutes did not explicitly address prodigality until 1565. Here the statutes of 1473 were expanded to include care and active intervention in the affairs of "furiosi, mentecapti, the demented, the prodigal and squanderers of patrimony and financial resources."[67]

From this point on litigants seem to conflate the categories of prodigality and mental incapacity more readily. If one wanted to deprive a patrimonially dangerous relative of legal personhood, dual attribution theoretically increased the chances of achieving that result. An allegation of prodigality might succeed where that of mental incompetence failed and vice versa. Either way, the remedy was the same. Dual attribution was possible because Florentines saw economic prudence as a defining feature of the rational person. It was useful because it gave families wishing to invalidate ill-advised contracts made by prodigal kin a powerful and effective legal remedy. Since a mentally incompetent person was barred from contracting, having a person judged as such in court called into question the validity of any contracts made after the first sign of incapacity. This was not a common strategy relative to other types of guardianship cases; families who chose this route were usually engaged in last-ditch efforts to put a stop to behavior that threatened financial ruin or to force a prodigal relative to fulfill his (rarely her) financial responsibilities.

The Florentine state had a stake in these cases, too. Civic authorities saw the financially incompetent or reckless as a threat to social order. The collapse of great families because of poor financial management brought dishonor to the entire community. Spendthrifts who ended up in the courts had often made illicit or highly controversial contracts, something Florence's commercial court, the Mercanzia, did not usually pursue. The ability to overturn such contracts on the basis of mental incapacity allowed civic authorities to police certain types of economic activity. Sixteenth-century cases in which petitioners sought to curb the reckless spending of their kin illustrate how the users of the courts leveraged the flexible definitions of mental incapacity and prodigality to protect the financial integrity of their households. They further shed light on the delicate balancing act the court performed in making such remedies available without introducing legal anarchy or allowing petitioners to profit unduly from them.

In February 1575, two of four sisters from a dying branch of the old and affluent Carnesecchi family implemented the dual attribution strategy to stop the rampant spending of their brother Bernardo. In their words, Bernardo was "of little sense and intellect. He goes around wasting his [wealth] to the serious detriment of his own goods and property, but also to that of the honor of his household." "Every day," they continued, "he ran up debts through *scritte private* (private contracts) preceding from *scrocchi*." Without intervention, Bernardo's sisters feared that his reckless spending would "utterly ruin them and that he would end up dying in some hospital or prison."[68]

Both the sisters and the Pupilli had an interest in putting a stop to Bernardo's pernicious spending. The types of contracts he made were damaging to the family and marketplace as a whole. *Scritte private* were private as opposed to public contracts. They were conducted between parties without the services of a notary and therefore often made without payment of the contract tax (*gabella dei contratti*). The Florentine government disliked them because they offered people a way of hiding taxable assets.[69] Although Florentine legislators did not ban *scritte private*, they took some of the wind out of their sails by declaring them inadmissible in court unless the contract tax had been paid on the full monetary value of the contract.[70]

Particularly insidious types of *scritte private* were the *scrocchio* and *barochio* or *barrocholo*. I have been unable to find an actual example of either instrument, but they appear to be types of loans designed to conceal high interest charges. We can imagine a situation in which one person gives another person something in place of money—an object or a debt receipt—but at a value superior to its actual worth. The borrower would sell the item, receiving less than expected, often having too little money to pay back the debt.

Credit was an important fact of life in Florence. Harder to square were excessive interest charges, the secondary credit market, and predatory lending. *Scrocchi* and *barocchi* were exploitative loans made to people who needed fast and easy credit. Certainly the desperate poor were a target. So, too, were young propertied men who had lost their fathers, presumably cooler heads who would have curbed their spending. In 1568, three years after a massive overhaul of Pupilli statutes, the Pupilli asked that the Duke add a clause about predatory contracts. According to the Pupilli, certain of their wards between the ages of eighteen and twenty-two were in the habit of liquidating immovable goods (*beni stabili*), *monte* credits, or borrowed money to purchase "horses or livestock of whatever kind" in order to "pay off *scrocchi* and *barroccholi* that they were making daily."[71] These young men often ended up in jail because of such contracts. The Duke's office replied that this was a "matter of great importance." Surely these vulnerable boys needed protection from the deceitful influence of vicious men.[72] In practice, this law extended to men over the age of twenty-two as well. In these cases, prodigality was pitched as madness.

The financial peccadilloes of Lorenzo and Tommaso Cambi furnish a good example. In January 1578 Guglielmina Albizi, the widow of Antonio Cambi, asked the Pupilli to assume the care of her sons Lorenzo and Tommaso: "They were not able to conduct their affairs or maintain their property. After the death of their father they ill spent a good amount of money wasting and destroying their patrimony through dishonest practices and with men of questionable reputations."[73]

By that point, Lorenzo was thirty years old. Guglielmina described him as a *prodigo* who, in a short span of time, racked up debts with Jews and others who trucked in *scrocchi* for thousands of scudi. Tommaso, still considered a minor though over eighteen, was of "little judgment and not really capable of governing himself." Several witnesses confirmed Guglielmina's report, including Lorenzo himself. The court decided that Lorenzo was publicly considered "weak-minded (*debole di cervello*) . . . and incapable of managing himself or his estate." Witnesses said that Tommaso was even more "senseless (*più insensato*) than his older brother and also incapable of managing himself or his estate." When the Pupilli interviewed Tommaso, however, they found him to be reasonable enough, though suffering the pains of youth and bad example. Lorenzo's business dealings had brought shame; the Pupilli referred to the "indignity of his obligations (*indignità delli oblighi*)."[74] Such behavior had to be stopped. The Pupilli assumed his care and Lorenzo lost his legal personhood.

As for Bernardo Carnesecchi, his case went to the Magistrato Supremo, which officially declared him out of his mind (*alieno dalla mente*), *insano*, and a spendthrift (*dilapidatore*).[75] This decision was a potential coup for Bernardo's sisters. As a legally recognized *prodigo*, Bernardo could no longer make damaging contracts. Even more useful, because he was also a legally recognized *mentecatto* some of those injurious *scrocchi* might even be invalidated if it could be proved that he had made them while he was mentally incapacitated.

In Roman law, the legal categories designating madness and prodigality operated on different timelines.[76] Madness was considered an objective state of natural incapacity that was recognized immediately after the first external evidence of such an internal state. Any legal transactions made after that first moment of madness were theoretically subject to question given the importance of a person's state of mind during the act of contracting. Prodigality, by contrast, was an artificial juridical category designed to provide *ad hoc* intervention. This category could only be applied to a person by an authority after a legal proceeding. This meant that, in the case of prodigality, a person's inability to contract began after a legal ruling, so any transactions made prior, however ill conceived, were still valid. On this principle, the Magistrato Supremo gave the Pupilli the authority "to change, correct, modify, alter or completely annul all contracts, pacts, and obligations made by Bernardo as they saw fit."[77]

Thus when Bernardo's sisters asked the Pupilli to assume his care as *prodigo* and *mentecatto*, they were likely hoping to prevent Bernardo from entering into ill-advised contracts in the future while rendering invalid his improvident legal acts of the past. This outcome was of great importance since the casualties of Bernardo's spending were the dowries they were promised by their grandfather. In order to provide for his granddaughters, Bernardo Carnesecchi the elder named his son Piero universal heir on the condition that "no part of the estate could be alienated unless it was used to fund the monacation or marriage of his daughters. Otherwise it was necessary to obtain permission to alienate property from the officers of the Monte comune."[78] When Piero died, control of the estate fell to Bernardo the younger, the *mentecatto* and *prodigo* in question. Control brought responsibility. Bernardo was supposed to manage the patrimony so that his sisters would have the means of either making a good match or entering a convent. According to his sisters, Bernardo was not equal to the task. At least two of them were married and another appears in a later case in a convent, but none of them had seen anything of their dowries.

The sisters' successful petition of 1575 opened the door to other claims against Bernardo's estate. Their victory in court was particularly galling to one Benedetto Chiavacci who claimed that he was in possession of a "contract (*scripta*) worth 179 lire written in [Bernardo's] own hand on November 18, 1575."[79] Bernardo's relative Francesco Carnesecchi had acted as guarantor to the loan, pledging that it would be repaid in five months. That time had come and gone and the debt remained unpaid. Benedetto asked the Pupilli to recognize Francesco's responsibility as guarantor to pay him. From Benedetto's point of view, if the Pupilli's mandate allowed them to overturn past contracts, surely they could not invalidate one that had been guaranteed by one of Bernardo's sane male relatives.

Benedetto had a point. Francesco's surety gave the contract undeniable legitimacy. Bernardo spent some time in prison for defaulting on the loan he made with Benedetto, but after examining the contract, the Pupilli decided that he was not liable for the full amount. When Benedetto petitioned the Pupilli again in January 1582, the Pupilli informed him that Bernardo had been forgiven part of the loan. The total amount he had to pay was reduced from 179 to 42 lire. Cristofano Carnesecchi, Bernardo's paternal cousin and new guarantor, would pay this amount. If Benedetto wanted to pursue the remainder, he would have to get it from Francesco, Bernardo's guarantor in the original contract. The Duke's office accepted this settlement.[80]

It is worth pausing for a moment to try to sketch the character of the man behind these documents. It is easy to assume that the mentally or physically impaired were inert or invisible figures, that they existed on the margins of society locked away in secret rooms. But incapacity was a large tent. It covered a diverse range of people from the severely mentally or physically incapacitated to people like Bernardo who functioned in society more or less normally were it not for certain habits that did not conform to socially and culturally defined notions of rational behavior. Unlike Girolamo Passerini or Francesco Martelli, men who spent most of their lives out of the public eye, Bernardo was a man about town. The record does not describe what he spent his money on, but it is clear that he spent heavily and was often on the hunt for more credit. Having defaulted on debt in the past, only the most exploitative loans were available to him.

This did not stop Bernardo from cultivating a social life. In January 1577, he petitioned the Pupilli informing them of his wish to marry. He was about thirty-two years old, but as a ward of the Pupilli he had to ask their permission before he entered into any contracts. The same Cristofano who helped Bernardo settle his debt with Benedetto vigorously protested the marriage. Cristofano reminded the Pupilli that Bernardo had a young sister of marriageable age still living in Bernardo's household who should be married first. It did not seem "honorable to him that [Bernardo] take a wife until his youngest sister had left the house" either as a wife or a nun.[81] The only real check on Bernardo's spending was his legal status as a *mentecatto* and *prodigo*. Marriage was a contract that could only be entered into by two mentally competent people. License to marry was tantamount to an admission of his mental capacity. It thus opened the door to any creditors the Pupilli had denied full repayment based on Bernardo's incapacity.

In May 1577, another of Bernardo's sisters, Maria, a nun, also advised the Pupilli to observe caution when considering this marriage. Her concern was less with the marriage as such than that the Pupilli prevent Bernardo from doing something "unworthy" (*indegna*) of their house, for they suffered shame (*vergognare*) knowing the weakness (*debolezza*) of his judgment (*cervello*) and the methods of his governance."[82] She concluded by saying that "he did not possess that prudence (*prudentia*) nor that judgment (*discorso*) required for something as important [as marriage]."[83] Bernardo possessed none of that *economica prudentia* that Bartolus da Sassoferrato considered the defining feature of the good paterfamilias.

Lack of prudence was only half of it. In the eyes of his relatives, Bernardo's self-interested behavior was also disgraceful. Having no children of his own, his primary responsibility was to manage the property set aside by his grandfather for his sisters' dowries. Bernardo completely shirked this duty, conduct that Cristofano deemed dishonorable and "not befitting his station."[84] Bernardo's "methods of governance" as Maria called it did not conform in any way with patrimonial rationality. Whatever Bernardo spent his money on, he had no regard for how it affected his sisters. By spending against resources that were intended to furnish their dowries, he reduced their social value as potential wives or nuns and imperiled their future well-being as well as that of their children.

These petitions seem to have foiled Bernardo's marriage plans. The outcome alleviated some of the strain on Bernardo's estate. Still, his sisters remained unappeased. Their part of the case picked up again in May 1580. The court confirmed that Bernardo had been declared *mentecatto* but that his estate was in good shape (*ha buone et idonee facultà*). "If it weren't for the debts he owed his relatives on account of the dowries of his two married sisters," they continued, "his affairs would be fine; his estate would permit him to live freely according to his status."[85] His sisters, however, further claimed that Bernardo owed them around four or five thousand scudi in unpaid compound interest on the principal of their dowries for an unspecified number of years. The Pupilli told the Duke that "creditors hounded (*molestato*) them because of this interest." In order to put an end to the sisters' demands, the Pupilli decided to liquidate some of Bernardo's holdings to resolve these debts once and for all.[86]

Surely Bernardo's sisters were owed their dowries. The Pupilli was required by law to protect such legitimate claims. It would not, however, countenance abuse of its court. They told the Duke that it was "not honorable or reasonable that their ward Bernardo, while he was in their care, suffer [claims to] interest. The Pupilli shouldn't have to put up with them either."[87] When the Pupilli had taken on the case in 1575, they had published bans notifying any and all creditors that Bernardo was no longer liable for interest. The bans required all creditors "to appear before the Pupilli and state their claims within one month so that they might receive payment according to a just estimate of what they were due."[88] If such protocols were followed, the Pupilli believed that it could "clean up [Bernardo's] mess (*disordini*) and all creditors would be satisfied." According to the Pupilli, Bernardo would remain sufficiently well-off (*facultuoso*) and "with the remaining he could live the rest of his life quietly and comfortably (*largamente*) according to his status and nobility (*secondo il grado et nobilità sua*)."[89] They did not doubt that Bernardo must provide for his sisters' dowries. But the Pupilli considered claims to interest a step too far and a distraction in their efforts to settle Bernardo's estate.

Although the Pupilli was not inclined to award the sisters interest on the unpaid dowries, it was very much working to make them whole. Bernardo's thoughtless management had put one of them in a real bind. In July 1583, the Pupilli wrote to the Duke relating crucial details of the case. Before Bernardo had been declared *mentecatto* and put under the care of the Pupilli, he had married his sister Aurelia to one Benedetto Rucellai. The marriage contract drawn up by Bernardo and Benedetto and approved by their relatives set the amount of the dowry at three thousand fiorini. This amount was to be deposited in the Monte comune. It could only be drawn on for reinvestment in immovable goods, a stipulation designed to secure the dowry.[90]

After Bernardo made this contract, the Pupilli told the Duke that he became "like one of those men of little judgment (*poco cervello*), although not to the point that he was completely *mentecatto*."[91] In this condition and without the consent of his relatives, he allowed Aurelia's husband, Benedetto, to persuade him to add another condition to the marriage contract. Bernardo agreed to pay Benedetto the dowry in cash (*liberamente*) without any security or reinvestment. The record does not entertain the possibility that Benedetto sweetened the second contract by promising Bernardo a kickback for making the change. Instead, the Pupilli and his relatives chose to read this conduct as the height of folly; the Pupilli even referred to it as an act of madness (*pazzia*). If the dowry were to be paid in cash, it would dissolve into Benedetto's patrimony with hardly a trace. If Benedetto died, restitution of the dowry from his estate would be extremely difficult for Aurelia. Reinvestment of the dowry either in immovable goods like property or in Monte credits made it easier to track and return.

Bernardo's relatives and the Pupilli saw such a disadvantageous contract as a definitive fall from reason. When Bernardo made the first marriage contract, he was clearly in his right mind (*in cervello*). When he was induced by Benedetto to make the second he was clearly *mentecatto*.[92] Prodigality shaded into madness here because Bernardo acted against the interests of his sisters. Whether in so doing he was expecting to profit himself is impossible to say. Either way, he flouted the social rules governing patrimonial rationality.

The Pupilli categorically denied the validity of the second contract. They did not do this lightly, admitting that the "foolishness and lunacy" (*sciocchezze e pazzie*) of the second contract should be examined by a legal expert (*savio*) in formal consultation. They elected one Messer Alessandro di Messer Antonio Melegonnelle for the job. He, in turn, supported the decision to annul the second contract. Benedetto, he insisted, had to guarantee the dowry through some kind of traceable reinvestment.[93]

At this point in the game it would seem that the sisters had won. Certain details, however, conspired against awarding the women their dowries outright. Two years previously, in January 1581, the Pupilli acknowledged the terms of Bernardo the elder's will, which prevented the alienation of property destined to support the dowries. They recognized, too, that Bernardo's spending had made liquidation of certain properties necessary. Thus the Pupilli asked the Duke's office for permission to make the requisite sales. After all, the Pupilli observed, "the testator [Bernardo the elder] could not have known that he would have a *mentecatto* for a grandson who would someday end up in the care of the Pupilli."[94] The Duke, "not wishing to deprive the Pupilli officials of their authority," instructed them to act in accord with their statutes, thus giving them permission to administer Bernardo's property as they saw fit.[95]

The only matter remaining was which properties to sell and to whom. These were not easy questions to resolve and involved the Pupilli in litigation connected to the case from March 1581 to September 1583.[96] The property battle was waged primary between Bernardo's cousins Cristofano and Francesco, both of whom wanted to purchase Bernardo's property and add it to their own. Could Francesco have stood surety for Bernardo's bad loans in the hopes that default would force the Pupilli to sell property he very much wanted to buy? Could Cristofano have had similar designs in repeatedly discrediting Bernardo in court? Evidence is suggestive rather than conclusive, but the motives of both cousins arouse suspicion.

Cases like these show Florentines trying to inscribe in law the idea that good economic decisions were those that took into account the honor and interests of an entire household, not merely the whims of the individual. These considerations also shaped the judgments of the Magistrato Supremo and the Pupilli. In some cases, the Pupilli was compelled to act on behalf of the victims of spendthrifts. In December 1584, for example, the Pupilli petitioned the Duke on behalf of one Cosimo Guidetti to reverse contracts that he had made. In accord with statute, the Magistrato Supremo had declared Cosimo *pazzo* and *prodigo* for having entered into *scrocchi* and *barocchi*.[97] Dual attribution here gave the Pupilli the authority to check imprudent future contracts and overturn those of the past.

Cosimo's contracts were undoubtedly problematic. The real source of concern, however, was the welfare of his five young children. When

the Pupilli reviewed Cosimo's contracts to see where they could intervene they encountered a matter of some delicacy. Other courts had
handed down sentences on Cosimo's debts, judgments the Pupilli did
not believe it had the authority to overturn. They asked the Duke
on behalf of Cosimo if they could invalidate these judgments so that
the money Cosimo lost through his ill-advised contracts would be
restored to him and, more important, to his children. The Duke
responded in the affirmative; he ordered that the Magistrato Supremo
grant the Pupilli the authority to recover all of Cosimo's losses, one
can imagine, much to the chagrin of his creditors.[98]

Through the courts, families could in some contexts exercise broad
powers of intervention over the economic behavior of their family
members in the name of patrimonial rationality. That said, the dual
attribution strategy did not always work. It was certainly less successful in the case of the allegedly mad spendthrift Vincenzo Micceri, who scuttled the attempts of his family and the Pupilli to save his
estate from his repeated efforts to spend it out of existence. In November 1581, Vincenzo's paternal uncle together with one of his cognate
relatives informed the Pupilli that he was living far beyond his means.
In four years he had squandered more than half of his wealth. They
asked that the Pupilli intervene "on the grounds of his wild (*disordinato*) and extravagant (*stravagante*) mode of spending." Witnesses
confirmed that Vincenzo was publicly considered a spendthrift for
often buying horses, dogs, and birds at exorbitant prices and then selling them at great losses.[99]

Witnesses also recounted a bizarre and shocking incident. One day
Vincenzo placed a hawk (*astore*) he had purchased for three scudi
in a piazza and, for no good reason, shot it into oblivion before an
awestruck crowd. To this gruesome and senseless act, the witnesses
added many other undefined examples of behavior that was not only
prodigal but, in their eyes, truly mad.[100] With the Duke's consent, the
Pupilli declared Vincenzo *prodigo* and *mentecatto* and undertook his
care. As statute required, they published bans throughout the city
that prohibited people from contracting with him.[101]

Vincenzo, however, remained a step ahead of his relatives and
the court. Eleven months after the petition, he became the subject
of another Pupilli communication to the Duke. The Pupilli wrote
that immediately after the publication of the bans, Vincenzo, eager
to spend money, sought out credit from anyone who would give it to
him. Since he could find no legitimate lender, he "procured a *cautela*

(a surety) which through *scritte private* identified Vincenzo as the debtor to priests, friars, and other religious persons for money and [unspecified] things (*robe*)."[102]

These *scritte private* were a real problem. Vincenzo borrowed from clerics, a category of people outside civil jurisdiction. The clerical lenders had gone "to the court of the Archbishop and there obtained judgments against the person and goods of the *prodigo*."[103] As a secular court, the Pupilli could not intervene in these transactions. "What was worse," Pupilli officers wrote to the Duke, "although they believed that Vincenzo had made the *scritte private* while he was under their care, they could not prove it."[104] Vincenzo himself had admitted to making them while being in the care of the Pupilli. He further alleged that he had sought out ecclesiastical lenders because he knew the Pupilli had no jurisdiction over them. The Pupilli believed it was their duty to inform the Duke of this fraud, but they remained powerless to do anything.

Viewed through a cultural lens, the spending habits of Bernardo Carnesecchi, the Cambi brothers, Cosimo Guidetti, and Vincenzo were the opposite of magnificence, an acceptable way of spending lavishly. There was nothing virtuous, dignified, or honorable about their accumulation of luxury goods because they were obtained at the cost of patrimony and by means of shady contracts. In the case of Vincenzo, consumption served no purpose save his own amusement. All of these men spent to serve their own rather than their families' interests. Such behavior is unlikely to go over very well in any culture. These men, however, broke the social, cultural, and, by the fourteenth century, legal rules that promoted patrimonial rationality.

The dual attribution strategy that associated mental and economic incapacity served pragmatic ends. Families and the state used the wedded categories to stop kin from utterly destroying their patrimonies and to invalidate infelicitous contracts. In Florence from the fourteenth through sixteenth centuries social rules and practices increasingly governed economic behavior. It was reasonable to spend money in ways that would enhance the honor, reputation, and wealth of the family. Anything that threatened its fragile social and financial well-being was tantamount to madness. By the late sixteenth century, Florence had well-articulated institutions that protected families from financial incompetence and recklessness. In this context, the person who performed a public and incendiary renunciation of patrimony and parentage was more likely to share Zanobi's rather than St. Francis's fate—a brief stint in prison followed by close supervision by court and family. Then, obscurity.

CHAPTER 4

From Madness to Sickness

. . . as the sea waves, so are the spirits and humors in our bodies, tossed with tempestuous windes and storms.

—ROBERT BURTON, *The Anatomy of Melancholy*

In April 1598, one Faustina Galeotti of Pescia petitioned the Pupilli on behalf of her son, Domenico. For nearly a decade, she told them, he had struggled with a disease called melancholy. Its first visitation nine and a half years before was dramatic: "he was so out of his mind he had to be tied up." After being "cured . . . he returned to himself for seven years and thirty months." But lucidity was not to last. Two and a half years before Faustina's supplication, Domenico "fell back into the same sickness."[1]

Faustina traced her son's relapse to three things. First, Domenico's father had died, leaving him to assume the reins of household management. He was also saddled with a marriage he had only reluctantly agreed to. Then the swelter of summer arrived and Domenico cracked. Weighed down by domestic discontent, the heat of June and July "drove him from his senses." His judgment was compromised, his behavior altered. In particular, he exhibited "embarrassing" spending habits. On one of his escapades he traveled to an inn about ten miles away in nearby Lucca where "400 scudi—[a rather hefty sum]—were taken from him." Faustina did not tell the Pupilli how Domenico lost the money; she said only that he could not recuperate his losses via the courts.[2] In April 1598, she asked that the Pupilli assume his care, surely in anticipation of the wild days of summer.

The chief official of Pescia interrogated Domenico's relatives as well as other witnesses from the region. Everyone agreed that he "suffered from melancholy humors" during the summer followed by long lucid intervals. While in the grips of the disease, he acted imprudently despite being a man of high esteem under normal circumstances. In a letter to the Pupilli, the official concluded that the onset of heat during the summer drove Domenico mad.[3]

The fight in court was not about whether or not Domenico was melancholic; on that point everyone agreed. What they objected to was Faustina's solution. They admitted that he needed someone to supervise his behavior during the summer, but, as a later iteration of the case reveals, a family solution had already been arranged. Domenico was not to sell property or contract without the intervention and consent of one of his cognate relatives.[4] Despite counterclaims, the Duke's office instructed the Pupilli to take on his wardship. Whether care was contingent on the season was not addressed.

Domenico's case offers only a fleeting glimpse of his life and the people he shared it with. Still, it relates a familiar tale. At the heart of the matter lay concern over a person's failure both to manage property and patrimony and to protect family honor and reputation. Domenico cut a poor figure as paterfamilias; his shameful and imprudent behavior threatened the material and social standing of his household. It also started a battle between his relatives over who would control his estate during those critical summer months.

Thus far, in comparison with other cases involving mental or physical incapacity prosecuted in Florentine courts between the fourteenth and seventeenth centuries, Domenico's is ordinary. What makes it extraordinary is Faustina's claim that her son's behavior was not merely incompetent or irresponsible but pathological. Medical explanations for mental and physical impairment like this one did not appear in the records of Florentine courts until the mid-sixteenth century. Prior to reforms of the 1540s, traditional Roman law categories for incapacity sufficed; the mentally incapacitated were generically referred to as *furiosi, mentecapti, fatui*, and *dementes* in Latin and, in Italian, *pazzi, matti*, and *mentecatti*. After 1540, the faces of the melancholic, manic, frenetic, and epileptic emerge in the records of the Pupilli and the Otto di Guardia from among an otherwise amorphous group of men and women, young and old, rich and poor who were considered mentally or physically incompetent.

From this point on, lay petitioners explicitly and increasingly linked abnormal thought and behavior to well-known physical illnesses that adversely affected brain function. What was more, though rare relative to the caseloads of the Pupilli and the Otto, court records show that medical explanations tended to work. Of the thirty or so cases of this type brought before the Pupilli and the Otto between roughly 1550 and 1630, two-thirds were granted in whole or in part. Medical explanations had, in a sense, arrived. Petitioners understood and used them; the courts understood and accepted them and they did so without recourse to expert medical testimony.

But why did Faustina resort to what sounds like a medical explanation in the first place? What did she mean by melancholy? And what did she gain by using it as the basis of her legal argument? What did it offer that traditional categories did not? This book has shown that as early as the fourteenth century, people like Faustina had at their disposal legal remedies for dealing with Domenico's destructive behavior. They also had an array of legal terms that activated these remedies in court. Why not simply say that Domenico could not manage his estate? Why not merely refer to him generically as "pazzo" or "matto," "furioso" or "mentecatto"? Why not call him a prodigal? All of these ways of speaking had the power to mark Domenico as a person in need of legal supervision. All of them could have carried the day in court. Faustina chose rather to tether her son's behavior, from wild outbursts to poor spending habits, to a specific disease and one that had complex social and cultural connotations. This chapter seeks to explain why.

Thus far we have explored the ways in which families dealt with, or perhaps profited from, the mental or physical incapacity of their kin. We have also observed the important but limited role courts of law and the increasingly centralized, absolutist, and interventionist Florentine state played in the process of helping desperate families and communities restore order to households and neighborhoods and find workable solutions to the problem of long-term care. We embark now on the history of how madness became a physical disease in Florentine society.

This is not a simple story to tell. The medical turn in Florentine courts is itself part of the long and complex history of the medicalization of European society. It begins in the thirteenth century as a southern European phenomenon with the institutionalization of a specific brand of medical knowledge in the new faculties of medicine at the universities of Salerno, Bologna, Montpellier, and Paris.[5] It takes off in the fifteenth and sixteenth centuries, when an increasingly large part of the European lay public were becoming conversant with the principles of academic medicine in a popularized, nontechnical form.

It rises to the surface in sixteenth-century Florentine court records when petitioners explicitly turned medical language to their own use in the courts.

How medicalization spread has long been a subject of debate, but historians no longer see it as a top-down progress narrative, tracing the rise of learned physicians, who, as a coherent professional group, successfully imposed medical norms on European society.[6] University-trained doctors were key engines in the process of medicalization, but, as consumers of health care and health care services, so were ordinary men and women. Recent work in the history of medicine has shown that learned physicians operated in a competitive socioprofessional marketplace that did not automatically privilege their proprietary claims to medical knowledge or practice.

Scholarship has shown that social and cultural factors were important engines of medicalization in European society. Social and cultural values, attitudes, and practices shaped how physicians explained sickness and health in their medical treatises at the same time that learned medical thinking gave laymen and women a way of identifying, understanding, explaining, and labeling certain types of behavior, contributing to what we might call disease vogues. In the sixteenth century, the disease melancholy seemed in and on many European minds.[7] So widespread was its appeal in philosophy, theology, art, and the European national literatures that scholars have dubbed the second half of this century the "age of melancholy" or even the "golden age of melancholy."[8] The disconsolate lover, the eccentric artistic, the brooding scholar, and the frenzied hero could be pathological bodies in the European imagination, their fraught psychic suffering traced back to underlying physiology. To put it another way, where some might have seen Domenico's melancholy as a bad thing, culture sometimes gave it a more noble hue. Melancholy's greatest virtue was its plasticity; once the breadth of its meaning and significance was generally grasped, petitioners could shape it into whatever form best described a relative's condition in court.

Faustina's case and others like it offer an excellent starting point for understanding the engines of medicalization and how they interacted so that petitioners in Florentine courts came to see madness as a physical illness and then successfully to use it as a legal strategy. But they also show how central ordinary men and women were in that process of medicalization. People like Faustina impressed onto plastic disease categories like melancholy their own social and cultural expectations. Thus the focus here is not on medical practitioners but lay petitioners and their creative use of medical concepts and language to attain desired legal outcomes.

THE WORLD BENEATH THE SKIN

Faustina, her relatives, court officials, and ducal secretaries shared common assumptions about health and illness. Environmental factors like climate had a profound effect on the body; the body, in turn, had a profound effect on the mind. The external world played upon a complex internal world. Here the humors reigned. Humoral doctrine maintained that the body was composed of four qualities— hot, cold, dry, and moist—which, in turn, made up the four primary elements—blood, phlegm, yellow bile, and black bile.[9] These four elements or humors took their natures from the qualities that governed them: phlegm was the coldest and moistest of humors, blood the hottest and moistest, yellow bile the hottest and driest, and black bile the coldest and driest. Humors were more or less prevalent in the body depending on season. Since blood was hot and moist it diminished in the autumn, a cold and dry season in which melancholy thrived. The correct balance (*eukrasía*, literally "good temperament") of these internal qualities and humors at play with the conditions predominating in the external world constituted health. Conversely, their imbalance (*dyskrasía*) in the body caused pain and illness. In this system, health and illness were not distinct conditions but relative states of greater or lesser equilibrium.[10] Since the body constantly teetered between states of sickness and health, prophylaxis was just as important as therapy.

The doctrine of the humors first appeared two millennia before Faustina pondered her son's condition in a collection of early Greek medical writings associated with Hippocrates of Cos (ca. 460–ca. 370 BCE); it was most famously assessed and augmented by Aristotle and the Roman physician Galen (129–199/217). It was subsequently systematized and repackaged by Muslim natural philosophers like Rhazes (d. 925), Avicenna (980–1037), Haly Abbas (fl. tenth century), and Averroes (d. 1198) before it reemerged in Italy to flourish anew during the eleventh and twelfth centuries in and around the southern city of Salerno and the monastery of Montecassino.

Salernitan texts together with the products of similar translation efforts in Spain formed the basis of the early medical curriculum in the new medical faculties cropping up at Bologna, Montpellier, and Paris during the twelfth and thirteenth centuries.[11] By the late thirteenth century, the curriculum had grown to include what scholars have called the "New Galen," an enormous collection of Galenic texts, many of which were Arabic commentaries on Galen's writing.[12] From the late thirteenth through the fifteenth century Italian medical faculties built a more or less uniform curriculum around this multilayered Greco-Arabic tradition. The cornerstone of university education was Avicenna's *Canon*, a massive five-book compendium of medical learning.[13]

In the late fifteenth and sixteenth centuries, medical humanists demanded critical editions of the Hippocratic corpus and Galen's works, asserting that centuries of translation from Greek into Arabic and Arabic into Latin had degraded the study of genuine Greek medicine.[14] Rail though they might against Avicenna and his ilk, their efforts to cleanse the Greek medical tradition were philological rather than substantive.[15] The doctrine of the humors remained the central organizing framework for understanding the natural world as well as health and illness until the seventeenth century, when new ways of imagining the body contributed to its slow demise.[16] For two millennia a humoral view of the body reigned.[17]

Humoral doctrine suggested two ways of thinking about the body. Hippocratic authors tended to envision it as a leaky container in which humors and the vapors produced by them intermingled, burbled, broiled, and seethed.[18] All substances entering the body—food, drink, and *materia medica*, odors, vapors, fumes, and smoke—had to be balanced against those exiting—sweat, urine, feces, mucus, tears, menses, semen, milk, and blood. The English author of *The Anatomy of Melancholy*, Robert Burton (1577–1640), evocatively imagined this world that lay just beneath the skin as a continuous churning seas of liquids sloshing and clouds of vapors meandering about from head to toe. More recently, Barbara Duden has observed that such a view of the inner body as "unstructured, osmotic space" encased within a thin, porous shell was extremely long-lived. It persisted through the eighteenth century even when the humoral system had lost its explanatory power.[19] Galen, by contrast, imagined the body as a "system of solid organs ranked by purpose and function."[20] The humors and the vapors they produced still sloshed about but tended to marinate organs in ways that either promoted health or induced illness.

The primacy of Avicenna's *Canon* in university *curricula*, especially as propaedeutic for approaching the unsystematic nature of Galen's enormous collection of writings, predisposed learned physicians to a more Galenic or organ-centered way of talking about disease. In their scholarly output and medical practice, they cast the humors as antagonists in complex disease narratives focused on specific organs or organ systems. When talking about diseases that affected thought, feeling, and behavior they spoke mainly about pathological humors and their noxious by-products originating from anywhere in the body to coalesce in the brain, where Galen and, following him, Avicenna located the seat of reason.[21] Once there these materials caused all manner of mayhem.

Whether one tended toward a more Hippocratic or Galenic way of thinking, the key to health was equilibrium. The two complementary aspects of medicine, prevention of disease and cure of disease, worked toward the same goal; the former sought to preserve, the latter to restore the body's balance through careful management of what medieval and early modern physicians classified as the six non-naturals: environment and climate, diet, evacuation and retention of bodily substances, exercise and rest, sleep and waking, and the passions of the soul.

Ordinary men and women like Faustina accepted that the head and brain were the seat of reason and that madness resulted when pathological material converged there. But they tended toward a more Hippocratic way of imagining the body as an unstructured vessel containing both healthy and pathological materials in constant flow. Humors that had been corrupted for any number of reasons carried sickness with them throughout the body. Serious illness resulted when these pathological flows could not be expelled through the body's many openings. The obstructed body was a sick body. The eruptions of carbuncles, abscesses, blisters, or tumors, the dramatic movement of the bowels, bouts of coughing or vomiting, flows of tears, gaseous bursts from either end—these could be interpreted and felt to be great salutary expulsions of sickness.[22] But relief was always only temporary; the humors churned and their vapors wandered without end until the body was no more.

"EVERYBODY MAKES MEDICINE HIS BUSINESS"

The complex learned textual tradition provided people like Faustina with the framework for explaining her son's behavior in medical or at least material terms. But how did she come in contact with it? It is safe to assume that Faustina never skimmed the Hippocratic works, perused Galen's enormous corpus, or thumbed through Avicenna's *Canon*. To be conversant with humoral medicine, she didn't have to.

Beginning in the thirteenth century, the fundamental principles undergirding dietetics and hygiene were slowly passed on to laymen and women in simple, easy-to-follow manuals for healthy living typically referred to as regimens of health.[23] These practical medical manuals flourished first in Latin, but versions in a variety of European vernaculars quickly followed.[24] The first example of this genre with the distinction of being written in, not translated into, the vernacular came from the pen of Aldobrandino of Siena, an Italian physician living and working in the French royal court. Sometime around 1256 he produced, in French, the *Régime du corps*, a manual in four books, outlining the day-to-day steps a person could take to prevent disease.[25] The purpose of the *Régime*, Aldobrandino informed his audience, was not therapeutic but prophylactic. It taught its readers not how to cure disease but only how to guard the body against it. He communicated the basic rules of dietetics and hygiene in simple, unadorned, nontheoretical language, giving his lay readership the fundamental tools to preserving health. More important, he based his advice on the most cutting-edge medical knowledge the universities had to offer.

At first, learned physicians like Aldobrandino tended to dedicate regimens of health to individuals of high standing. They quickly came to reach and serve a larger population.[26] During the late thirteenth and first half of the fourteenth century some of Europe's most illustrious doctors wrote them. The regimen of health that Arnald of Villanova (1240–1311) addressed to James II of Aragon subsequently became the most widely diffused dietetic text in Latin during the Middle Ages.[27] From the middle of the fourteenth century to the end of the fifteenth, regimens of health were plentiful in Europe. Demand for them was fed in part by the growth of an urban audience eager for prophylactic health strategies as well as by the arrival of plague and its cyclical occurrence.[28]

The great divide between academic and domestic medicine was not so much conceptual as it was practical. Therapeutics was the province of learned physicians in their academic and professional milieus. By contrast, prophylaxis was largely a domestic affair. It took place mostly in the household and involved all the hygienic, dietetic, and lifestyle choices an individual made in the course of his or her day. Proper application of the six non-naturals, which could be easily adapted in daily dietetic and hygienic routines, served both prophylactic and therapeutic ends. Their regulation prevented disease; their adjustment cured it. Ordinary men and women were responsible for fending off disease; physicians, for treating it.[29]

The demand for preventive health manuals and recipe books accelerated in the sixteenth century when a range of health-related material could be disseminated quickly and cheaply in print. Beginning in the 1520s, printed vernacular popular health books, especially those that passed on therapeutic and prophylactic recipes, were flying out of books stalls in great numbers across Europe. The most successful of these recipe books by far was the *Secreti del reverendo donno Alessio piemontese* of 1555. Compiled by Girolamo Ruscelli, a hired pen for one of Venice's most preeminent publishing houses, the *Secreti* would appear in seventy editions in almost every European language, including Latin by the end of the sixteenth century, and over a hundred by the close of the seventeenth.[30]

By Faustina's day a veritable cascade of preventive medical literature in the vernacular, including herbals, recipe books, regimens of health, collections of medical aphorisms, plague treatises, lapidaries, and electuaries, flooded sixteenth-century European book markets. Recent scholarship that explores this burgeoning market in vernacular medical literature has not only revealed a larger, more diverse audience for medical information, products, and services but also shone light on new sites of knowledge production, adding household and convent gardens and kitchens to traditional academic settings.[31]

But Faustina need not have scoured family bookshelves to learn about humoral medicine. Outside the confines of her home, she moved about in a society that had long demanded university-trained physicians and their expertise.[32] In the thirteenth century, a number of Italian cities had begun to employ *medici condotti*, salaried physicians retained by city governments to care for the sick poor often at civic hospitals. They treated injuries resulting from state-sanctioned punishment or torture, provided medical evidence for trials or investigations, and offered their expert medical opinions to anyone who requested them. In the fourteenth and fifteenth centuries, religious corporations, confraternities, and guilds followed suit, keeping their own physicians on retainer.[33]

What was more, in the piazzas of her town, Faustina was likely to find a pluralistic and competitive market for health care products and services sold by a range of healers to male and female clients from different social classes. This motley group included university-trained physicians and surgeons who often worked closely with apothecaries as well as empirics, cunning men and women, alchemical, astrological, or occult healers, remedy sellers, tooth drawers, snake charmers, and charlatans.[34] She may even have enjoyed the pleasure or perhaps suffered the irritation of watching troupes of charlatans decked out in colorful costumes prance across makeshift stages to hawk a special syrup or promote a miraculous pill.

Efforts to regulate this thriving market in health were not uniform across Europe, but a number of Italian municipalities did try to impose some measure of order on it. As one might expect, learned physicians and their associated corporations dominated medical licensing regimes. In republican Florence, the guild of doctors, grocers, and apothecaries set the standards for medical practice and regulated the sale of remedies. Like other Italian licensing bodies, they awarded licenses to all manner of practitioners provided their methods accorded with the principles of learned medicine. Regulatory bodies may not have been able to eradicate all forms of rogue healing, but they did manage to ensure some consistency in treatment since practitioners who lacked formal training had to play by their rules in order to get a license.[35]

In the wake of plague beginning in the fourteenth century, matters of health were connected to environmental concerns like the effects of climate and the quality of air and water. The internal world of humors and their by-products was extremely susceptible to the world outside. Air, the first non-natural, was an enormous category, representing the entire external environment and the effects it had on bodily health. City statutes issued in response to outbreaks of plague illustrate well the connection late medieval and early modern people made between sickness and the environment. Many of the ordinances promulgated by the city of Pistoia in 1348, for example, were designed to improve the quality of the air on the assumption that corruption entered the body through the mouth and nose in the form of smoke, vapor, or odors. Malodorous industrial processes like tanning and the slaughter of animals were banned outright or heavily regulated to prevent the creation and spread of foul, disease-bearing stenches.[36] Similarly, sixteenth-century printed popular health books were full of recipes for scented pastes, perfumes, waters, powders, and oils that people could use to create healthy environments. And they applied them liberally to their bodies, clothing, and furnishings.[37]

But medical language and concepts were also available outside medical arenas. Faustina could have absorbed humoral analogies, for example, from sermons. Since the thirteenth century, Dominicans, Franciscans, and Benedictines had used medical language in their sermons to instruct their lay audiences. They likened the disordered soul to the imbalanced body and bad habits (*mali mores*) to bad humors (*mali humores*). The six non-naturals as prophylactic and therapeutic strategies for preventing and curing diseases of the body had spiritual counterparts that were seen to prevent and cure diseases of the soul. The regulation of diet could be compared to abstinence from sin, exercise could represent the performance of penance, physical purgation like bleeding, enemas, and vomiting were similar to confession.[38] The famous moralizing archbishop of Florence, Antonino (1389–1459), also likened physical and spiritual healing strategies. "Penance," he wrote, "is a purging of ill humors, that is, an evacuation of vices . . . confession is like a rhubarb of decoction, which causes vomiting."[39] In other words, humoral language had long been spoken in households, shops, and public squares throughout Italy by the time Faustina went to court.

Perhaps as early as the fourteenth century and certainly by the sixteenth, an urban center like Florence and its Tuscan domains shared a common though admittedly fluid medical culture largely though not exclusively based on the principles of Greek humoral medicine.[40] Learned physicians and ordinary men and women alike consistently drew from the same Greek medical tradition particularly in the realm of preventive medicine.[41] To put it another way, a simplified version of learned medicine was mainstream medicine. As a propertied woman in an affluent Tuscan town, Faustina very well might have called on the expertise of every medical practitioner money could buy from the most eminent of physicians to the lowest of empirics. She may have called in spiritual healers from her parish priest to the local exorcist. Still, if she wanted to make a medical argument in court, it had to conform to the principles of Greek humoral medicine even if only in the most rudimentary fashion.

THE TEXTS BEHIND THE CASE

Faustina's debt to academic medicine is clear if we compare her explanation of Domenico's disease to consultations that university-trained physicians wrote on behalf of mentally disordered patients. Take, for example, the *consilium* written by the Italian physician Bartolomeo Montagnana (ca. 1380–1452) for the melancholic and "pitiable" Battista Vincentino. According to Montagnana, Battista incorrectly believed that he was "a prelate and most devoted servant of God and a great law-giver for all people, although he neither had the disposition for this nor the skill, training, or power to achieve such things for himself." Montagnana connected these delusions to sediments of melancholy material that had gathered in Battista's brain, compromising the proper functioning of his "powers of imagination and cogitation."[42]

The effects of melancholy were written into Battista's flesh; his skin had taken on the color of lead. Other signs revealed themselves in gastrointestinal distress, limpid and watery urine, a slow, faint pulse, and a recent history of troubled sleep. The signs most obvious to the lay observer were those communicated by behavior. Battista persisted in his delusions of the priestly life by praying, preaching, and delivering sermons. The sick man further experienced instantaneous and obsessive bouts of fear. At other times he was plagued by grief.[43]

It was not Battista's brain that was the ultimate source of his troubles. Rather, a complicated series of events were at play in his body. The root cause of his malady, Montagnana explained, was an excess of melancholy matter. Under normal conditions this substance, known as black bile, from *melaina chole* in Greek (*cholera nigra* or *atra bilis* in Latin), was a natural part of the body's constitution. Black bile became toxic in surplus quantities and led to a particular manifestation of the disease of the same name.

As Montagnana described, bodies that were naturally cold and dry were particularly good breeding grounds for black bile, which was itself of the same quality. If important organs like the heart and brain were cold and dry by nature and circumstances conspired to exacerbate these qualities, these organs became black bile factories, inundating the body with surplus matter. The liver, whose main function was to regulate the balance of humors, was weakened by its unsuccessful efforts to purge black bile from the blood; it passed the excess on to the spleen. In its turn, the spleen failed to disperse or redistribute black bile to the organs that were naturally disposed to expel it. From there, black bile infiltrated the entire body. Soon all the organs, despite contrary efforts, manufactured the noxious stuff until they assumed the harmful characteristics of black bile itself, which in Montagnana's words was dark and tangled like a wood (*sylvestris*).

It was in this wild environment that Battista's rational faculties were ensnared. Once these dark humors ascended to his brain, Montagnana noted, they laid siege in particular to the powers of imagination and cogitation located there, the faculties in the brain that collected, interpreted, and made judgments about sensory data. This was the immediate cause of Battista's false ideas about the world and his role in it.

Faustina's explanation of Domenico's illness conforms to the general principles outlined in Montagnana's *consilium* but contradicts certain details. How could her son Domenico suffer an excess of melancholy humors, which were cold and dry, in the hot and dry months of June and July? If he were truly melancholic wouldn't he be more likely to fall prey to melancholy during the autumn or the winter? And if Domenico's sickness had something to do with heat instead of cold, why wasn't he sick in August, the hottest month of the year? The simple answer is that melancholy was a capacious disease category. It was caused by more than merely the superfluity of black bile.

A *consilium* written by Giovanbattista da Monte (1498–1552), professor of medicine at Padua and renowned for his clinical teaching, accords more with Faustina's argument. In consultation with two other physicians, da Monte offered his opinion on a case of a Jewish man who had "gone out of his senses" (*venit extra rationem*). His friends claimed that prior to this episode work had been particularly taxing, he was often fearful, and the smallest things drove him to anger. He did a tremendous amount of business and made long trips to northern European climes where he was exposed to extremes of heat and cold. When he returned to Italy after one such trip, he exhibited strange and violent behavior: "his eyes moved without his control, [he had] an expression of rage, he wished to strike those around him, [and] he rolled himself from his bed."[44]

All three physicians decided that he was in the grips of melancholy. According to da Monte, the patient's habits and lifestyle had caused it:

> his temperament, age, and the time of year all contributed to the generation of these symptoms. [The patient] went on a very long journey, during which his head suffered great heat, and then after the heat, cold. He worked a great deal without stopping; he ate rich, heat-producing foods as is the custom in Poland and northern Europe. He

consumed more rich food in a day than we eat in a year. He drank
strong wine, and ate all manner of substance that produced dryness
and heat.[45]

The patient, da Monte concluded, was suffering from too much heat
owing to a superfluity of corrupt blood. This type of blood could
cause melancholy even where no melancholy substance existed. One
would think that the return to Italy, a climate that da Monte suggested suited him, would have recalibrated his complexion. Instead,
yet another alteration of his environment shocked his system so violently that he suffered severe mental distress.

Generally speaking physicians used the humoral system of medicine to tell stories about an individual body's struggle and often failure to maintain a workable balance between the worlds inside and
outside the thin layer of flesh. That story was not merely descriptive
as modern psychiatric and neurobiological classification systems are;
it was explanatory.[46] Medieval and early modern physicians believed
that Greek humoral theory described objective bodily states, which
could be accurately read from physical and behavioral signs. They
also believed that body and soul were intimately connected. Just as
the physical world significantly affected a person's thoughts and feelings, one's emotional reactions to events or situations profoundly
affected the body. These features of academic medicine appear in
court cases even if the technical details of diseases and brain anatomy
do not. Petitioners explicitly linked abnormal cognitive, emotional,
and behavioral states to material causes and believed that the most
precarious moments in a person's life were those involving change
in environment, climate, diet, or habits. For Faustina's son and da
Monte's patient, stress coupled with vacillations between hot and cold
weather generated pathological humors and then disease.

"INFINITE ARE THE SPECIES OF MELANCHOLY"

Nebulous borders create at once confusion and opportunity. The
mutability of humors made distinguishing between diseases difficult
at the same time that it provided medieval and early modern Europeans with a powerful framework for parsing the full range of human
behavior and accounting for the individual experience of disease. One
disease could easily turn into another depending on the quality, quantity, and location of the humors together with environmental conditions acting on the body. Diseases that affected brain function were

an especially tangled wood since the humors could trigger what Avicenna admitted was an infinite number of abnormal cognitive, emotional, or behavioral states.[47]

He tried to make juggling the sundry manifestations that his Greek forebears had identified more manageable by classifying them according to the qualities that caused them in concert with how those qualities affected cerebral structures and operations.[48] Still, learned physicians from the thirteenth through the seventeenth century who followed Avicenna's nosology were met with a dizzying array of conditions that affected cognition and behavior. Excessive cold was especially detrimental to mental activities like memory and reasoning, causing *lethargia*, a deep drowsiness dulling sensation and perception. When sufficient moisture was added to excessive cold, somnolent or stuporous diseases like *apoplexia* resulted.[49] Where cold and dry qualities dulled the mind, hot and wet diseases excited it. At the opposite end of the spectrum, excessive heat or burning caused violent or aggressive diseases like *mania*.[50]

At the same time that proper classification in clinical situations could be a real challenge, the flexibility of the system gave physicians—and for that matter petitioners—ample latitude to explain an enormous range of behavior. The impulsiveness of Domenico and the violence of da Monte's Jewish patient were better captured by hot humors like blood, yellow bile, or burnt black bile while Battista's nonviolent delusions were better explained by a surfeit of black bile in its natural cold and dry state. Yet all of these men were said to suffer from melancholy. How could one disease embrace three completely different humoral and behavioral states?

Learned discussions of diseases that caused madness in practical medical literature from the thirteenth through the seventeenth century betray a general flattening of Greco-Arabic categories from myriad diseases of the brain to a lumping of all mental illnesses and impairments under three or four easily recognizable conditions like melancholy, mania, frenzy, and epilepsy.[51] The melancholy disease generated by excess black bile presented in unprovoked fear, sadness, and false ideas accompanied by isolation and antisocial behavior. Mania represented the opposite end of the spectrum, revealing itself variously in violent or aggressive behavior. Frenzy (*phrenitis*) indicated raving with fever. Epilepsy was among the diseases that interfered with motion. Corrupt or surfeit humors originating in the nerves caused blockages in the head that in turn caused spasmodic movements of the limbs.[52] As early as 1300, melancholy had begun to subsume mania, too, embracing the full spectrum of abnormal behavior from sadness with no cause to unprovoked rage.[53] Physicians contributed to this trend by increasingly addressing mania as a subspecies of melancholy in their learned treatises.[54]

Cases from the Pupilli and Otto di Guardia reflect the thinking and tendencies of this tradition. Lay petitioners accepted and parroted the view that madness had somatic roots and, though it may have originated somewhere else in the body, generally targeted the brain. Petitioners also exploited the tremendous diagnostic overlap that characterized disease categories. The case of the woolworker Marco illustrates the commonly held belief that mental incapacity was caused by an illness located in the brain. In 1549, the Otto fined Marco for having sold a *scrocchio* and then imprisoned him for failure to pay the entire amount of the fine. For reasons that are not clear, Marco's brother-in-law Piero petitioned the Otto, asking that the Duke forgive Marco the debt and release him from jail. According to Piero, everyone who knew Marco also knew that he "was bothered exceedingly by the falling sickness (*mal caduco*), which was located in his brain in such a way that he's absentminded and acts as if he [has no] memory."[55] The problem was not Marco's refusal to comply with the court's demands but his inability to do so. He was not criminal so much as he was sick; it was his brain not his will that prevented him from paying the fine. Unfortunately the outcome of the case was not recorded so we do not know how the court ruled. At the very least, we can say that Piero considered an argument connecting Marco's behavior to an underlying illness plausible enough to warrant using it as the foundation of his plea.

Other cases demonstrate that Piero's strategy could work even though detail was thin on the ground. Faustina's petition on behalf of her son Domenico is one of the more descriptive of these types of cases. In others, the mere evocation or repetition of a disease category with little description sufficed. Take, for example, the case of Pierantonio and Ridolfo Guasconi, two purportedly melancholic brothers. In 1585, Paolo Guasconi, a knight of Malta, asked that the Pupilli assume the care of his younger brother Pierantonio who, "had succumbed to melancholy humors."[56] Since Paolo had been called to Naples to take the helm of a galley, he was not available to supervise Pierantonio himself. Once consent of their relatives was confirmed, the Duke's secretary granted Paolo's request and the Pupilli took up Pierantonio's care.

A continuation of the case later that year adds a twist to the story. In this petition, we meet another melancholic brother. Here Paolo Guasconi told the Pupilli that melancholy humors had assailed his brothers, Messer Ridolfo and Pierantonio, for many years. "Many cures and different remedies" made them better for a time, he added, but "they soon grew worse and needed supervision." Pierantonio was the more violent of the two, acting "furiosamente," as Paolo put it. The Pupilli had by that time assumed the care of Pierantonio and his property. In order to avoid the "disordini" that tended to follow in his wake and particularly "to flee greater damage and shame," Paolo asked that the Duke keep him in the Stinche prison. He asked, too, that Ridolfo, presumably the more manageable of the two, "be put in a religious community (*monasterio di frati*) or in another appropriate place where he would be held and cared for until it pleased God to free him from these frenetic humors (*humori frenetici*)." The Duke again agreed, leaving the final decisions up to the Pupilli in the case of Pierantonio and the *frati* of whichever community Paolo wished to put Ridolfo in.[57]

Ridolfo disappears from the record after this petition while Pierantonio spent the next twenty-five years in and out of prison. In 1594 he was released at the request of Paolo, who insisted that his brother "had returned to his right mind (*ritornato in cervello*)." In the same breath, Paolo told the Pupilli that he "wanted to give him [Pierantonio] a wife in the hopes that he would have children." If the Pupilli thought this request suspicious they did not let on. Instead, they interviewed the priest of the Stinche and several other Stinche functionaries. All of them assured the Pupilli that Pierantonio "had sufficiently returned to his senses, performing all the acts befitting a sane man."[58] The Duke permitted Pierantonio's release but only on the condition that his relatives take him to a villa and keep him there. But Pierantonio, it would seem, could not stay out of trouble. He was captured and returned to prison in 1599 and again in 1608 for being "pazzo" and "furioso." The record finally closes on his story in 1610. This last petition found him suffering malarial fever (*febbre terzana*) while confined in a fortress of Borgo San Sepolcro, a small town about seventy miles southeast of Florence.[59]

Detail in this case is too scant to paint a back story. We know little other than that Paolo, the statutory caretaker of his unruly brothers, spent most of his time in military service away from Florence. Relatives agreed that the brothers needed supervision and were content to let the Pupilli assume the job. Exactly what was wrong with Pierantonio and Ridolfo is unclear. We can only speculate about what that behavior might have been, but to Paolo and his relatives it was an embarrassment. Not only did it threaten "disordini" in the household, but it also brought shame (*vergogna*). The phrase most often repeated of the brothers is that they "had succumbed to melancholy humors which made them frenetic." As Paolo said, he had sought "cures" and "remedies" to no avail. The sickness always returned, causing behavior counter to what their families wanted or expected of them.

Language here is slippery. The men were said to have succumbed to "melancholic humors" and "maninconic humors that made them frenetic," suggesting that they suffered the more aggressive forms of melancholy.[60] This was shorthanded to "frenetic humors" in one instance. Strictly speaking, there were humors that generated the disease frenzy (*phrenitis*) as well as humors causing frenetic behavior. There was no frenetic substance existing naturally in the body. The slippage between disease category and behavior was common in these cases. It in no way imperiled outcomes; in this case as in others, the court accepted the imprecise labels and the petition.

PATHOLOGIZING BEHAVIOR

Laymen and women used the protean melancholy, frenzy, and *mal caduco* interchangeably to explain and, more pointedly, to find legal solutions for behavior that had traditionally warranted court intervention, namely, the mismanagement of patrimony, reckless spending, the accumulation of debt, unprovoked or excessive violence, and behavior that flouted social norms. The language may have changed, but the problematic behavior remained the same. Even gross simplification of disease categories in no way compromised a petition's outcome. The court's response was pragmatic. Judges and magistrates usually accepted highly generalized language since their concern was less the technical precision of the argument than the ability of the outcome to maintain order in families and communities.

In her petition of 1598, Faustina claimed that her son lost his fortune only when in the grips of melancholy. Relatives and neighbors agreed. When free from melancholy, Domenico was an able businessman; when sick he went on spending sprees. The adverse effects of *mal caduco* on the brain were similarly held responsible for Marco's *scrocchio* of 1549. Faustina and Marco's brother-in-law were not alone in using medical language to explain financially ruinous behavior. In October 1562, Giovanni Dellosso had his eldest brother, Michele, imprisoned in the Stinche for being *mentecatto* on account of various dark humors (*diverssi omori chchorsso* [*sic*]).[61] A year later Giovanni together with his brother Battista petitioned the Pupilli, claiming that Michele had proven himself incapable of managing his affairs for about a year. The greatest concern seemed to be the integrity of their mother's dowry, which Michele controlled after the death of their father. The brothers asked that Michele relinquish that control and that the Pupilli assign him a guardian.

Over the next month, the Pupilli conducted an investigation only to find that the exact nature of Michele's condition was in dispute. The guards of the Stinche testified that they had "heard him speak and hold rational conversations." Moreover, they did not think the term "mentecapto" was appropriate since "he did not go around doing crazy things." In their view, "one could say that he was of feeble mind and brain, but to such a minor degree that he could be released from prison."[62] Unfortunately the paper trail ends there with no evidence of resolution.[63]

Since the dowry of Michele's mother was on the line, we can imagine a scenario in which the Magistrato Supremo granted the petition even if there existed conflicting testimony. As we have repeatedly seen, Pupilli cases tended to hinge on how problematic behavior affected vulnerable members of a household. The case of Gino Capponi is a good example of this propensity. In April 1578, his brother Luigi petitioned the Pupilli together with their nearest relations to say that Girolamo, who had recently finished a six-month term as Podestà of Empoli, "was suddenly struck by melancholy humors." According to Luigi, Girolamo "showed evident signs of it" while he was Podestà. Once he returned home "it was necessary to seize him and lock him up at home." Reckless spending habits were again offered as evidence of an underlying pathological condition. Luigi asked that the Pupilli "prevent Girolamo from making any more loans or other contracts without their express permission so that he did not reduce himself, his little children, and his wife to extreme misery, which would surely follow were he not supervised." The Duke's office immediately granted the petition, instructing the Pupilli to "ensure that this Girolamo does not ill manage his estate."[64] The following month, the Duke's office promulgated a ban publicly identifying Girolamo as a person who "continually wasted and consumed his estate . . . and had racked up debts with various types of people . . . to his ruin and dishonor."[65] The compelling detail in Girolamo's case is mention of his wife and children. His behavior threatened their well-being and thus the future of his line. In this case as in many others, the Pupilli decided in favor of relatives against troublesome kin.

Supplicants and magistrates also used medical categories to explain criminal behavior in the hopes of reducing sentences and punishments or negotiating settlements between parties. As we learned in an earlier chapter, Florentines sometimes argued that poor judgment accompanying youth was a kind of mental incapacity. This connection was made in several cases to defend young men caught in the city with illegal weapons. In some of these cases, petitioners or court personnel posited melancholy or *mal caduco* as a contributing factor to this type of malfeasance. In February 1578, Antonio di Alesso, a boy of fifteen, found himself in prison. He had been fined twenty scudi and sentenced to three drops of the rope by the Otto for being in possession of a concealed dagger within the confines of the city of Florence. Antonio asked that the Duke grant him grace for this punishment since "he erred because of an innate weakness."[66] He further claimed that his mother was a poor widow with other young children to care for. His predicament would only bring them trouble. In the Otto's version of this supplication they confirmed that Antonio had indeed been fined and sentenced, though they claimed that it was because he was found crossing a piazza with a firearm (*pistolese*). They added that he suffered from *mal caduco*, a fact his fellow workers confirmed.[67] The Duke responded by commuting the corporal part of the sentence to imprisonment, which would presumably end once Antonio had paid the fine. Antonio was forgiven in part for his misbehavior; his physical condition was one of the mitigating factors of the case. On the one hand, it served Antonio's family by sparing them the humiliation of his corporal punishment. On the other hand, the court did not hold him fully responsible for his illegal behavior. He broke the law not because he was wicked or criminal but because he was mentally ill at the time.

The judicial calculus that went into a case like Antonio's was straightforward. The assertion that he was sick unto madness took some of the social sting out of punishment, but the safety of family and community was the paramount concern. So far as we know, Antonio was a first-time offender and his crime was relatively small. Leniency was in the best interest of Antonio's family while simultaneously being of little cost to the community at large. Such a solution satisfied justice; it was restorative rather than disruptive, the chief aim of civil and criminal litigation from the judge's or magistrate's point of view. In cases where petitioners or magistrates posited a somatic cause of troublesome or illegal behavior, the point was not to quibble over medical details but to make households, litigants, and the community whole.

THE USES OF DISEASE NARRATIVE

Medical arguments gave some measure of temporal specificity to conditions that seemed unpredictable and admitted the possibility of lucid intervals. Because sickness in humoral medicine was tethered to season and the stresses of life, work, family, and love, savvy petitioners fashioned plausible stories about how a specific disease had influenced a person's behavior. There is no better example than that of Domenico, whose melancholy came back without fail every June and July in the context of a difficult home life. Melancholy gave Faustina a timeline that helped her understand her son's episodic outbursts and explain why they might be keyed to certain seasons. Melancholy also explained when and why Domenico experienced lucid intervals. Most important, it warned court officials that those lucid intervals were not likely to last. As someone susceptible to climate, Domenico would surely succumb again. Where acute disease like melancholy, mania, or frenzy helped explain why a person might be stark raving mad at one time and completely sane at another, chronic diseases like *mal caduco* helped take lucid intervals out of the equation. The behavior of a person who had it was always subject to question.

In a case that took place between 1564 and 1574, for example, several people petitioned the Pupilli about Bernardo Guasconi for allegedly not being able to conduct his affairs because of "a defect of mind . . . and some impediment particular to those people vexed by mal caduco." In case anyone tried to pinpoint exactly when *mal caduco* compromised Bernardo's behavior, the record adds, "he was vexed by mal caduco almost continuously in such a way that it made him insane and alienated from his mind."[68] The implication here is that this was not a man who could ever be trusted to conduct business.

Interestingly enough, he was allowed to marry and have children but was prevented from managing his estate or making any decisions about how it was to be passed on. As people who lacked intent, the mentally incompetent were not supposed to marry. In practice, law and society recognized degrees of incompetence. Bernardo seems to have been mostly competent to function in social circles but tended to make poor financial decisions. We have seen over and over the importance of patrimonial rationality as constitutive of the legally competent person. Here, Bernardo's relatives associated his poor judgment with a chronic illness to strengthen their claim that he could be married but still needed the supervision of more prudent kin.

Petitioners could also use medical categories to fix sharper temporal boundaries for incidences of somatically induced madness by claiming that they had sought medical treatment that ultimately failed. Domenico fits this bill since his mother, Faustina, mentioned that he had been successfully treated when the disease first struck but subsequent attempts to mitigate its effects failed after it reappeared. The stresses of Domenico's life—an unwanted marriage, the pressing needs of family, household, and work—were so acute that, in the end, neither his body nor treatment could fend off melancholy. The disease became a permanent, predictable, and highly destructive part of his life. Faustina emphasized in her petition that at certain times of the year, Domenico was simply beyond treatment; this was why he needed supervision and more supervision than the family could provide on its own. Despite opposition from relatives, Faustina believed only court intervention could adequately protect Domenico's estate. The court agreed.

Paolo Guasconi used a similar strategy when claiming that his brothers Ridolfo and Pierantonio were melancholic in such a way that neither was fit for society, one sent to prison and the other put in a religious community. Treatment for their sicknesses had succeeded at first, but ultimately failed. Even if a petitioner used medical categories indiscriminately, making little distinction between melancholy and frenzy or giving little shading as to how a person experienced *mal caduco* throughout the course of life, he or she was still adding a sense of temporal precision based on observable phenomena.

MADNESS, MEDICINE, AND CULTURE

Lay litigants successfully used medical explanations—and sometimes rather imprecise medical explanations at that—to explain and excuse the problematic behavior of their relatives. They singled out melancholy as a useful catchall disease that accounted for a range of behaviors from poor judgment to unprovoked violence. But when exactly did Tuscans begin to do that and what made melancholy so appealing? The year 1540 is an artificial milestone. Our ability to see melancholy, mania, frenzy, and other like diseases in Florentine court records after that date is the result of changes in official documentary practice that, as so often happens with legal records, reflects a preexisting lay mentality. The move from Latin to vernacular and Romano-canonical to summary procedure in the 1540s surely unveiled some of the language petitioners had been using when they brought cases to court before notaries packed their phrasing into Roman law boxes. Had Faustina lived at the end of the fifteenth rather than the end of the sixteenth century she might have told the Pupilli that her son was melancholic, but the nature of record keeping in the republican courts would have masked this language.

Other types of evidence suggest that the change in thinking occurred earlier. Fifteenth-century Florentine tax records written in the vernacular show that when Florentines had the chance to describe the mental and physical disabilities of their relatives they tended to maintain traditional social or Roman law language. In the Catasto of 1427, for example, Florentines typically referred to their mad kin as *pazzo, mentecatto, non sano della mente, non è in suo sentimento, non ha buono sentimento, fuori di sé*, and in one instance *sciocco*.[69] That said, one Florentine included among his household a son "sick in body and mind" and "mal maestro," the vernacular term for a motor disease like *mal caduco*.[70] Other than this brief instance, no specific diseases appear. Melancholy surfaces in one record but only to describe the desolation that a father felt when he realized that none of his sons wanted to stay and work with him in his shop.

We step onto firmer ground if we turn to interactions between medicine and culture to fill in some of these gaps. Case upon case in the civil and criminal courts of Florence demonstrate that what constituted mental or physical incapacity was in part socially constructed. Petitioners and court personnel often placed behavior that threatened commonly held values or practices outside the bounds of reason to protect the social status or economic integrity of a family. Madness in late medieval and early modern Italian society was a cultural construct, too, exercising the imaginations of natural philosophers, theologians, physicians, and poets alike. Moreover, between the thirteenth and sixteenth centuries it was increasingly medicalized in a wide range of literature.

More and more over the course of this period, physicians and *literati* identified certain lifestyles as susceptible to mental illness and certain types of people as emblematic of specific pathologies. We might call this the medicalization of sociability. The lovesick suitor, the suicidal hermit, the pensive scholar, the physiologically inspired genius, the fool for Christ, the melancholy monk or nun, and the divine or demon possessed—all of these characters fit into a psychobiological framework that associated particular somatic constitutions with specific personalities or behaviors. By the sixteenth century, melancholy had emerged as the organic wellspring from which these conditions originated. Understanding behavior through medical terms or concepts, however, was not ideological so much as it was descriptive or explanatory. Despite the disturbances melancholy wrought, in cultural contexts, it was a double-edged sword, having acquired both positive and negative connotations. Its particular valence was wholly contingent on context.[71]

The medical tradition saw little romance in mental illness. Diseases like melancholy and mania caused cognitive and behavioral defects with serious moral implications. Both of these conditions cut a person off from the intellective soul, the immaterial, immortal, and noble organ of abstract thought. The intellective soul used the brain as its instrument. If this instrument was damaged or compromised the process of moral reasoning and the performance of moral action were inhibited if not curtailed.[72] Melancholics and maniacs could really only operate on the same cognitive level as brute beasts since they lacked commerce with the part of the soul that identified them as rational and thus human.

It is not surprising then that melancholics, but especially maniacs, were likened to animals. Borrowing from Galen via Avicenna, physicians identified two forms of mania: a mild jovial kind called doglike mania (*mania canina*) and a violent kind called wolflike mania (*mania lupina*).[73] According to the famous Florentine physician Niccolò Falcucci (d. 1411/12), anger, fury, and rapacity characterized wolflike mania. Giovanni Arcolani (ca. 1390–1458), professor of medicine at Bologna and Padua, maintained that those afflicted with "wolfiness" (*lupinositas*) often lashed out at those around them. They acted as if they "were not men but demons and wolves," and in their "agitation, jumping around, constant inquiries, lupinosity . . . and appearance, they did not seem to have the look of men."[74] In mania, the ability to exercise reason, the defining characteristic of the human as opposed to the animal soul, was conquered by irrational anger. *Mania canina*, or doglike mania, was less serious than the lupine variety. As Guainerio described, instead of snarling these types of maniacs smiled incessantly and pranced around like dogs.[75] Arcolani added that *mania canina* was associated with "friendship accompanied by obedience and acquiescence."[76] The canine maniac rejoiced constantly when it was not appropriate to rejoice and submitted himself to the will of other men.

The interplay between medicine and culture is evident in the adoption of the term *tripudiare* in Latin translations of Avicenna by physicians to describe the behavior of a canine maniac. *Tripudiare* originally denoted a pagan dance in triple time. It came to mean exuberance and in the context of fourteenth- and fifteenth-century Italy, if not before, excessive exuberance. This word appeared not only in medical treatises but in theological literature as well. Roberto da Lecce (1425–1495), a famous Franciscan preacher of the fifteenth century, dedicated a Lenten sermon of 1455 to the subject of tripudiators and when it is permissible to tripudiate. You could tripudiate, Roberto proclaimed, "when your brother took a wife, or if news came that Italy was pacified . . . and that she had armed herself against the infidel." He then admitted that he himself had "tripudiated for the space of one Ave Maria when Saint Bernardino was canonized."[77] Outside of these cases, which illustrate love of family, country, and God, tripudiation was the path to sin. In less pious contexts, it evoked the servile and libidinous gyrations of loose women before men in search of indiscretion.

In the medical sense, tripudiation was a type of conduct, more or less nonthreatening, that broke codes of social propriety. On the one hand, it showed a certain pathological lack of control. On the other hand, it showed a slavish tendency to subservience. Just as dogs do not necessarily distinguish between masters, so the canine maniac, who pranced about in a continuous state of exultation, was considered without the will or the ability to make a rational choice or exercise self-control. In this case, as with all presentations of melancholy and mania, the physical change brought on by these illnesses was a process of moral degradation. Melancholics and maniacs of any variety were suffering simultaneously from physical and moral illnesses. In some cases the spirits in their cognitive faculties were rendered chaotic, in others these sufferers became something less than human in their appearance and conduct. Their commerce with reality was impaired, they could not know themselves, and in their low and bestial state they could not know or understand the good.

In the sixteenth century Tomaso Garzoni, that inveterate cataloguer of the mad and their madnesses, folded lupine mania into his description of melancholic and savage people. In general, he claimed the usual characteristics for melancholy (*maninconia*); it was caused by an abundance of the melancholy humor (*humore melancolico*) and presented with sadness, fear, an inordinate desire for solitude, and excessive weeping. But melancholy humors could also create a type of melancholy that, Garzoni noted, "the Greeks called lycanthropy and the Romans wolf madness (*insania lupina*)." In this state:

> Men leave their house in the month of February, and, like a wolf, go wandering around burial places, howling and pulling the bones of the dead from their graves, dragging them into the streets, striking fear and terror in all those who meet them . . . melancholics of this type have pale faces, dry and sunken eyes, weak vision, and shed nary a tear. Their tongues are dry, they are extremely thirsty, and they produce very little saliva.[78]

For learned physicians as for Garzoni the descent into bestiality was not an ontological but a perceptual problem. Galen's *De locis affectis*, which came into the hands of medieval physicians through a Latin translation of an Arabic abridgement of the work known as *De interioribus*, furnished several examples of the types of delusions melancholy caused. Melancholics, for example, imagined themselves to be kings, wolves, demons, birds, or artificial instruments.[79] Echoing this tradition, the Milanese physician Giovanni da Concoreggio (1380– ca. 1448) noted that certain melancholics think that they are lords, some wolves, and others roosters and so they extend their arms like wings and sing.[80] In cases of doglike, wolflike, or demonic mania, a human being did not change into a dog, a wolf, or a demon but rather, as a result of a severely damaged imagination, assumed the characteristic appearance and behavior of such beasts. As the Florentine physician Lorenzo Bellini (1643–1704) saw it: "lycanthropy, which is recognized as the first species of mania, is nothing other than the false belief of being a man changed into a wolf."[81] Damage to the imagination was serious. The consequent melancholy or mania could significantly alter a person's behavior and appearance. Though the body was sick, it remained human and in need of medical treatment.

Still, the fear of demons and demonic possession were very much part of melancholy's baggage train. Some forms of melancholy looked a lot like possession; it was often difficult to tell the difference. For many physicians, from Falcucci and his ilk in the late fourteenth and early fifteenth centuries to the famous Girolamo Mercuriale (1530–1606) in the late sixteenth, regulation of the six non-naturals played a critical role in battling hostile supernatural entities on the principle that demons had to work through natural means to infiltrate a body. Falcucci averred, for example, that the problem was not so much the demon but the deleterious physical alterations such a creature wrought in the body. Demonic possession was really nothing more than the manipulation of bodily humors to create pathological bodily environments. Falcucci argued that physicians were equally capable of manipulating bodily humors. They could set right the imbalances created in a body by a demon through the six non-naturals.[82] An informed application of learned medicine was capable even of that.

Theologians accepted the idea that the devil might induce madness by making the body sick. In some people he impressed the human imagination with sin-inducing ideas or fantasies.[83] In others he set in motion humoral imbalances that ultimately damaged the brain. But theologians also conceded that because melancholy and mania disrupted the rational faculties more generally, these diseases could lead a person to wrong belief without demonic intervention. In 1599, for example, word got out in Siena that Daria Carli, a well-heeled nun of about thirty at the convent called Santuccio (Santa Maria degli Angeli), was spouting heretical things with no regard for the consequences. Moreover, she had refused the sacrament of confession for nearly a year. The ecclesiastical and secular authorities in Siena called the young woman before them to see what she had to say for herself. To their horror they found that she thought the incarnation was a sham. Daria told her stern yet solicitous audience that she simply could not believe that God would have lowered himself in such a way. The whole idea of hell seemed dubious, too. She called it a "fabricatione"—an invention of men. It seemed to her "against the goodness of God to create souls if they were to be damned and unreasonable that God would want people to pray since he already knew what needs they had."[84] Daria was willing "to debate the matter up to a certain point, but she could not bring herself to believe many articles of faith." The inquisitors were deeply concerned. Daria's unconventional thinking had also stoked the ire and invited the hatred of her fellow nuns. They threatened her so vehemently that she "had amassed a good collection of stones and stored them in her room to defend herself."[85] There was more at stake, of course. Such thinking and behavior threatened the well-being of those who lived around her as well as her own immortal soul.

The officials of the inquisition were not quick to condemn Daria, however. They entertained the idea that the problem might not be so much heresy in the mouth of a sinner as misunderstanding in the mind of a melancholic. In his letter to the inquisition in Rome, Thommaso Malaspina, the governor of Siena, remarked that it had yet to be ascertained whether Daria said "these things because of *furor* and some humors that required treatment by hellebore," a common remedy for melancholy.[86]

When the case moved on to Rome a year later, the office of the inquisition ordered that she receive instruction in orthodoxy with particular focus on the articles of faith that she misunderstood willfully or otherwise.[87] In February 1601, the inquisition in Rome ordered that the convent separate Daria from the rest of the nuns and put her in prison cell that was outside of the cloister but still on convent grounds if such a place existed.[88] Hope remained that proper religious instruction might turn her onto the right path, but she should not disrupt the harmony of the community in the meantime.

There was reason to think that Daria's real problem was the conventual life in the first place. The medieval medical and theological tradition had long acknowledged that certain lifestyles could be pathological. Monks and nuns were especially susceptible to mania and melancholy because they (presumably) did not have ways of naturally purging damaging humors from their bodies through sexual intercourse. The resulting blockages could cause *acedia*, a state of spiritual lassitude and religious indifference in which a monk or nun turned away from or felt alienated from God.[89] In the mid-fifteenth century, theological writers plugged the concept of *acedia* into the humoral framework. Antonino of Florence, for example, spoke about *acedia* in humoral terms, claiming that both melancholics and phlegmatics were inclined to *acedia* because of their pathological humoral complexions.[90]

Physicians also talked about how unhealthy the life of the religious could be. Guainerio marked the Pinzochere, religious communities of women, as particularly susceptible to mania, having himself witnessed the great stress they put on their bodies during long bouts of forced starvation in their desire to serve God.[91] He claimed, too, that some religious who spent long hours in solitude, practicing extreme asceticism, tended to experience profound sadness. Others were plagued by constant fear of God and future judgment.[92] More than a century later, Mercuriale sang the same tune. Melancholy was common among nuns, he insisted, since they spent "the greater part of their lives in quiet and meditation."[93] Sharon Strocchia has shown that nuns in sixteenth-century Florence frequently suffered psychological and physical conditions they identified as melancholy using Greek humoral, religious, and supernatural interpretive frameworks. Nuns worked with priests and physicians to diagnose and treat melancholy. But, like petitioners in Florentine courts, they relied a great deal on their own experience to define, diagnose, and treat the condition.[94]

MELANCHOLY TRIUMPHANT

By the fifteenth and sixteenth centuries, people like Faustina grasped the material humoral underpinnings of diseases that adversely affected the rational faculties and recognized how serious they were. In their worst forms, these diseases reduced the human soul to its basest, bestial form. More insidiously, they could induce states of spiritual indifference, wrong belief, and heretical behavior thus imperiling the immortal soul. But if melancholy and mania were associated with such wretched people, why would petitioners fearing for the honor of their families apply the term in court? The simple answer may be that they were desperate. But cultural attitudes to madness were not uniformly negative; some thinkers gave melancholy in particular a positive spin. In the late twelfth century, for example, learned physicians outlined a conceptual framework for lovesickness, a pathological form of love with organic roots, at the same time that scholars and poets were elaborating the conventions of courtly love in vernacular literature.[95] Before Avicenna's *Canon* was translated into Latin in the late twelfth century, lovesickness was described in a section of Constantine the African's (d. ca. 1087) *Viaticum*, a handbook for travelers who lacked access to medical care while on the road. The *Viaticum* was subsequently adopted in universities as a medical textbook, but its influence was felt beyond the medical classroom. By the thirteenth century, it had generated a lively commentary tradition, revealing the complex interactions between medical, poetical, and theological ruminations on the subject of passionate love. Early on, the *Viaticum*'s commentators likened lovesickness to melancholy. They also maintained that it was typical among the nobility, whose lives of relative wealth, comfort, and leisure did not provide the body adequate opportunity for purging black-bile inducing by-products of digestion.

The etymological associations in this commentary tradition between the terms *eros* (erotic love), *heros* (hero), and *herus* (lord) linked up with another literary tradition taking off at the same time. Sometime before 1210, the Parisian master David of Dinant translated the pseudo-Aristotelian *Problemata 30.1*, which explicitly associated melancholy and greatness. *Problemata 30.1* opened with the question: "Why is it that all those who have become eminent in philosophy or politics or poetry or the arts are clearly of an atrabilious (melancholic) temperament, and some of them to such an extent as to be affected by diseases caused by black bile, as is said to have happened to Heracles among the heroes (*de heroibus*)?"[96] The three crowns of Florence, Dante, Petrarch, and Boccaccio, fed the tradition of ennobling lovesickness in their works, but the Italian incarnation par excellence of heroic love was Ariosto's *Orlando Furioso* (1516; 1521; complete edition 1532), whose obsessive quest to win the love of Angelica drove him mad.

Traces of the tradition of lovesickness are found in the case of one Lorenzo Galigaio from 1572. In this petition, Lorenzo asked that the Duke release him from prison. He had been put there four years earlier for being "pazzo." Lorenzo countered that "he was bothered by melancholy humors of the sort that did not cause him to harm anyone except for a particular woman whom he followed around." So great was Lorenzo's humoral condition that he harbored two false ideas: first, that he had been "made a person of standing," and second, that the woman he was pursuing "would consent to his [sexual] desires." He stood vigil at her house day and night until he was finally captured and put in prison. Lorenzo assured the Duke via the Otto that since his incarceration he had not "returned into the humor since he had successfully purged it together with some of his other sins."[97]

When the Duke's secretary looked into the matter he found inconsistencies in Lorenzo's account. Lorenzo had in fact on numerous occasions "hovered around the wife of Girolamo Giudacci." He would follow her to their house where he then "laid siege" to it, loitering all day long. Girolamo's wife was not the only target of his attentions either. Lorenzo was also in the habit of hanging around the courtyard of the

Duke's Pitti palace. When the Duke appeared, Lorenzo would cling to his carriage and "bug his Serene Highness insisting that all he really wanted was to serve him." The secretary wrote to the Duke, perhaps somewhat wryly, that Lorenzo now said he had returned to sanity and asked that he be released from prison. His Serene Highness, the Duke, did not grant Lorenzo's request.[98] Surely Lorenzo fell far short of the epic hero, but his behavior would have resonated with an audience familiar with pathological love. Had Lorenzo not also marked the Duke as one of his obsessions, his strategy might have worked. In the end, the Duke remained unmoved.

The ennobling qualities of melancholy found especially fertile ground in the work of Marsilio Ficino (1433–1499), renowned Florentine Platonist, erstwhile medical student, and son of an eminent Florentine physician, who popularized the theory of melancholy genius in his De vita of 1489. Divided into three books, "On a healthy life," "On a long life," and "On obtaining life from the heavens," this treatise was essentially a manual of health for scholars whose lifestyles made them particularly susceptible to diseases involving black bile or phlegm. In the fifth chapter of the first book, Ficino draws explicitly on the pseudo-Aristotelian Problemata 30.1 to associate melancholy with greatness rather than spiritual despair or pathology. He went a step further by connecting black bile to Platonic notions of divine frenzy, the sine qua non of genius. The melancholic complexion was known to produce a range of pathological personalities from the despondent to the volatile, but in the right quantity and quality it produced extraordinary people, not least of all those Sybils and soothsayers who had commerce with the divine. Not all forms of melancholy created heroes or inspired genius, he cautioned. Melancholy produced by the combustion of black bile, yellow bile, or blood compromised judgment while the residue such burning left behind made people dull and stupid.[99]

Ficino's marriage of the pseudo-Aristotelian Problemata 30.1 and Platonic notions of divine frenzy became a popular theme in elite male intellectual circles.[100] The Neoplatonist Angelo Poliziano (1454–1494) and the Venetian humanist Ermolao Barbaro the Younger (1453–1493) claimed that melancholy was the sure path to the sublime, compelling even ordinary people to create great works of art and literature.[101] One Cipriano Giambelli, a sixteenth-century Veronan canon, put a positive interpretation of melancholy in the mouth of one of the protagonists in his dialogue Il diamerone ove si ragiona della natura.

The character Il Padre Teologo claimed that melancholy's tendency to drive the sufferer to seek out solitude could, in fact, ease and stabilize the mind: "Very useful are both solitude and melancholy, in such wise that the solitary life holds the mind recollected so that it does not wander hither and thither in quest of sensible things, and melancholy, which is born from an abundance of coldness and dryness, has the effect of fixing and stabilizing our thoughts, and renders us, as it were, stable and firm in sweet and delightful contemplation."[102] Torquato Tasso (1544–1599) also maintained that poets of great genius, who were often worked into fits of poetic frenzy as they composed their verses, tended to be melancholic. This type of melancholic madness was not so much pathological as it was inspirational. Despite being a physical illness or potentially unfavorable complexion that caused people to make bad judgments, on the eve of the sixteenth century, melancholy began to absorb the odor of nobility, becoming the premier disease of scholars, artists, and prophets. In sixteenth-century England and Spain, melancholy was the favored disease of aristocrats, who wore its symptoms like badges of honor and status.[103] Far from being a scarlet letter, melancholy could suggest positive traits like rare and extraordinary talent.

It is this version of melancholy that might have softened the social impact of a claim that someone was mad in a court of law. If, to mitigate some of the shame associated with Domenico or Girolamo Capponi's spending habits or Ridolfo and Pierantonio Guasconi's unruly behavior, their relatives had to label them mad, so much the better if that madness was of an exalted or aristocratic type. Protean melancholy could suggest many things, not least of all demonic possession. In elite and, as Sharon Strocchia has argued, particularly elite male circles, however, it donned noble raiment.[104]

Historians of northern Europe have observed that melancholy in England and the German lands tended to have diabolical or spiritual connotations. Erik Midelfort, for example, drew a parallel between the increasing incidence of melancholy and rising instances of demonic possession in Germany in the wake of the Protestant Reformation.[105] In this narrative, fear of the devil trumped medical ways of understanding madness. Melancholy was not a disease of the body but one of the soul. It was not until the eve of the seventeenth century that melancholy lost its demonic or religious luster and became widely considered an organic disease. A similar story holds for scholars of

English history, who have viewed Renaissance attitudes to melancholy as a reaction to sectarian controversies in England.[106] According to these historians, the reception of Greek medicine as an authoritative explanatory framework came late to German and English society.

But Greek medical ideas were never a dead letter between the thirteenth and sixteenth centuries in Italy. When melancholy entered the courts of sixteenth-century Florence it did so as a medical disease rather than as an example of demonic possession or religious anxiety. Moreover, it was only one among other humoral conditions that were recognized as potential causes of mental illness. This does not mean that petitioners discounted the possible spiritual consequences of disease. Melancholy was, after all, an iridescent thing; its meaning often changed depending on the light in which it was viewed. In domestic spaces, it was seen simultaneously as a physical and spiritual illness that demanded the ministrations of doctors of the body as well as of the soul. In social spaces, heroic, genial, or aristocratic melancholy might have been the more desired aspect of the disease, but fear of demons was surely never far from medieval and early modern minds. In courts of law, the medical or somatic aspect of madness was the most useful. It could explain and excuse bad or ill-conceived behavior. It could better anchor that behavior to a specific timeline, giving the impression that madness could be predictable or at least less unpredictable. Mainstream humoral medicine was the operative language that got results. Savvy petitioners like Faustina successfully exploited it to the fullest in court and they did so with no apparent prompting from medical personnel.

CHAPTER 5

The Curious Case
of Forensic Medicine

The Dog That Didn't Bark in the Night

Ah, how much care men ought to exercise
With those whose penetrating intellect
Can see our thoughts—not just our outer act!

— DANTE, *Inferno*

"There is scarcely another disease more easily and more frequently feigned than insanity and no disease more difficult to discern."[1] So remarked Paolo Zacchia (1584–1659), personal physician to two popes and legal advisor to the Rota Romana, the highest appellate tribunal of the Catholic Church.[2] Between 1621 and 1659, he issued the *Quaestiones Medico-Legales*, a monumental compilation of medicolegal topics and case studies that would continue to appear in multiple editions throughout Europe until 1789.

Medicine rather than law, he argued in this treatise, was the discipline best equipped to answer a wide range of legal questions that involved the body in court. The body was, in a manner of speaking, its own witness; it spoke in the language of physical signs.[3] Who better to interpret the body's "testimony" than the physician who knew it intimately? In cases of madness, who better than the physician understood the somatic origins of abnormal behavior, or was best equipped to determine when, how, and in what situations the infinite varieties of mental illness were likely to manifest themselves and what that meant for the law? Above all, who better than the physician could make a body testify against itself to expose those fakers and frauds who feigned madness in the hope of overturning a contract or denying criminal liability? Surely physicians were the best judges of the body as witness. But jurists, judges, and civic officials could learn this language, too, so long as they took the time to acquire some measure of medical expertise. The *Quaestiones Medico-Legales* was a good place to start.

A now defunct grand narrative once celebrated Zacchia as the codifier of what modern readers would call legal or forensic medicine, that is, the application of medical knowledge to legal problems by medical experts in courts of law.[4] More recently, historians have better situated Zacchia's work in a much longer conversation taking place in medieval and early modern Europe that examined the relationship between the two disciplines.[5] Beginning with the revival of Roman law in twelfth-century Italy, jurists and, by the fourteenth century, civic legislators debated the role medical practitioners might play in criminal litigation. Fifteenth-century Italian humanists disputed the relative merits of medicine and law as truth-seeking disciplines.[6] Which of the two, they wondered, was of the greatest social and political use and who, the doctor or the lawyer, should enjoy higher social status? Interactions between medicine and law intensified in the sixteenth and seventeenth centuries throughout Italy, Germany, and France.[7] Doctors were accorded a more visible and regular role as expert witnesses in continental courts, and physicians and surgeons began to write manuals, instructing their peers on how to give medical testimony.[8]

But social historians have advised against reading too much into claims to special authority that physicians began to make on the eve of the seventeenth century.[9] A very different picture emerged when they entered the courts of seventeenth- and eighteenth-century Europe through case records to observe medical practitioners in the act of giving medical testimony in both continental legal and English common law arenas. They found that the meaning and authority of medical expertise in Europe have varied a great deal from time to time and place to place. Behind statutes that *seem* to have privileged the professional expertise of physicians, surgeons, and midwives lurks a great deal of ambiguity about the exact nature of that expertise and how it was to function in court. In many respects, the origins of forensic medicine belong not to the seventeenth but to the nineteenth century.

I want to add further shading to this discussion by placing Zacchia in a much longer history of the medicalization of European society understood specifically as a sociocultural process. The court records that form the basis of this study are, at best, artifacts of judicial processes and, at worst, dim fragments of much larger dramas playing out in families, communities, and courts. Civil and criminal cases tend to speak most effectively as a chorus. And so, throughout this book, I have sought patterns among the nearly three hundred cases involving madness that appeared in Florentine courts between the fourteenth and seventeenth centuries. But we are fortunate to have some cases for which enough detail remains to permit a solo performance. Our study ends on one such case.

In addition to several extant summary reports, nearly one hundred and forty folio pages of witness testimony survive, giving us a rare glimpse of the architecture underlying incapacity suits. We capture litigants in the act of building a case both for and against madness from the ground up. The strategies they employed to prove their allegations implicitly reveal, too, the criteria judges and magistrates performing judicial functions used to determine the soundness of that argumentative architecture. From this privileged vantage point, we can also ask to what degree if any the medicalization of European society influenced their decision-making process.

The case ultimately tells us three things. First, despite the great institutional and administrative changes than accompanied Florence's transition from republic to duchy, the key features of Romano-canonical process persisted. Roman law continued to shape how litigants and judges determined when people were to be held responsible for crimes or contractual obligations, under what circumstances they were released from liability, what constituted proof of incapacity, and how they distinguished genuine from fraudulent claims of incompetence. Second, expert witnesses played only a limited role in these proceedings; they had no binding authority on the judge. The final outcome of a case rested with the autonomous discretion of a court official whether he was a citizen-judge, a bureaucrat with legal training, or, in the sixteenth century, the Duke or his secretary. Finally, much more than the bare facts of a case influenced final decisions. The courts took into account how a sentence would affect the social and material circumstances of a family and, in some cases, the republican or ducal treasury. Judges proved themselves willing to compromise so long as the law was not abused and public peace was maintained. What triumphed in the end was not special medical expertise but the enduring values expressed by patrimonial rationality.

From the perspective of Tuscany, the history of legal medicine in seventeenth-century Italy is not unlike the curious case of the dog that didn't bark in the night. Academic discussions about the role medicine might play in legal matters did not impose medical ideas and medical experts on Tuscan courts. The evidence from Florentine court records tells us that lay petitioners and court officials were at home with medical explanations for mental incapacity two generations before Zacchia was born. The evidence from culture tells us that this was likely an even earlier development. When ordinary laymen and women from all walks of life made medical arguments, even in the most hotly contested of cases, courts accepted or rejected them without certification by a medical practitioner or explicit recourse to expert medical testimony. Zacchia and his ilk were trying to carve out a well-defined professional space for physicians in a culture not only familiar with but fluent in the fundamentals of humoral medicine and in which efficacy not status or occupation still determined a medical practitioner's success.[10]

MAD NORTH-NORTH-WEST: THE CASE OF MARIA

Shakespeare's Hamlet admitted to feigning madness when he told his erstwhile university chums Rosencrantz and Guildenstern that he was "but mad north-north-west: when the wind is southerly I know a hawk from a handsaw." After reading the case of Maria de' Placidi, one gets the sense that Maria could have said the same thing of herself. Her madness seems suspect, her motives opportunistic.

The case begins conventionally enough. In 1567, Maria's sister brings her before the Pupilli claiming that she is "vexed by melancholy humors" and unable to manage her affairs or care for her person. For proof, Thommasa tells the court that Maria had made a gift of her entire estate to one Piero Mellini, a man with no discernible social or political ties to their distinguished family.[11] In other words, the gift flouted rules governing patrimonial rationality.

Thommasa's allegations fell on deaf ears. When the Pupilli interviewed Maria they found her speech and conduct reasonable. Maria admitted to promising her property to Piero but on the condition that she enjoy its fruits until her death—a standard arrangement. The property in question was in Rome where she had lived for many years, twice a wife and twice a widow. She added that she had no use for her sister's meddling; as a widow, she could dispose of it as she saw fit. When the Pupilli bumped the case up to the Duke, his office replied that "nothing further was required."[12] Maria's gift to Piero warranted no legal intervention.

Now here's the rub. When the case reappeared before the Pupilli six months later, Maria sang a very different tune. This time she petitioned the court herself, insisting that as a widow of "a certain age who was often vexed by melancholy humors," she was "incapable of caring for herself or maintaining and managing her estate." She asked that the Duke grant the court the authority to assume her guardianship to stave off financial ruin.[13] After a second interview, the Pupilli also changed its tune. Where before Maria seemed competent, now she seemed "rather unstable, ill-humored, and poorly suited to self governance." In this new estimation, she needed a guardian. The Duke agreed, ordering that Maria's care revert to her closest relative. Thommasa fit that bill. The record does not explicitly state that she took legal control of Maria's estate, but it is reasonable to assume that she did so with the requisite male supervision.[14]

The case took yet another turn a year later. Maria petitioned the Pupilli again this time to invalidate the gift to Piero. She had managed to convince the court of her mental incapacity the year before to get a guardian. Why not claim, too, that she had been of unsound mind in the very moment she made that contract, thereby abrogating it altogether? She asked the Pupilli "to annul the gift since it was made to the detriment of herself, her sister, and her unmarried niece, the daughter of her [presumably deceased] brother."[15] She repeated her claims of the previous year but added that "she had been induced to make the gift only after Piero had made her great promises."[16] What those "great promises" were, the record does not say.

Enter Piero, who, not surprisingly, launched a countersuit. Maria, he argued, entered into the contract with her eyes open and with both her personal interests and social obligations in mind. The reservation of usufructory rights was strong evidence of her capacity for rational thought. Plus, it bore the imprimatur of a court; Maria herself "wished that [it] be executed correctly with the approval of a judge of the Campidoglio and with all the requisite solemnities." There was also nothing rash or impulsive about it. Maria's long years in Rome had seen her immersed in a morass of litigation. Piero claimed that he had helped her navigate these turbulent waters. Finally, he said that Maria made the gift on the condition that he marry her niece. The gift of her estate then served doubly as a dowry for that niece and payment for Piero's legal services.[17] Surely no person of questionable mental capacity would have had the presence of mind to craft such a prudent contract and execute it to the letter of the law. By the same token, surely no notary worth his salt would attach his name to a contract in which the mental capacity of one of the parties was in doubt.

It was only when Maria and Piero arrived in Florence so that he could meet and marry her niece that everything changed. Piero had no doubt that some collusion between the sisters had taken place. He reminded the Pupilli of how "at another time, when Maria was not on good terms with her sister . . . she claimed the opposite, namely, that she was sane and prudent." Whatever passed between the sisters, the plan they devised to invalidate Piero's claims to Maria's property worked. The Duke's office was prepared to side with Maria and Thommasa against Piero, the unrelated interloper. The Pupilli was instructed to "examine the gift because, [with Maria] being *mentecatta*, it is not reasonable that it took place."[18]

From March to August 1569, the consul of Florence at Rome and a representative from the Pupilli deposed witnesses based on questions (*articuli*) prepared and submitted by the two opposing parties.[19] Maria's side sought to prove her incapacity to invalidate the gift, Piero's side, her capacity to make it stand. So began the manufacture of Maria's madness, on the one hand, and the manufacture of her sanity, on the other. Roman law and the long tradition of commentary it generated in medieval and early modern Italy had a shaping influence on the way the two sides framed their articles and chose their witnesses. And so, the extant witness depositions reveal a larger and longer debate in the Roman law tradition on how to prove madness on the one hand and sanity on the other. But though Roman law inclined, it did not govern; it offered guidelines rather than concrete structures and clear answers. Proving mental incapacity was a problem for Roman jurists, it bedeviled the medieval heirs of that tradition, and, despite the efforts of someone like Zacchia who believed medicine could bring more certainty to the endeavor, it dogged his contemporaries as well. Where formal legal structures dropped the tune, social and cultural norms and practices picked it up.

Maria's side had the greater amount of ground to cover before her incapacity was established to the court's satisfaction. In order to protect the sanctity of contracts, the viability of criminal law, and fend off false or frivolous claims of incapacity, Roman jurists and their later Italian counterparts built safeguards into the process of examining such allegations. Soundness of mind was to be presumed unless proven otherwise and the burden of proof rested with the party claiming incapacity.[20] Moreover, it was not sufficient to claim that a person had been mad for all of his or her life. It was easy enough to muster witnesses who would say as much. Since Roman and Italian jurists recognized the possibility of lucid intervals, mental impairment had to be linked to the specific time in which a contract was made or a crime was committed. But how did one prove madness at a specific time and how did the judge evaluate that claim? The Roman law tradition offered two standards for proving capacity or incapacity: witnesses who could attest to a person's behavior over the long term and at specific moments, and the quality of the legal act—was the legal instrument made for good reasons, in the appropriate manner, and approved by a recognized legal authority. Maria and Piero made full use of both strategies.

THE TROUBLE WITH WITNESSES

Roman law passed on to Italian jurists the idea that mental incapacity was legible to most ordinary people through external behavior, especially speech. That meant that witnesses played an important role in helping a judge determine a person's state of mind. Some of Italy's most famous jurists, including Bartolus da Sassoferrato (1313–1357) and Angelo Aretino (d. 1472), argued that incapacity could be sufficiently proved if a witness had seen someone rave and generally carry on like a mad person.[21] On this principle, Maria produced witnesses willing to say that she was crazy while Piero produced just as many to say the opposite—hardly stable ground on which to make a decision. In contested cases like Maria's where each side contradicted the other, witness testimony might seem of little use.

But Italian jurists had long pondered the trouble with witnesses testimony.[22] They had no illusions about its reliability. Few witnesses were good witnesses. Even if they were bent on telling the truth, which was not at all guaranteed, witnesses rarely did a very good job of it. They were often mistaken in their relation of the so-called facts; they tended to make judgments rather than simply to convey what they saw or heard; and their judgments were often tautological—the hypothetical person Titius was crazy because he did the types of things a crazy person would do. Or they were based on assumptions—a witness who saw a man in chains might assume he was mad because mad men often ended up in chains.[23] Witnesses were also known to make false judgments based on insufficient knowledge of context. Perfectly sane people sometimes found themselves insulting those around them or lashing out. Such behavior was not mad in itself. In some cases, it might have been a rational response to provocation.[24] Moreover, witnesses were rarely impartial; they tended to give testimony that served their own interests. Finally, witnesses were sometimes suborned; if testimony appeared to be too good to be true, it probably was.

Some forty or fifty years before Maria's case, the celebrated Milanese jurist Filippo Decio (1454–1535) exploited the weaknesses of witness testimony in an undated *consilium* he wrote on behalf of one Giovanni de Zuchano.[25] Like Maria, Giovanni had made a gift of his entire estate while retaining usufructory rights for himself until his death. Also like Maria, the choice of recipient raised the hackles of an unnamed relative who felt unjustly excluded from a share of Giovanni's patrimony. The unnamed relative resorted to the common legal fiction that the testator, Giovanni, must have been mad to have denied a legitimate heir the fruits of inheritance.[26]

The plaintiff set out to prove that Giovanni's mental incapacity was a substantial limiting factor on his legal status. From boyhood until his death, he argued, Giovanni habitually ran amok through streets and alleyways speaking in the manner of fools and mad men.[27] He could not respond to questions put to him and continually exhibited the demeanor, conduct, and speech of a *mentecaptus*.[28] People who knew Giovanni, be they family, friends, or acquaintances, commonly held him to be *mentecaptus*, *stultus*, and *fatuus*.[29] Three witnesses explicitly confirmed these allegations.

But Decio made quick work of dismantling their testimony on two grounds. First, the plaintiff's articles were too general and seemed written to lead witnesses to provide specific answers. They were prepared, Decio claimed, with a "particularly extensive, excellent, and rare diligence by most expert men, who wished to instruct the witnesses in the hopes of proving [Giovanni's] *dementia*."[30] Such singular diligence aroused suspicion. Even more damning was the fact that the testimonies of the witnesses were uncannily similar, suggesting premeditation and coaching. Citing Bartolus on this point, Decio argued that they must have been suborned.[31] Second, the witnesses did not inspire confidence. They claimed to have directly observed Giovanni's aberrant behavior for the entire period of *his* life. But they were under twenty-five at the time of testifying whereas Giovanni himself would have been nearing the age of seventy. How could they possibly offer insight into the state of Giovanni's mind or the nature of his actions over the course of his life when for most of that time they were children? To accept their testimony was unwise if not absurd.[32]

Weak testimony did not mean that Giovanni was a model of rational thinking. Witnesses for the defense admitted that he was coarse and slow-witted (*grossolanus*). But he was not, in their estimation, a *stultus* or *mentecaptus*. Decio agreed. Stupidity or loutishness, though not prized qualities in a man or woman of property, was not tantamount to insanity and thus not a bar to contracting. At issue was the presence or absence of judgment, not whether it was good or bad. As Aretino observed, a mad man could not make a will because, having no judgment, he could not understand the consequences of his actions. A *grossolanus*, by contrast, who did have judgment, ill-advised though it might be, was fully capable of expressing his material wishes in a will.[33] It is worth remembering here what examples from applied law have taught us; the difference between lack of judgment and bad judgment hinged on social or cultural values coupled with what the litigant wanted to accomplish in court. In Maria's case, her side argued that her affront to patrimonial rationality demonstrated a complete lack of judgment and full-blown melancholy. In the cases of young men carrying illegal weapons from Chapter 2, petitioners also spoke of a lack of judgment but one that was understandable in the young. The young were, by definition, foolish in so far as their rational faculties had not yet fully developed. There was good reason to hope they would grow out of it.

LUCID INTERVALS AND THE QUALITY OF THE CIVIL OR CRIMINAL ACT

What litigants needed most in cases of mental incapacity were witnesses who could help them link madness or sanity to the specific time a contract was made or a crime was committed—the biggest challenge in a legal tradition that recognized the possibility of lucid intervals. This was no easy task. Bartolus asked his readers to imagine a situation in which witnesses said that a person was mentally impaired (*fatuus*) because they heard him speak like a mentally impaired person. But what if that allegedly impaired person sometimes peppered normal speech with vain and senseless chatter?[34] Was he only partially mad but mostly sane or mostly mad but partially sane? If the course of a person's life stretched out along a timeline, how did one distinguish between lucid and mad phases?

Jurists knew only too well the difficulties in establishing specific markers along that timeline; in some cases they exploited them to serve their clients. Take, for example, a *consilium* written by the Sienese jurist Mariano Sozzini (1401–1467) that questioned whether the alleged incompetence of a man named Giovanni Vernelli impinged on the validity of a contract he made. According to his lawyer, it was null because Giovanni was *mentecaptus* at the time of making it. Witnesses confirmed these allegations. Giovanni, they said, was clearly not of sound mind and *mentecaptus* before, during, and after the contract was made. Three witnesses even claimed that Giovanni himself wanted to be called *mentecaptus*.[35]

But, like Decio, Sozzini was not easily moved to invalidate a legal instrument. That Giovanni was mad for a long period of time was not, in his mind, sufficient proof that he was mad at the time in question. Plus, witnesses for the opposing side argued that he seemed sane to them. As proof, they pointed to the fact that he had practiced his trade without event. He also had a wife of good stock. Neither the successful performance of one's occupation nor a favorable marriage typically belonged to anyone but a person of sound mind.[36] The whole business about Giovanni wishing to be called *mentecaptus* also struck Sozzini as highly suspicious. It demonstrated cunning rather than incompetence since, in Sozzini's phrasing, the foolish (*fatui*) generally labor under the misapprehension that they are wise.[37] In other words, Giovanni undermined his case by using a rational argument to claim that he was, in fact, not rational.

Cases like these appeared in Florentine courts and aroused similar suspicions. Domenico di Girolamo from the tiny Tuscan town of Starda, for example, was already in the care of the Pupilli as a poor madman (*povero mentecatto*) when he petitioned the court for the second time in March 1584. In 1579 he had sold some property, but the buyer had cheated him out of half the money he believed he was owed. Or so he said. In his first petition he asked that the Pupilli countermand the sale and award him the "just price." His petition fell on deaf ears; the Duke and his officers refused to invalidate the sale. In the second petition, Domenico asked that the court help him recoup his loss from the sale together with returns on its yield. The Duke found this request highly suspicious, responding, "this is not the supplication of a madman."[38] We might wonder how Maria convinced the Pupilli of her own madness when she, too, used a rational argument to prove her irrationality. Again, legal remedies followed both social and legal logic. If Maria's gift did not adversely affect a network of kin, the court may have responded differently to the case. Here the logic of patrimonial rationality was stronger than suspicions about her motives.

The fact remained that it was relatively easy to dismiss claims to madness amid conflicting accounts; the possibility of lucid intervals made both sides in a suit right at different times. If witnesses for one side saw a person act like a madman it did not necessarily follow that they *always* saw him act that way.[39] And it hardly mattered if a person was said to be mad *near* the time the contract was made. A bout of madness that occurred close to the act of contracting did not speak to the contractor's state of mind during the act of contracting.

Since witness testimony was not good at reliably interpreting a person's state of mind at a specific time, jurists needed another standard of proof for determining a contract's validity. That standard, according to Bartolus, was the quality of the act itself.[40] The very act of contracting produced a concrete document subject to systematic analysis. If the person in question made the contract for good reasons, in the proper way, and with the approval of a notary, the law presumed soundness of mind.[41]

This reasoning applied to criminal acts as well. In cases where people were accused of killing someone, the Roman jurist Prospero Farinacci (1554–1618) advised examining the reason for the act and the perpetrator's behavior immediately afterward to divine whether it bespoke madness or sanity. In his opinion:

> if someone publicly and in the open killed someone else with whom there existed no enmity or reason for killing, and, furthermore, if he killed this person suddenly and without any prior dispute, and after he killed the person he did not hide himself or flee, but acted in a way that announced his *furor* or *insania*, then I should think that . . . he committed the crime in a time of *furor*. If on the other hand, he wounded and killed the person circumspectly for some particular reason be it bad blood, or a previous dispute, and after the incident he fled or went into hiding knowing full well that he had committed a crime, or he sought to conceal his crime, then he demonstrates that he was of sound mind at the time of committing the crime.[42]

Presumably a person in the grips of madness would do what no sane person would—namely, kill without reason or provocation and remain on the scene once a crime had been committed.

Bernardo Carnesecchi's case from Chapter 3 offers a good example of how the quality of the legal act principle worked in court. There the Pupilli closely examined how he contracted and on what terms to determine whether or not he was sane when he did so. The court considered the first marriage contract he made with one of his sister's prospective husbands reasonable on the grounds that it was executed properly and on conventional terms. By contrast, Bernardo made the second contract in secret, without the consent of his relatives, and according to terms that were injurious to his sister. In order to settle the matter, the Pupilli elected a jurist to write a formal opinion. That jurist agreed that where the first contract demonstrated sanity, the method and content of the second were an affront to reason and so signaled madness. In the end, madness was in the eye of the judge or jurist. That decision, however, was not an arbitrary one. It rested on witness testimony, close study of a person's behavior, sometimes an examination of his or her contracts, and often the court's own interview.

In his dispute with Maria, Piero used the quality of the civil act to help manufacture her sanity. His side submitted articles arguing that Piero had become an important source of material and legal support to Maria as she advanced in age and declined in health. Thirteen of Piero's witnesses confirmed that Piero had been living with Maria for a number of years. A few of them were unsure about the nature of the services he performed for her, though most suspected it was in some supportive capacity. The more informed described a situation in which Piero doubled as an accountant and legal advocate. Maria's neighbor, Antonio de' Cavi, had seen Piero at Maria's house doing her errands, though he could not be sure who was paying for them. He was a little clearer on Piero's legal role in Maria's life. "Several times before Maria made the gift to Piero," he said, "perhaps some time in the year 1567, he spoke with Piero who told him that Maria's income (*entrate*) was in shambles, seized and tied up." For this reason, Antonio recounted, "Piero had to represent her interests in court and spend his own money on her behalf for food and other necessities." It was for this reason that Maria decided to give Piero her estate, an arrangement that other people who received similar services from him seemed inclined to do. If that were not enough to paint Piero in noble hues, Antonio mentioned that he often saw the frail Maria "holding onto Piero's arm" as she left or returned home.[43] Piero was not kin, but, in light of his services, the gift was not unreasonable.

Piero's articles also argued that Maria showed good judgment during the making of the gift and that it was formally sanctioned by the appropriate authorities. He produced seven witnesses who were present at the making of the contract and were generally impressed by her conduct. She seemed to be "rather well in her mind" and "a wise woman." She knew what the contract stipulated and "signed it in her own hand according to the Roman custom."[44] The other witnesses followed suit save one who could not read or write. Witnesses also claimed that Maria did not sit idly by during the proceedings. According to one witness, "while the notary was drafting the gift contract, Maria reminded him of many things and argued with the judge."[45] Another witness said Maria "quarreled with the judge and the notary [because] she wanted to understand [the process] step-by-step, making them repeat [what they said] when she didn't understand [something]."[46] Yet another witness said that "while the contract was being drawn up, Maria asked that it be read several times by the notary, telling him: "'Io voglio intendere bene ogni cosa (I want to understand each thing well).'"[47] Once it was signed, the judge and notary validated it. As far as the law was concerned, everything was in order; the gift should stand.

Or at least Piero's side made a robust argument that it should stand. Although proof on the basis of the quality of the civil act did a relatively good job of demonstrating a person's ability to act rationally while contracting, it was not foolproof or, for that matter, family-proof. Maria's side undermined it on two counts: the reason for the gift showed lack of judgment and the officials who validated it may have overestimated her abilities. Maria's first allegiance should have been to her family and Piero was not natural kin. Against Piero's claims, Maria and Thommasa argued that a gift of her entire estate to some "extraneo" (neither an agnate nor cognate relative) that deprived her, her sister, and her unmarried niece of their just portion was a compelling reason to question its validity. Showing gratitude was well and good, but not if it contravened patrimonial rationality. This principle explains why the Pupilli awarded the estate and care of Francesco Martelli from Chapter 1 to his mercenary cousins despite his mother's court-sanctioned request that they go to a less proximate but more trustworthy relative.

One of Maria's witnesses was also a Roman notary, who "had heard from different people that she was vexed by certain humors." These humors, he believed, made her crazy (pazz[a]). It was "as if [she were] possessed (*spiritata*); and she remained for some time under such an influence."[48] Maria's side used the notary's testimony to suggest that Piero's notary validated the gift contract under false pretenses or without sufficient information, a strategy other litigants had used in Florentine courts. In 1546, for example, the nephew of Jacopo Barga claimed that his uncle was insane after he made a particularly unfavorable contract with Marchuccio Pagnini. Jacopo's nephew insisted that Marchuccio knew of Jacopo's *dementia*. Most of the notaries in town knew about it too and refused to sanction his contracts. But Marchuccio managed to find a green, young notary whom the record called "not very experienced" to officiate.[49] The outcome of the case was not recorded, but the deck was stacked against Marchuccio. Maria's side likely hoped that her notary cast similar doubts on the validity of the gift she made in Rome. They argued implicitly that any notary who knew her personally or remotely through rumor would have known she was not competent to make a contract. But notaries abounded in Rome. It would not have been hard to find one who was ignorant, inexperienced, corruptible, or perhaps all of the above.

FIXING THE TIMELINE WITH MEDICINE

Unlike jurists, physicians trained in the humoral tradition of medicine were at home parsing the infinite species of mental illness. They excelled, too, at making plausible predictions about when they were likely occur. Moreover, by the mid-fourteenth century, medicine had arrived on the academic scene as a theoretical discipline on par with law and theology.[50] But in spite of its careful study of madness and its entry into the scholastic mainstream, jurists rarely employed medical knowledge or categories in their own treatises. Whereas ordinary laymen and women—perhaps in consultation with medical practitioners—used humoral language to build their cases as early as the 1540s in Florentine courts, medical knowledge and arguments were slow to breach the precincts of academic law. Until the seventeenth century, they remained autonomous disciplines.

This is not to say that jurists ignored medicine as an important epistemological framework. Baldo degli Ubaldi (1327–1400), in fact, said that the two were both valid methods for seeking truth:

> You should know that the judge is like a physician who detects disease in three ways. He observes disease, first, notionally and imperfectly through the examination of urine. In this instance he sees

sickness in the same way that a man sees something in a mirror, as if through a kind of shadow. The judge does a similar thing when he sees by examining and comparing plausible things with things that are close to the truth in order to know the truth. Secondly, the physician sees by touching the pulse. The judge does likewise when he, so to speak, touches on the truth through open testimonies. Thirdly, the physician sees by making predictions based on things that are removed from sight. In like manner the judge supposes things concerned with a case, which do not pertain to the verdict at hand.[51]

Physicians and judges both had their diagnostic tools, direct and indirect, for sniffing out disease on the one hand and truth on the other. The physician catches the first glimpse of disease obliquely through the examination of urine, the judge, the truth through analogous cases or situations. Similarly the pulse is to the physician what witness testimony is to a judge, a more direct way of laying bare the nature of a disease or the details of a legal case.[52] However methodologically similar medicine and law were, their objects of knowledge were distinct. Medicine could not solve legal problems and the law had no business treating the body.

In some respects, the law had little need of specific medical knowledge. The Roman legal tradition predisposed medieval jurists to recognize the somatic origins of mental impairment. Late Roman law spoke of it as a physical disease (*morbus*) or a defect (*vitio*) and one that could be of either long or short duration.[53] A person who was sane most of the time might occasionally fall prey to an illness of the body that affected the mind and its ability to function properly, as in the case of fever. By the same token, mental defects due to chronic sickness were not always legally incapacitating. Medieval jurists adopted this view and its accompanying language, making medical categories seem extraneous. They knew that madness might be the result of a disease and that it might affect a person's ability to contract or be held liable for a crime. But they seemed to see no need for a doctor to confirm or disconfirm madness; abnormal behavior remained a sufficient indicator of it.

In the fifteenth century, the language of humoral medicine began to penetrate legal discourse. When Bartolus tackled the problem of lucid intervals in the fourteenth century, he argued that prior episodes of mental disturbance could be significant limiting factors on a person's capacity to contract. Madness authoritatively established in the past was presumed to persist into the future until it was proved otherwise.[54] In this discussion, Bartolus referred to the mentally impaired person as a *furiosus*. By contrast, a century later, Aretino inserted medical-sounding language into the debate. As he put it, "someone is presumed *furiosus* since sufferings of humor (*passiones humori*) are thought to last unless it is proved otherwise."[55] In a *consilium* written to prove the mental incapacity of one of the parties in a property dispute, the Imolese jurist Alessandro Tartagni (1424–1477) similarly likened the *furor* of his client to suffering (*passio*) or sickness (*morbus*).[56] The traditions of medicine and law independently concluded that madness could be the result of disease. But it was medicine rather than law that referred to it as suffering (*passio*) or sufferings of humor (*passiones humori*).

Some sixteenth-century Italian jurists employed medical categories in their learned treatises, but references continued to be few and far between. In his discussion of criminal responsibility and mental incapacity, Giulio Claro (1525–1575) referred to a case of 1454 in which a certain Iacobina Ferraria beat a three-year-old girl to death with a stick. It was discovered that she was suffering from the effects of black bile and that she had previously spent time in the hospital of San Vincenzo as a *mentecapta*. She was subsequently absolved of liability and sent back to San Vincenzo presumably so that she could not harm anyone else.[57] Similarly, in a treatise on criminal law published in 1606, the jurist Farinacci included *phrenetici*, another category drawn from learned medicine, among those who could not be held responsible for crimes. Like Claro, and possibly borrowing from him, Farinacci cited the case of the melancholic Jacobina. Claro and Farinacci name the illnesses they believed were the cause of a person's mental incapacity, though there is little detail beyond that.

It was Paolo Zacchia who integrated medicine and law in the most substantive and comprehensive of ways by explicitly applying the form and content of medical knowledge to cases in secular and ecclesiastical courts.[58] Zacchia addressed madness most comprehensively in book 2, a third of which was devoted to mental defects. Here he rolled out an impressive catalogue of conditions impinging on the faculties of reason, including an exhaustive list of the various forms of mental incapacity, a comparison of their similarities and differences, attendant physical signs and behavioral manifestations, and their duration.

Most important for the problem of proof in cases of madness and of particular use for judges trying to adjudicate them was Zacchia's discussion of how to tell if a person was feigning his or her condition.

"There is scarcely another disease," he claimed, "more easily and more frequently feigned than *insania*; and no disease more difficult to discern."[59] As he saw it, a person who knew well what physical and behavioral signs accompanied each disease would be less prone to mistake madness for dissimulation.

The biggest problem was that varieties of madness were legion. Zacchia enumerated no less than fifty distinct species and subspecies of damage or disease that adversely affected the rational faculties. As physicians had done before him, he collapsed all of these categories into two principal forms of illness, namely melancholy and *furor* on the one hand, and a category representative of simplemindedness (*fatuitas*), often accompanied by physical disabilities like deafness or muteness, on the other. Most melancholics—though, of course, not all—tended to suffer largely in silence; they were fearful, sad, and dejected. In contrast, sufferers of *furor* labored in perpetual motion without end; they were reckless and full of wrath.[60] Physicians read these diseases from signs inscribed in the flesh and manifest in behavior. The judge ought "first to consider the face," Zacchia instructed. "In people who were truly melancholic or suffering *furor* the face tends to the color of the earth or is slate-colored. In *furentes* the face is uncommonly ruddy, but it can also have a certain grayness if it is mixed with melancholy." The eyes, he added, were indeed windows onto the soul. "In melancholics," he maintained:

> the eyes are dark . . . and an abundance of the melancholy humor is visible; the eyes of the melancholic, in fact, are held transfixed to such a degree that those suffering from it seem to be senseless. In others, however, the eyes are cavernous and sunken into the eye cavity as if they had withdrawn and swallowed themselves. This latter condition is even more likely to occur in the raving mad.[61]

Physical signs had to be evaluated alongside behavior. People in whom blood has mixed with melancholy, for example, will "avoid those who are stronger than they are; they become angry and are consumed by rage at the least provocation; they scream and shout; they threaten those present as well as those who are absent. With savage countenance and violent motion of the body, they are terrifying."[62]

These manifold indicators were by no means easy to fake. According to Zacchia, "if a prudent physician looks into the mind (*animus*), without too much trouble he can recognize from all the aforementioned signs when *furor* or melancholy are truly at play versus when a person is poised to dissemble."[63] He encouraged his readers to consider insomnia, a characteristic feature of *furor* and often one of melancholy as well. Several factors contributed to wakefulness: "dryness of the humor itself, which caused blockage in the brain," or a defective imagination that could not properly receive data from the senses.[64] The Roman physician Celsus, Zacchia said, rightly pointed out that "as much as sleep is difficult for these sufferers it is still necessary. A person feigning *furor*, then, can be found out; for it is impossible that this person not be seized by sleep. Wishing to remain awake for a long time is against his habit when there is no internal cause forcing him to stay awake."[65] The prudent physician knew to check for certain signs of disease that simply could not be aped by healthy people for the simple reason that their bodies could not physically do such things. Moreover, even if some melancholics were said to be able to fall asleep, Zacchia claimed their sleep would be fitful and troubled.[66] Good luck to those trying to feign madness in their sleep!

Physicians and court officials could use clever tricks to unmask pretenders. Zacchia related the story of a physician—"most learned and skilled," in his words—faced with a disputed case of madness. The physician "ordered that the madman (*insanus*) was to be struck with many blows, though he had no intention of actually carrying out such a threat. If the man were truly insane he would have turned to the parts being beaten by those many blows, but if he were in fact pretending to be mad, he would have recovered his senses by virtue of not wishing to receive the blows."[67] In other words, the doctor was able to scare the pretense from the pretender. A truly mad person would not have registered the threat as a mentally competent person would.

But Zacchia's systematic and exhaustive treatment of the legal implications of madness was a distant echo of a conversation that had long been taking place in the households and courts of Florence for at least a century. Jurists may not have incorporated medical knowledge and categories into their learned treatises, but litigants and court officials were using them explicitly in the courts nearly fifty years before Zacchia was born. Judges were already looking for the physical marks of madness in the faces of the allegedly impaired. In a case of 1576, for example, the Pupilli ruled that a certain Giovanni Mingorlioni was *crazy* (*matto*) and in need of a guardian after observing his physical condition and listening to him speak. His appearance did little to help. According to the Pupilli he had hair down to his shoulders, had terror-stricken eyes (*li ochi spaventati*), and was of a sickly pallor.[68]

The Pupilli read madness from these physical signs. Witness testimony confirmed it. For one, Giovanni's sanity was discredited when it came to light that he had given over part of his house for the enjoyment of several wool washers, left two workshops vacant, and allowed mice to have the run of them. He even bought food for them to eat. Between sixteen and eighteen witnesses from the neighborhood, including merchants from the prestigious wool guild, supported these allegations and agreed that he generally led the life of a "pazzo."[69] The fact that his economic behavior was also eccentric if not bizarre convinced the Pupilli that Giovanni was mad. Clearly he needed a guardian. The Duke's office granted Lionardo's request.

Giovanni's physical description resembles that of the melancholic Girolamo Passerini, whom we met in Chapter 1. When court officials interviewed him in 1579 they concluded that he also seemed "terror stricken (*spaventato*)." His hands trembled and he had trouble speaking. All these things, they said, "proceeded from melancholy humors."[70] Without explicit recourse to medical experts, court officials recognized that the appearance and behavior of the two Giovannis marked them as sick enough to warrant legal intervention. In short, the process of medicalization was felt in applied law long before medical language infiltrated academic legal literature.

ASKING THE EXPERTS

That brings us to the question of expertise. Jurists knew that witness testimony was necessary but unreliable. They did not, however, consider it equally unreliable. Instead they entertained the possibility that some witnesses were better than others because they had special knowledge or skills. Roman procedure recognized two types of expert witness: the land surveyor (*agrimensor*), who determined the boundaries of property after natural events like floods had destroyed or obscured them, and the midwife, who certified pregnancies.[71] Both experts in these instances played a forensic role since recourse to their expertise was under certain circumstances mandatory. They did not, however, cede the same forensic role to medical practitioners that they had to land surveyors or midwives.[72] Judges were free to consult with medical practitioners, but their testimony was neither mandatory nor binding. Medieval jurists were similarly receptive to the testimony of medical experts. In a treatise called *De percussionibus* (On wounding), written by the Bolognese jurist Odofredo (d. 1265), and another called *De vulneribus* (On wounds), by the Mantuan jurist Guido da Suzzara (1225–1293), the two authors argued that surgeons and university-trained physicians had the special ability to make causal connections between wounds and death.[73]

Some medieval jurists set great store by medical experts, conceding even that they should sometimes be considered "as if they were judges" (*quasi iudices*).[74] In the treatise on witnesses attributed to Bartolus, the author asserts that theoretically doctors, midwives, and the like "were not properly speaking witnesses, but rather to be regarded as judges" for their capacity to offer judgment on specific points of a case.[75]

Contemporary lawmakers also recognized the ability of medical practitioners to establish causal relationship between wounds and death. In the statutes of various Italian cities, legislators increasingly urged judges to employ medical experts in criminal proceedings. The statutes of Bologna of 1288 required judicial authorities to provide two doctors in cases of homicide or severe wounding.[76] Perugia likewise arranged for the hiring of at least two doctors, one of whom was to be skilled in surgery.[77] Other cities followed suit, namely, San Gimignano (1314), Padua (1316), San Miniato al Tedesco (1337), Mirandola (1386), Bassano (1389), Florence (1415), Verona (1450), Brescia (1470), Milan (1480), Ferrara (1506), Genoa (1556), and Urbino (1556).[78]

The law's receptivity to expert medical testimony in criminal cases, in canonization proceedings, and to help resolve questions surrounding paternity, pregnancy, and abortion did not mean that doctors and surgeons were a necessary part of the adjudication process. And where medical practitioners may have increasingly appeared in criminal trials to explain causes of death, in Florentine courts, they moved like shadows through a negligible number of cases involving mental incapacity even when litigants were making medical arguments or judges were basing their decisions in part on the physical "testimony" of the body. I have found seven cases in the Pupilli or the Otto di Guardia between the fourteenth and seventeenth centuries in which a medical practitioner (*fisico* or *medico*) was called as a witness for his special expertise.

If someone asked a medieval or early modern Italian jurist who he thought most reliably proved a person's state of mind at a specific time he might say a doctor, but he was more likely to say a priest. Performance of the sacraments demanded soundness of mind. The

sacrament of confession, for example, required that confessees distinguish right from wrong and recognize the consequences of their
wishes and actions. Who better to judge a person's ability to receive
the sacraments than the one who bestowed them? In his *consilium* for
Giovanni de Zuchano, Decio claimed that the testimony of three clerics who said they had heard Giovanni's confession was a good indication of his sanity.[79]

In the case of Maria, her side included the testimony of a doctor
to prove that she was melancholic while Piero included the testimony
of a priest to prove that she was sane. But the value of the doctor and
the priest in this case did not lie in their ability to offer to the court an
accurate reading of Maria's state of mind—one through the body, the
other the soul. They were intended to link her state of mind to the act
of contracting. They were Maria's and Piero's respective ways of fixing the timeline. This was an innovative argument that came not from
learned law or medicine but the medicalization of daily life in Italy.

Both testimonies were important to their respective sides; neither was mandatory; neither was privileged. The judge took both
into account; he was legally bound by none. Moreover, Maria's doctor, specifically called a *fisico*, "practiced in recognizing melancholy
humors," was not her only medical witness.[80] He was one among three
other witnesses who lacked medical expertise but added their own
interpretations of her physical condition based on their lay knowledge
and experience of the melancholy disease.

Maria's first witness, one Marco degli Ambrosini, did just that.
Although he could not claim medical expertise, he still freely commented on her medical condition and offered justification for his
assessment. As Maria's neighbor in the Piazza Catinara for some
twenty-five years, Marco had long been a familiar face in her household. He was also on intimate terms with her son Agnolo. In the time
that he knew her, he said that "he had always seen her full of melancholy humors, doing and saying crazy things." Maria's list of mad
moments was longer than he could possibly recount in one sitting.
She acted like a "fool" (*sciocca*), an "idiot" (*balorda*), and a moody
or ill-humored person (*humorista*).[81] On more than one occasion,
for example, she had gone after her son and husband brandishing
a knife while spewing scandalous things that had no bearing on the
topic at hand.[82] At another time, Marco said, she "spent the whole
night without going to bed or sleeping. A great madness persisted in
which she spouted a good deal of nonsense and said rude things."[83]

This behavior was, in his opinion, the norm rather than the exception. It was also public. Marco and several other of her neighbors knew that she frequented the apothecary shop of one Messer Gisberto Tedesco, a "fisico" for "similar humors."[84] Marco also claimed that she consistently showed reckless disregard for her own health. Several times and for no apparent reason she ordered that barbers and other medical practitioners of low to middling status draw her blood without there being any need and without the permission of her physicians (*medici*).[85] For Marco, all of these things pointed clearly to melancholy.

Marco was not, as the record stated, "skilled in recognizing melancholy humors except through its effects," namely, that Maria said and did things that no sane person would. But he was no stranger to the disease. Marco told the court that "he had never seen a person who suffered from melancholy humors remain in his mind for very long." When such humors took hold, "they altered a person's mind and brain." What was more, he did not have far to look for examples of melancholy's cruel effects. Maria's son Agnolo suffered from them, too, and so vehemently that, according to Marco, sometimes he had to be bound and locked up. If that was not enough, Marco added that one of Maria's cousins suffered from similar humors that drove her to do crazy things.[86] Maria, it would seem, was mired in melancholy.

Marco was not the only layman willing to comment on Maria's alleged sickness. Onesto de' Nobili, a fellow Florentine, had his own views on the matter. During the 1550s, Onesto lived with Maria and her late second husband in the Piazza Catinara, serving as amanuensis. From his secretarial perch within the household he was able to observe Maria's behavior. He found her to be "a mercurial (*variabile*) and ill-humored person (*humorista*) of little mind." He saw madness in the "variety of gestures she made." Moreover, nothing she said made sense. Onesto had to admit that, like Marco, he was "not skilled in recognizing the melancholy disease." Still, he did not believe Maria's humors were melancholic. Whatever humors they were, they seemed to be of the kind to induce "fickleness" (*leggerezza*), foolishness (*sciochezza*), and a "type of madness" (*spezie di pazzo*), suggesting a frenetic rather than a depressive condition.[87]

Petitioners throughout this study repeatedly applied the term *pazzo* to mentally disturbed people of all types from *mentecapti* to *furiosi*, melancholics to frenetics. In this instance, Onesto connected the term to aggressive behavior to distinguish it from the stereotypical dejection that characterized melancholy in its strictest sense as a disease that caused profound sadness and a penchant for solitude. But humors were beside the point. In Onesto's opinion, Maria was so pathologically changeable in speech and behavior that he could not consider her a woman of sound mind. He was not alone in his thinking. Whatever people thought of Maria in Florence, Onesto maintained that in Rome she was considered "half mad and foolish."[88]

The third witness, Sebastiano de' Caccini of Pistoia, was of a similar mind. His acquaintance with Maria and her late second husband went back to 1540, twenty-five years before Maria made the problematic gift contract. Even then he considered her a "foolish woman without a mind."[89] The many occasions Sebastiano saw Maria speak and behave as no sane woman would confirmed his view that she was crazy (*pazza*). Like Marco and Onesto, Sebastiano was "not skilled in recognizing melancholic humors." That did not stop him from testifying that the humors Maria suffered were not so much melancholic as wild and frenzied. Like Onesto, he invoked the more hostile sense of the term *pazzo*. Maria, after all, did not "experience sadness." But the particulars mattered little. Even if Sebastiano could not say what the causes of her humors, melancholy or otherwise, were he could attest to the fact that "he had never seen her in her [right] mind."[90]

After a good deal of talk about Maria's purported melancholy by laymen who claimed intimate acquaintance with her and her household, the fifth witness was finally a physician. In the words of the record, Sebastiano Capano was "practiced in recognizing diseases from melancholy humors being himself in the profession of physic." Capano had known Maria for three years. During that time, he had tried to treat her specifically for melancholy.[91] When asked how he knew that she was melancholic he said that while speaking with her he noticed that her brain tended to wander. She would flit from one thing to another, often losing track of what she was trying to say. This testimony differs little from that of Marco, Onesto, or Sebastiano de' Caccini. Unlike these earlier witnesses, however, Sebastiano *fisico* could justify his claim that she was suffering from melancholy rather than another disease based on his medical knowledge. Perhaps to underscore his expertise, Sebastiano spoke in Latin, saying that "burnt yellow bile ascending to her brain, that is, to her cogitative faculty," was at the root of her illness. He had no doubt that melancholy was running its course, adding that "during the year between 1565 and 1566 he had treated her, prescribing [medications]."[92] His experience of medicine and his examinations of her body and behavior led him to conclude that she was indeed melancholic, that burnt yellow bile explained her aggressive tendencies, and that she was suffering its ill effects during that critical year of the contract with Piero.

Sebastiano Capano's testimony was an important addition to that of the lay witnesses who preceded him. As insiders they had ample opportunity to observe those countless moments, erratic and strange, that were otherwise hidden from the eyes of casual acquaintances who lived beyond the walls of Maria's household. At least one of them confidently attributed her behavior to melancholy. Two others demurred, claiming that humors were surely in play though probably not those that induced melancholy per se.

Expert medical testimony helped explain some of the confusion that witnesses expressed in trying to connect her behavior to a specific disease, but again, the particulars were beside the point. Maria was mad; they all agreed. The question was when. What Sebastiano *fisico* did was help fix her madness in time. Melancholy humors were responsible for Maria's aberrant behavior, he claimed. But what really mattered was that he was treating Maria for this disease during the year of the contract. This testimony fit nicely with that of Marco, who mentioned that he and several of Maria's neighbors had often seen her at Messer Gisberto Tedesco's pharmacy at that time as well. Why was she there? To fill the prescriptions that Sebastiano had given her, of course. Why did her condition not improve? As Marco said, for all her capriciousness, the one thing Maria was certain to do was disregard good advice. She had been ignoring the counsel of concerned physicians for years. When she was supposed to be listening to Sebastiano Capano she was off getting bled by barbers and quacks.

Maria's remaining witnesses were those of *public voice and fame*. They were less intimately connected to her but important for establishing that Maria's mad behavior and melancholic condition were generally known and considered to be true among her neighbors. One witness was a Roman notary who could say little more than that he "had heard from different people that she was vexed by certain humors of the kind that she seemed to have had earlier." These humors made her crazy (*pazz[a]*). It was "as if [she were] possessed (*spiritata*); she remained for some time under such an influence."[93] The testimony of a notary challenged the judgment of the Roman notary who validated the gift contract. Although it was important to uphold the authority of notaries to safeguard the sanctity of contracts, it was not impossible to imagine a scenario in which inexperience or incompetence led a notary to misjudge the capacity of a contracting party to enter into a valid contract. Maria's notary witness suggested the possibility of such an occurrence without having to say so explicitly.

Another witness who had known Maria for nearly ten years confirmed that she was a "woman lacking in mind, but whether such a defect proceeded from melancholy or some other humors he did not know."[94] He was, however, aware that Maria had tangled with her dead husband's family in court even if he could not describe the particulars of that litigation. The last witness said nothing at all about humors, melancholy or otherwise, but could confirm that during the twenty or so years that Maria was married to her second husband, Francesco Serragli, she was never "in her right mind nor a woman of sensible speech or sound judgment. During that whole time, everyone who knew her thought as much."[95] The rumors wending their way through Rome's winding streets to be whispered in crowded squares was the same; Maria was mad. Was she melancholic? Manic? Frenetic? No matter. Some kind of noxious humors were choking her brain. The gift she made to Piero was yet more proof of her insanity. What person, after all, would sign away all she had to some stranger when she had a sister and an unmarried niece to think of?

The construction of Maria's mental incapacity was a collaborative effort. The pieces fell into place only when all testimony, particularly that of Marco, Onesto, Sebastiano de' Caccini, and Sebastiano *fisico* were taken in concert. The first three confirmed Maria's instability over the long term. They were not present at the making of the contract with Piero, but Marco at the very least could say that he knew Maria was being treated at the time by both legitimate and questionable medical practitioners. Enter Sebastiano *fisico*. His testimony more firmly fixed Maria's mental incapacity to the time of the contract. He confirmed that he had indeed been treating her throughout the year of 1565 and 1566 specifically for melancholy. Marco's testimony gave further weight to these claims since he said that he saw her often at Gisberto Tedesco's pharmacy in search of a cure for her humors. Sebastiano *fisico*'s testimony was purely strategic for the temporal shading it added to Maria's case. It was not required by the court.

THE MANUFACTURE OF SANITY

Maria's alleged sanity was no less constructed than her alleged madness. It, too, was a collaborative effort though witnesses for Piero presented to the court a horse of a very different color. To connect her sanity to the time of the gift contract, Piero's side ignored medical matters altogether and conjured up an image of Maria as a pious and practicing Christian. The key witness here was Maria's parish priest, who could attest to the fact that she was receiving the sacraments from him during the time she made the contract. The image of Maria the good Christian did not conform perfectly to the other portrait Piero's side painted of her, namely, the freeloading ingrate who broke her bond to serve her own interests. Still it was plausible enough and it fixed her sanity to the time of the contract.

The rector of San Paolo, Maria's parish church, was Piero's first witness. He testified that he had known both Maria and Piero for three or four years in Rome. He could not speak in depth about the nature of their relationship, but he had seen Piero in Maria's house on numerous occasions. Since he had not witnessed the gift contract he was also unable to say anything about her state of mind at that particular time. He could, however, confirm that in the time that he had known Maria, and more important during the time of the gift contract, he heard her confession, administered communion to her, and visited her at her house when she was sick.[96]

Maria seems to have been ill rather often. Not only had the cleric seen her sick in bed a number of times, but he claimed that whenever she went to church she was helped along by two people whose names escaped him. Physical frailty proved no obstacle to devotion. "Every Saturday for one year," he told the court, "Maria sponsored masses he delivered at the church of San Cesareo, even donating lamp oil for Saturday mass many times."[97] Such heroic efforts in the face of illness proved to him that she was "a good Christian."[98] At no point did melancholy enter the fray. As far as the cleric was concerned, Maria's physical state did not compromise her mind. When he spoke to her and reasoned with her he recognized her to be a "prudent woman of sound mind."[99]

When Piero's other witnesses were asked to weigh in on Maria's status as a Christian, those who could comment on it supported the priest's testimony. Maria was a devout Christian. As such, she was a sane person with full rational capacity. Maria's neighbor, Antonio de' Cavi, for example, claimed that he saw her "go countless times to the church of the Trinità to attend services. Afterward she would go to visit those convalescing in the church's hospital in the manner of all sane people and good Christians."[100] Here was a woman widely known for energetically performing good works all with the appropriate "fear of God." Seven other witnesses added their voices to the chorus singing Maria's praises as a model Christian. Among them, Pietro Alfonso de' Tabia was not sure which church Maria frequented, but he knew that she went regularly. He claimed that he saw her "go to church every morning to hear mass and that he considered her a good Christian who made confession and received communion often."[101] He was certain that others of her acquaintance shared this view of her.

The young Sienese matron Adriana who had rented a room in Maria's house with her first husband was more voluble on the subject of Maria's piety. She said that Maria often made confession and received communion and went nearly every week to the church of the Trinità where she heard mass and the holy offices. Adriana frequently accompanied Maria to that church, but even more often—"infinite times"—the ladies "went to a little church near the river where Maria had masses said," presumably on behalf of other people. She was, in Adriana's estimation, "an honest person and a devout and good Christian."[102] Anyone who knew her thought as much as four other of Maria's neighbors could attest.

Together the testimonies of the priest and seven of Piero's carefully chosen witnesses suggested that concerted and consistent efforts to care for the soul demonstrated Maria's grasp of what really mattered in Christian life. If she proved herself to be a tough operator when it came to managing her estate, squabbling with the relatives of her dead husband over property, then she was in good company. Protracted battles with kin over patrimony were the norm in Italian society, accounting for a great deal of civil litigation. The demands of patrimonial rationality did not ensure peaceable transfers of property. If anything, they seem to have caused a good deal of squabbling among those who thought their claims were more pressing or more compassionate.

We will soon see that the family of Maria's second husband considered her to be, to put it mildly, a meddling shrew. Be that as it may, when it came to the great metaphysical questions, Piero's witnesses maintained that Maria had her head screwed on straight. Medieval and early modern Europeans sometimes associated spiritual indifference or *acedia* with the melancholy disease or some comparable illness. By contrast, acts of Christian devotion regularly and properly performed could signal a healthy mind in which reason was intact. Still the testimony of the priest was only useful in the context of the testimony of several other lay witnesses who could also speak to Maria's impeachable character as a good Christian. Like the physician, the priest was important, but his testimony was not dispositive.

THE GHOST OF RELATIVES PAST

Whether Piero's contract stood or Thommasa and Maria's side carried the day is hard to know for certain. The Duke's reply to the Pupilli of December 17, 1568, instructing them to "re-examine this *donatio* because, [Maria] being *mentacatta*, it is not reasonable that it took place," is the last official judgment on the matter despite the fact that the lengthy witness depositions submitted to the court by the two sides in the case were not taken until the spring and summer of the next year.[103] Subsequent court proceedings indicate that, whether or not Thommasa took control of Maria's property and care, the gift was not executed. Rather, the drama continued.

In 1573, Maria found herself entangled once again in litigation. The family of her second husband, Francesco Serragli, disputed her claim to certain properties that they believed were part of his estate. This battle started in Rome when Francesco died back in 1564. Since there were no surviving children from the marriage, Francesco's family argued that an alternative (*substitutio*) heir had been named. This heir should take possession of the house in which Maria was living at that time and the two attached *bottegas* that earned her rental income.

But Maria was a step ahead of the game. She teamed up with Piero and Antonio Mellini, who as her lawyers asked that the court of the Campidoglio in Rome recognize her as "padrona" of these properties because they were part of her dowry.[104] The Mellini won their suit; the success of this litigation in 1566 must have been one of the reasons Maria made the gift to Piero. Maria was still in possession of the properties in 1573, and if Francesco's heirs could prove that the properties in question had never been Maria's in the first place, Piero could have no hope of claiming them as part of the gift contract.

I have been unable to find the outcome of this case; its interminable loose ends permit little more than speculation about what finally happened. What do remain are the questions that the two opposing sides prepared for witnesses and testimonies given on behalf of Francesco's heirs. We can piece together the claims Maria's side made but not the specific arguments her supporting witnesses made to defend them. Still, there is something to learn from these fragments. The questions coupled with the depositions that do survive bring yet another version of Maria to life. In the litigation of 1573, she is neither a melancholic madwoman nor a devout Christian but a tyrant and a harpy. Amazingly enough, one of the questions her side drew up questioned the mental capacity of her second husband, asking whether "he was a man of mind or really *mentecatto.*"[105]

According to witnesses for Francesco's heirs, Maria's first husband, who, like her second husband—to add yet another twist to the case—was also named Francesco Serragli, moved his family from Florence to Rome to live among the Tuscan community in the Piazza Catinara. According to witnesses, they lived in a palazzo estimated to be worth around a thousand scudi and rented out the two attached *bottegas.*[106] This first Francesco died in 1536. Two years later, Maria married the second Francesco Serragli. Francesco II moved into the palazzo Maria and Francesco I had shared and collected rent as his predecessor had done before him.

This second Francesco was reputed to be "rich and rather well to do."[107] When he married Maria in 1538 he brought to the table holdings in a leather company and a large warehouse (*magazzino grossissimo*) containing wine that was brought in from the countryside by his own muleteers on his own mules.[108] He also had money enough to purchase the palazzo of Francesco I together with all its furnishings and the attached shops when he married Maria.[109] What Maria brought to the marriage is less certain. The record is foggy about what Bartolomeo, Maria's son from her first marriage, gave to her if he gave her anything at all. Francesco I's estate was valued at around four thousand scudi and comprised two vineyards and several rental properties.[110] If she saw nothing of the proceeds from these properties, her husband left her with a good deal of "gems, pearls, rings, golden necklaces, and precious clothing . . . that she could sell for more than 1,000 scudi," if she so desired.[111]

The heirs of Francesco II tried to establish that Maria was, in Christiane Klapisch-Zuber's words, no more than "a passing guest" in these households and an unwelcome one at that. The house she lived in with her first husband did not devolve to her as part of her dowry upon his death. Instead her second husband had to buy it. Whether he bought it from her son, Bartolomeo, is unclear. None of the witnesses seemed to understand exactly who owned what and no one provided documents of ownership.

In the litigation of 1569, Piero Mellini had presented Maria as a paragon of womanly virtues. She ran an orderly house, she spent her time in worthy female pursuits like sewing, weaving, and praying, and she regularly performed the acts of Christian charity that adorned the characters of upright and desirable women. If she had been ungrateful in the end, surely it was because she had been swayed by her grasping sister. By contrast, Francesco II's side served up a Maria in possession of the worst female qualities, namely, greed, stupidity, and shrewishness. Several of the witnesses for Francesco II's heirs claimed that Maria was a "haughty woman who wished to have a hand in every aspect of household governance. When Francesco, her husband, opposed her, she started to shout at him, hit him, curse at him, and threaten him so vehemently that he was forced to do whatever she wanted." What was worse, her meddling destroyed Francesco II's fortune. According to witnesses, Maria made poor business decisions in the name of her husband that "in the course of time reduced Francesco to a weak, old pauper."[112] He entered their marriage a wealthy man, but, because of her "prodigality," he died "in extreme poverty and ruin."[113] Witnesses agreed that Maria was to blame. At no point did they represent her as mad or melancholic; she was, in their eyes, rather a conniving fishwife.

But Maria's side did not attribute madness of any kind to her either. They, in fact, suggested that the mind of her second husband had fallen prey to the ravages of time toward the end of his life. One of her questions asked "whether Francesco was and had been a man of mind or really *mentecatto*."[114] If advanced age had deprived him of his ability to run a household, Maria's interventions were justifiable; they made her responsible rather than controlling. But the witnesses in support of Francesco II's heirs would not take the bait. Those who could speak on this count generally agreed that Francesco was, in the words of one witness, "a wise, prudent and lettered man with good judgment until the very last moments of old age."[115] Another witness added that Francesco was lucid to the end, though he may have "lost his capacity to reason (*rimbambire*) a little before his death because of age and poverty."[116] For the most part, all his actions and business dealings made sense to those around him.

There is something absurd about this case. Maria marries two affluent men with the same name. After the death of husband number one, she marries a man who has the wherewithal to purchase her first husband's palazzo, its furnishings, and the *bottegas* attached to it. When husband number two dies, she enlists the help of Piero Mellini to retain hold of this palazzo and its attached *bottegas* despite counterclaims on it made by her second husband's kin. Piero seems to have persuaded the court that the property was Maria's. Maria rewards Piero with the gift of her estate for after her death and the hand of her niece in marriage. But something changes Maria's mind when she returns to Florence with Piero in tow. The cause of that change—the fury of her Florentine relatives, namely, her sister or a scheme the two women hatched to overturn what in hindsight may have seemed an imprudent contract—remains mysterious. Maria seems to have succeeded in having Piero pushed out of the picture, but she could not shake Francesco's heirs, who persisted in their fight to win the properties in Piazza Catinara at Rome that they believed Francesco had purchased and so rightly owned. So much for what the documents tell us.

***

No words ring more true about Maria's case than Lawrence Stone's now famous remark about marriage litigation: "the story of what really happened has to be pieced together from two semi-fictitious constructs created by the prosecution and defense, each buttressed by the often coached, and occasionally false, sworn evidence of their respective posses of witnesses."[117] Trying to get a grasp of Maria's character or the true nature of the situations that repeatedly sent her to court is like trying to capture the image of the moon on water.

The "Maria" that Thommasa and Maria herself presented to the court was a doddering, sick old widow—a lamb in the jaws of the wolfish Piero. Witnesses for Maria's side painted her portrait with a coarser brush, but the effect was more or less the same; she was moody and melancholic. Her behavior was often erratic and her language often inappropriate. In Piero's account, by contrast, we meet a good and reasonable Christian woman whose intention to fulfill her obligations to him had been hijacked by her grasping sister. Then there is "Maria" the conniving mastermind who played people against each other for her own benefit.

Even if the "real" Maria is lost to time, there is something to be learned about how petitioners in Italian courts leveraged the language of madness and particularly disease for all it was worth to build their arguments. There is also something to be learned about the history of the interactions between medicine and law in European history. Between the thirteenth and seventeenth centuries, humoral medicine increasingly penetrated the legal realm as it had households, market-places, and culture. But it entered the courts not as the privileged domain of medical experts. Instead ordinary Tuscans were comfort-able advancing medical arguments and court officials were com-fortable evaluating and accepting them without calling in a medical expert.

For the entire period of this study, at no point did one type of per-son or occupation acquire the sole authority to define madness or con-trol its use. An assortment of different hands shaped it into whatever form best served practical ends. For some families that meant protect-ing an individual by making arrangements for reliable long-term care, for others, curbing reckless spending, for yet others, excusing crimi-nal or socially aberrant behavior. It is true that courts of law increas-ingly sought the opinions of medical practitioners particularly in the realm of criminal law. But in the end, the interests and opinions of kith, kin, and community tended to win the day.

Zacchia's work codifies a development that had long been in the works. His argument that learned physicians constituted a unique, distinct, and, for their knowledge, training, and expertise, privileged occupational group is more properly a part of the professionalization of medicine. But that is the story of a later age.

Conclusion

Madness is perhaps the worst illness a man can have, first because
it deprives him of speech making him similar to irrational animals and leaving him nothing other than the appearance of humanity. Second, because, unlike other illnesses, it does not induce in
him the desire to free himself from it . . . therefore . . . by law of
humanity and of the Christian religion we are servants of compassion and relief, how much more ought we do in a case where the patient cannot help himself, not having at his disposal his own will?
—ASF, SDP, reg. 341, fol. 515r

It was not until 1643 that an institution devoted solely to the care
of the severely mentally disturbed was established in Florence. The
above epigraph was one of several justifications for its foundation.
Santa Dorotea dei Pazzerelli (of the mad) was the brainchild of Alberto
Leoni da Revere (1563–1642), a Carmelite originally from Mantova.
He had served for some time as the chaplain of the Stinche where
he observed firsthand the passage of mentally disturbed men and
women in and out of prison. Leoni secured the funds, permissions,
and real estate for its foundation, but his efforts were not rewarded
until 1643, a year after his death, when Santa Dorotea was officially
established on the eastern outskirts of the city, a few blocks down
from the Stinche prison itself. In 1688, Florence's famous old hospital
Santa Maria Nuova followed suit, creating a ward for poor mad men
and women, called the "pazzeria."

These Florentine foundations were by no means the first of their
kind in Europe or Italy. Already in 1375, a Muslim hospital for the
mad was founded in Granada perhaps on the model of similar institutions that existed in North Africa.[1] Similarly, a number of hospitals
throughout Europe had been admitting mentally disturbed men and
women into their general populations since the fourteenth and fifteenth centuries: the Hospital de Colom in Barcelona, the Hôtel-Dieu
in Paris, hospitals at Elbing and Erfurt in Germany, and St. Mary of

Bethlehem in London, otherwise known as Bedlam, to name a few.[2] The first European hospitals created specifically to house the severely mentally incapacitated appeared in fifteenth-century Spain: the hospital of the Nuestra Señora de Gracia at Saragossa and the Hospital de San Cosme y San Damián of Seville, commonly known as the Casa de los Innocentes and perhaps more commonly referred to as the "casa de los locos." Clerics from Seville took this model with them to Rome where they helped found Santa Maria della Pietà there in 1550. At the beginning of the sixteenth century, the hospital of San Vincenzo in Prato at Milan also took up the care of mad men and women or "pazzarelli."

In 1586, Tommaso Garzoni, a member of the Order of Regular Lateran Canons and prolific satirist, constructed a different type of hospital for the mad. His was an imaginary edifice described in the satirical work *L'hospedale de' pazzi incurabili* (*The Hospital of Incurable Fools*) published that year. In it, he took his readers through the "hospital's" rooms where they met a motley crew of mad men and women. For Garzoni, the "hospital" was really the world of his time, which he believed had become the "image of madness itself." Folly ruled as a tyrant over men and it was philosophers and intellectuals who had crowned her.

The problem of knowledge and what constituted the right type of knowledge had long exercised the minds of Europe's premier intellectuals when Garzoni imagined his fantastical hospital of fools. Like Erasmus's *Praise of Folly* (1511), he was adding his voice to what Michel Foucault rightly identified as a complex epistemological debate taking place in early modern Europe. But Garzoni's decision to place his collection of mad, bad, and dangerous to know in a hospital is not evidence of an early modern precursor to Foucault's "Great Confinement," or some emergent connection between madness and deviance in European minds, or new strategies of social and political control.[3] As Lisa Roscioni argued, there simply is no one history of mental institutions in medieval and early modern Europe, nor is there one narrative trajectory or paradigm that describes why they were founded in the first place.

The history of Santa Dorotea is both more mundane and more humane than the world of satire might suggest. In May 1642, the Auditore della Regia Giurisdizione (auditor of royal jurisdiction) noted that there were twenty-four people considered *pazzo* languishing in the Stinche. It was around this time that Alberto Leoni was chaplain there. Whoever these twenty-four *pazzi* were, they had nowhere to go. They cycled instead around a revolving track that went from the streets, to prison, to Santa Maria Nuova, where, if they were poor, they could receive temporary care, only to return to prison; their families, if they had them, had apparently abandoned them. Around 1642, Leoni conceived of a place "to be erected in our city of Florence where the mad (*pazzarelli*) could be cared for."[4]

A group of like-minded men took up where Leoni left off, claiming that the duchy of Tuscany needed "a hospital devoted to the care and compassionate treatment of the sick who suffered a kind of *mania* and the supervision of those incurables there."[5] These efforts were intended to remove the burden of care from the shoulders of Tuscan families and to provide some remedy to the many problems that "caused *furiosi* to be abandoned in public to wander the streets."[6] The goal was to furnish the Florentine duchy with an institution that could provide long-term care for the severely mentally disturbed. After four years of careful planning in which a governing board began the task of administering the institution, in 1647, Santa Dorotea admitted its first *pazzarello*.

At its foundation it had room for sixty patients who would be divided according to sex and station.[7] It tended toward inclusiveness and its founders were explicit on this point. Santa Dorotea was a place devoted to the care of "*pazzi* of whatever sort, men as well as women of every country, nation, people, state, social class and condition."[8] To cover the hospital's overhead and allow the poorest of its patients to stay for free, the cost of admission was assessed for each patient according to what he or she could reasonably pay. Careful attention was paid to diet—the most important preventive and therapeutic health strategy among the six non-naturals. On a daily basis, the patients were given good wine, but only a little of it with specific amounts of bread, meat, salad, and vegetable soup (*minestra*) in accord with season and the principles of Greek medicine.[9] The hope was that this regimen would if not alleviate at least not exacerbate patients' symptoms, most of whom suffered the most severe of mental illnesses.

What exactly the foundation of Santa Dorotea meant in Florence is hard to say. It could mark nothing more than the charitable vision of one man who was moved by the wretched lot of the mentally disordered languishing in prison to build a comfortable, clean place where they would be fed, clothed, and cared for. Gilabert Jofré, a

Mercedarian friar in Valencia, had done just such a thing in 1409.[10] Moreover, Santa Dorotea was not Leoni's first charitable foundation. Six years earlier he had established a Casa dei Catecumeni to convert Jews and other "infidels."[11]

From an administrative point of view it seems to signal an important change in attitudes to who should care for the mad even if it did not completely change the reality of madness in Tuscan society. The family remained the primary custodial institution for the mentally and physically impaired well into the eighteenth century. Santa Dorotea could not solve the age-old problem of how to provide long-term care for severely mentally disturbed men and women. Nor was it yet the first port of call for the mad. It was often the place that people ended up when all private and public solutions had failed.[12] A vulnerable person's fate still depended and would continue to depend on the resources, kindness, willingness, and presence of his or her relatives. Still, Santa Dorotea and the Pazzeria at Santa Maria Nuova offered Tuscans and their magistrates a different answer to questions they had been asking for centuries about what to do with the most severely disturbed among them. How well it met their needs in the coming centuries is a topic for another book.

***

For all of the great advances in neurobiology, madness was and remains a terra incognita. Its strangeness will continue to fascinate; its unpredictability will continue to arouse suspicion; its rare but explosive expression in unimaginable acts of violence will continue to cause fear and outrage. The study of how madness is represented, defined, and understood does indeed communicate a society's values, attitudes, and assumptions. What it fails to acknowledge is the great distance that often exists between thinking and doing, imagining and living. Whether the mentally disturbed or physically impaired were thought to be possessed by the devil, singled out by God for special sanctity, troubled lovers, or melancholy geniuses was quite literally immaterial to medieval and early modern men and women when family honor or patrimony was on the line or order was imperiled.

The shift from representation to action captures Tuscans trying to help or occasionally to exploit mentally or physically impaired relatives. In so doing it shows us how Florentines and their civic authorities mutually took on the task of ordering their society from household to street to marketplace. This is the society of makeshifts at work. By observing the legal, judicial, social, and cultural strategies Tuscans constructed and mobilized over the course of three hundred years and through three hundred or so civil and criminal cases, we gain great insight into the evolving nature of early modern families and their relationship to their governing arrangements, their attitudes to spending and domestic economy, their understanding of Greek medical ideas, and their use of medical practitioners in court.

The History House will always remain closed to the later generations that return to it. Documentary and material sources as well as categories of historical analysis help historians to crack windows and doors and listen through walls or peer through keyholes. But it is only by combining representations and actions that we can make sense of the whispering there.

ASI *Archivio Storico Italiano.* Florence: Olschki, 1913–.

Bart. *De test.* Bartolus da Sassoferrato, *De testibus,* in *Commentaria: Cum additionibus Thomae Diplovatatii.* Ed. G. Polara. Rome, 1996.

Bull. Hist. Med. Bulletin of the History of Medicine. Baltimore: Johns Hopkins University Press, 1939–.

C. *Codex Iustiniani*

D. *Digesta*

I. *Institiones Iustiniani*

Ius Commune Ius Commune: Zeitschrift für Europäische Rechtgeschichte. Frankfurt am Main: V. Klostermann, 1967–.

Nov. *Novellae Constitutiones Iustiniani.* Berlin: Weidmannos, 1895.

Stud. Hist. Phil. Sci. Studies in History and Philosophy of Science. Oxford: Pergamon Press, 1970–.

V.A.S. Vostra Altezza Serenissima

V.E.I. Vostra Eccellenza Illustrissima

Zac. *Quaest. Med. Leg.* Paolo Zacchia, *Quaestiones Medico-Legales.* Amsterdam: Johanne Blaeu, 1651.

NOTES

INTRODUCTION

Sophocles, *Ajax*, *The Complete Greek Tragedies*, ed. David Grene and Richmond Lattimore, trans. John Moore (Chicago: University of Chicago Press, 1957), 271–77.

1. Jerome Wakefield, "The Concept of Mental Disorder: On the Boundary Between Biological Facts and Social Values," *American Psychologist* 47, no. 3 (1992): 373.

2. Arthur Kleinman, *Patients and Healers in the Context of Culture: An Exploration of the Borderland Between Anthropology, Medicine, and Psychiatry* (Berkeley: University of California Press, 1980); Louis A. Sass, *Madness and Modernism: Insanity in the Light of Modern Art, Literature, and Thought* (Cambridge, Mass.: Harvard University Press, 1992); Ian Hacking, *Rewriting the Soul: Multiple Personality and the Sciences of Memory* (Princeton, N.J.: Princeton University Press, 1995) and idem, *Mad Travelers: Reflections of the Reality of Transient Mental Illnesses* (Charlottesville: University Press of Virginia, 1998).

3. Michael MacDonald, *Mystical Bedlam: Madness, Anxiety, and Healing in Seventeenth-Century England* (Cambridge: Cambridge University Press, 1981), 1.

4. James N. Butcher, Susan Mineka, and Jill M. Hooley, *Abnormal Psychology*, 14th ed. (Boston: Allyn & Bacon, 2010), 34. See also Franz G. Alexander and Sheldon T. Selesnick, *The History of Psychiatry: An Evaluation of Psychiatric Thought and Practice from Prehistoric Times to the Present* (New York: Harper & Row, 1967) and Gregory Zilboorg, *The Medical Man and the Witch in the Renaissance* (New York: Cooper Square Publishers, 1969). The now immortal and often cited quotation about presentism comes from E. P. Thompson, *The Making of the English Working Class* (New York: Vintage, 1966), 12.

5. Jerome Wakefield offers a useful guide through the extensive scholarly literature on this debate in "The Concept of Mental Disorder." The most famous attack on psychiatry remains Michel Foucault, *Histoire de la folie à l'âge classique: Folie et déraison* (Paris: Plon, 1961), published in English as

Madness and Civilization: A History of Insanity in the Age of Reason (New York: Vintage Books, 1973).

6. Foucault, *Madness and Civilization*, 8.

7. For accounts of this reorientation, see W. F. Bynum, Roy Porter, and Michael Shepherd, eds., *The Anatomy of Madness: Essays in the History of Psychiatry* (London: Tavistock Publications, 1985–88); Arthur Still and Irving Velody, eds., *Rewriting the History of Madness: Studies in Foucault's "Histoire de la folie"* (London: Routledge, 1992); and Colin Jones and Roy Porter, eds., *Reassessing Foucault: Power, Medicine, and the Body* (London: Routledge, 1994).

8. Notable studies within this enormous literature include Anne Digby's *Madness, Morality, and Medicine: A Study of the York Retreat, 1796–1914* (Cambridge: Cambridge University Press, 1985); Roy Porter, *Mind Forg'd Manacles: A History of Madness in England from the Restoration to the Regency* (Cambridge, Mass.: Harvard University Press, 1987); Colin Jones, *The Charitable Imperative: Hospitals and Nursing in Ancien Régime and Revolutionary France* (London: Routledge, 1989); Ann Goldberg, *Sex, Religion, and the Making of Modern Madness: The Eberbach Asylum and German Society, 1815–1849* (New York: Oxford University Press, 1999); and Lisa Roscioni, *Il governo della follia: Ospedali, medici e pazzi nell'età moderna* (Milan: Bruno Mondadori, 2003).

9. MacDonald, *Mystical Bedlam*; R. A. Houston, *Madness and Society in Eighteenth-Century Scotland* (Oxford: Oxford University Press, 2000); Jonathan Andrews and Andrew Scull, *Customers and Patrons of the Mad-Trade: The Management of Lunacy in Eighteenth-Century London* (Berkeley: University of California Press, 2003).

10. Roscioni, *Il governo della follia*, introduction.

11. Sara Tilghman Nalle, *Mad for God: Bartolomé Sánchez, the Secret Messiah of Cardenete* (Charlottesville: University Press of Virginia, 2001), 158–60.

12. Fourteen comparative essays for a later period show that histories of mental institutions are anything but teleological. See Roy Porter and David Wright, eds., *The Confinement of the Insane: International Perspectives, 1800–1965* (Cambridge: Cambridge University Press, 2003). See also Roscioni, *Il governo della follia*.

13. Olwen Hufton, *The Poor of Eighteenth-Century France, 1750–1789* (Oxford: Clarendon Press, 1974); Nicholas Terpstra, *Cultures of Charity: Women, Politics, and the Reform of Poor Relief in Renaissance Italy* (Cambridge, Mass.: Harvard University Press, 2013), 8.

14. Exceptions are Basil Clarke, *Mental Disorder in Earlier Britain* (Cardiff: University of Wales, 1975); Richard Neugebauer, "Mental Illness and Government Policy in Sixteenth- and Seventeenth-Century England" (Ph.D. diss., Columbia University, 1976); and Wendy J. Turner, ed., *Madness in Medieval Law and Custom* (Leiden: Brill, 2010).

15. Raymond Klibansky, Erwin Panofsky, and Fritz Saxl, *Saturn and Melancholy: Studies in the History of Natural Philosophy, Religion, and Art* (New York: Basic Books, 1964); Ernesto Grassi and Maristella Lorch,

Folly and Insanity in Renaissance Literature (Binghamton, N.Y.: Medieval
& Renaissance Texts & Studies, 1986); Winfried Schleiner, *Melancholy,
Genius, and Utopia in the Renaissance* (Wiesbaden: In Kommission bei
Otto Harrassowitz, 1991); Noel L. Brann, *The Debate over the Origin of
Genius During the Italian Renaissance* (Leiden: Brill, 2002); Jane Kromm,
*The Art of Frenzy: Public Madness in the Visual Culture of Europe, 1500–
1850* (London: Continuum, 2002).

16. For melancholy in Italian literature, see Gustavo Tanfani, "Il concetto di melancholia nel cinquecento," *Rivista di storia delle scienze
mediche e naturali* 39 (1948): 145–68; Bruno Basile, *Poëta melancholicus: Tradizione classica e follia nell'ultimo Tasso* (Pisa: Pacini, 1984);
and François Baruchello, *La folie de la Renaissance: Analyse de
"L'hospital des fols incurables" de Garzoni, 1549–1589* (Evrecy: Association France-Italie, 1998). For melancholy in English literature, see
Douglas Trevor, *The Poetics of Melancholy in Early Modern England*
(Cambridge: Cambridge University Press, 2004); Adam Kitzes, *The Politics of Melancholy from Spenser to Milton* (New York: Routledge, 2006);
and Angus Gowland, *The Worlds of Renaissance Melancholy: Robert
Burton in Context* (Cambridge: Cambridge University Press, 2006). For
melancholy in Spanish literature, see Javier García Gibert, *Cervantes y
la melancolía: Ensayos sobre el tono y la actitud cervantinos* (València:
Edicions Alfons el Magnànim, Institució Valenciana d'Estudis i Investigació, 1997); and Teresa Scott Soufas, *Melancholy and the Secular Mind
in Spanish Golden Age Literature* (Columbia: University of Missouri
Press, 1990); for melancholy in French literature, see Jacqueline Cerquiglini-Toulet, *La couleur de la mélancolie: La fréquentation des livres au
XIVe siècle, 1300–1415* (Paris: Hatier, 1993).

17. Walter Kaiser, *Praisers of Folly: Erasmus, Rabelais, Shakespeare*
(Cambridge, Mass.: Harvard University Press, 1963).

18. Maria-Luisa Minio-Paluello, *La "Fusta dei Matti": Firenze giugno
1514* (Florence: F. Cesati, 1990), 12.

19. MacDonald, *Mystical Bedlam*, 9; Schleiner, *Melancholy, Genius, and
Utopia*, 17.

20. MacDonald, *Mystical Bedlam*, 10.

21. H. C. Erik Midelfort, *A History of Madness in Sixteenth-Century
Germany* (Stanford, CA: Stanford University Press, 1999).

22. Marsilio Ficino, *De triplici vita*, trans. Carol V. Kaske and John
R. Clark (Binghamton, N.Y.: Medieval & Renaissance Texts & Studies,
1989).

23. See Klibansky, Panofsky, and Saxl, *Saturn and Melancholy*; Mary
Frances Wack, *Lovesickness in the Middle Ages: The Viaticum and Its Com-
mentaries* (Philadelphia: University of Pennsylvania Press, 1990); Brann, *The
Debate over the Origin of Genius*.

24. See Lauro Martines, *Lawyers and Statecraft in Renaissance Florence* (Princeton, N.J.: Princeton University Press, 1968); Andrea Zorzi,
*L'amministrazione della giustizia penale nelle repubblica fiorentina: Aspetti
e problemi* (Florence: Olschki, 1988).

25. There are excellent institutional studies of madness for late medieval and early modern Florence, but they tend to maintain Foucault's framework. See, for example, Graziella Magherini and Vittorio Biotti, *L'isola delle Stinche et i percorsi della follia a Firenze nei secoli XIV–XVIII* (Florence: Ponte alle Grazie, 1992); Vittorio Biotti, ed., *"È matto e tristo, pazzo e fastidioso": I saperi sulla follia, magistrati, medici, e inquisitori a Firenze e negli stati italiani del '600* (Florence: Nicomp, 2002); Graziella Magherini and Vittorio Biotti, "Madness in Florence in the 14th–18th Centuries," *International Journal of Law and Psychiatry* 21, no. 4 (1998): 355–68; Enrico Stumpo, *I bambini innocenti: Storia della Malattia mentale nell'Italia moderna (secoli XVI–XVIII)* (Florence: Le Lettere, 2000).

26. In May 2005 the University of Verona hosted an international conference dedicated to the study of Zacchia and the origins of legal medicine. For the conference proceedings, see Alessandro Pastore and Giovanni Rossi, eds., *Paolo Zacchia alle origini della medicina legale, 1584–1659* (Milan: Franco Angeli, 2008). See also Jacalyn Duffin, "The Doctor Was Surprised; or, How to Diagnose a Miracle," *Bull. Hist. Med.* 81, no. 4 (2007): 699–729.

27. Gianna Pomata, *Contracting a Cure: Patients, Healers, and the Law in Early Modern Bologna* (Baltimore: Johns Hopkins University Press, 1998).

28. Randolph Starn, "The Early Modern Muddle," *Journal of Early Modern History* 6, no. 3 (2002): 296–30.

29. Arundati Roy, *The God of Small Things* (New York: Random House, 2008), 51–52.

30. The most famous and revolutionary of these studies for Italy is David Herlihy and Christiane Klapisch-Zuber, *Tuscans and Their Families: A Study of the Florentine Catasto of 1427* (New Haven, Conn: Yale University Press, 1985).

31. More recent notable studies within this immense literature include Christiane Klapisch-Zuber, *Women, Family, and Ritual in Renaissance Italy*, trans. Lydia G. Cochrane (Chicago: University of Chicago Press, 1985); Thomas Kuehn, *Law, Family, and Women: Toward a Legal Anthropology of Renaissance Italy* (Chicago: University of Chicago Press, 1991); David I. Kertzer and Richard P. Saller, eds., *The Family in Italy from Antiquity to the Present* (New Haven, Conn: Yale University Press, 1991); Joanne M. Ferraro, *Family and Public Life in Brescia, 1580–1650: The Foundations of Power in the Venetian State* (Cambridge: Cambridge University Press, 1993); Giulia Calvi, *Il contratto morale: Madri e figli nella Toscana moderna* (Rome: Laterza, 1994); Anthony Molho, *Marriage Alliance in Late Medieval Florence* (Cambridge, Mass.: Harvard University Press, 1994); Trevor Dean and Kate J. P. Lowe, eds., *Marriage in Italy, 1300–1650* (Cambridge: Cambridge University Press, 1998); Stanley Chojnacki, *Women and Men in Renaissance Venice: Twelve Essays on Patrician Society* (Baltimore: Johns Hopkins University Press, 2000); Anne Jacobson Schutte, Thomas Kuehn, and Silvana Seidel Menchi, eds., *Time, Space, and Women's Lives in Early Modern Europe* (Kirksville, Mo.: Truman State University Press, 2001); Katherine A. Lynch, *Individuals, Families, and Communities in Europe, 1200–1800: The Urban Foundations of Western Society* (Cambridge: Cambridge University

Press, 2003); and Philip Gavitt, *Gender, Honor, and Charity in Late Renaissance Florence* (New York: Cambridge University Press, 2011).

32. Richard Goldthwaite, *Wealth and the Demand for Art in Italy, 1300–1600* (Baltimore: Johns Hopkins University Press, 1993); Carole Collier Frick, *Dressing Renaissance Florence: Families, Fortunes, & Fine Clothing* (Baltimore: Johns Hopkins University Press, 2002); Patricia Fortini Brown, *Private Lives in Renaissance: Venice Art, Architecture, and the Family* (New Haven, Conn.: Yale University Press, 2004); Evelyn Welch, *Shopping in the Renaissance: Consumer Cultures in Italy, 1400–1600* (New Haven, Conn.: Yale University Press, 2005); Jacqueline Marie Musacchio, *Art, Marriage, and Family in the Florentine Renaissance Palace* (New Haven, Conn.: Yale University Press, 2008); Isabelle Chabot, *La dette des familles: Femmes, lignage et patrimoine à Florence aux XIVe et XVe siècles* (Rome: École française de Rome, 2011).

33. Sandra Cavallo, "Secrets to Healthy Living: The Revival of the Preventative Paradigm in Late Renaissance Italy," in *Secrets and Knowledge in Medicine and Science, 1500–1800*, ed. Elaine Leong and Alisha Rankin (Burlington, Vt.: Ashgate, 2011), 191–212.

34. I am grateful to Christiane Klapisch-Zuber for sharing references to mad men or women that she found in *ricordanze*, unfortunately a tiny number. "Memoriale" di Domenico di Simone di Bartolo Cambini, 1458–1477, Innocenti, Estranei 238, fol. 20v: (6 janvier 1466). "Piero d'Angnolo di Berto Cecchi mio chongnato mi preghò che io tenessi in chasa mia la Chaterina sua sirocchia la quale non era sana che aveva manchamento del celabro . . . Stette la Chaterina sopradetta in chasa mia a mie spese circha d'anni tre e mesi, e di poi s'andò a stare chon Berto suo fratello."

35. Thanks to Klapisch-Zuber for also providing this reference. ASF, Acquisti e Doni, 20, fol. 78v, July 18, 1522: "la Agnoletta nostra sorella . . . che lei entrò in casa mia a Nuovoli inferma et pazza . . . perché non habbiamo ragionato del disagio mio che tutto decto tempo non sono mai ito in villa con la mia brigata nè anchora del guastamento della casa che continuamente ha fatto detta Agnoletta suo agio in su uno palcho dove la ho tenuta serrata."

36. Furio Diaz, *Il Granducato di Toscana: I Medici* (Turin: UTET, 1976), 465–524.

37. At the time this book went to press, Mariana Labarca Pinto was preparing a doctoral thesis titled "Madness, Emotions and the Family in 18th-Century Tuscany" at the European University Institute.

38. Antonio Anzilotti, *La Costituzione Interna dello Stato Fiorentino sotto il Duca Cosimo I de' Medici* (Florence: Francesco Lumachi, 1910), 32–35.

39. See Mario Sbriccoli, "Fonti giudiziarie et fonti giuridiche: Riflessioni sulla fase attuale degli studi di storia del crimine e della giustizia criminale," *Studi Storici* 29 (1988): 491–501; Arlette Farge, *Le goût de l'archive* (Paris: Editions du Seuil, 1989); and Trevor Dean, *Crime and Justice in Late Medieval Italy* (Cambridge: Cambridge University Press, 2007).

40. Historians of medieval Europe have long placed the revival of Roman law in the twelfth century in various regions of Italy, especially at Bologna.

See, for example, Hermann Kantorowicz, *Studies in the Glossators of Roman Law: Newly Discovered Writings of the Twelfth Century* (Cambridge: Cambridge University Press, 1938); Helmut Coing, ed., *Handbuch der Quellen und Literatur der neuren Europäischen Privatsrechtsgeschichte*, I (Munich: C. H. Beck, 1973); and Hermann Lange, *Römisches Recht im Mittelalter, I, Die Glossatoren* (Munich: C. H. Beck, 1997). Charles M. Radding has located the revival of Justinianic law even earlier in the eleventh century; see *Origins of Medieval Jurisprudence: Pavia and Bologna, 850–1150* (New Haven, Conn.: Yale University Press, 1988); and Charles M. Radding and Antonio Ciaralli, *The "Corpus Iuris Civilis" in the Middle Ages: Manuscripts and Transmission from the Sixth Century to the Juristic Revival* (Leiden: Brill, 2007). Anders Winroth, in *The Making of Gratian's "Decretum"* (Cambridge: Cambridge University Press, 2000), has argued, however, that the teaching of Roman law developed more slowly than scholars have previously thought. According to his study, the clumsy and imperfect application of Roman law by Gratian, a canonist thought to have been active in Bologna when the study of Roman law was supposedly flourishing, casts doubt on just how sophisticated the grasp of Roman law actually was in the twelfth century. Pivotal to this argument is Winroth's discovery that the *Decretum* was not one book but two. The earlier recension was Gratian's own work, which was later subsumed in a much larger version compiled by Gratian's students. The two recensions reflect different intellectual climates, one in which Roman law had not been thoroughly assimilated and the other in which a technical grasp of Roman law is clear and sophisticated.

41. According to the Roman jurist Paulus, an insane person (*furiosus*) could not obtain possession of property without the authority of his guardian. Although the *furiosus* could touch the property with his body, he was not thought to have the disposition (*affectio*) for holding it. Paulus likened it to placing something in the hand of a person fast asleep. D. 41.2.1.3.

42. D. 50.16.209; D. 50.16.246; D. 50.17.124.1 For language that suggests a synonymous relationship between the *demens* and the *furiosus*, see D. 1.18.14; D. 26.1.3; D. 2710.7.1. For examples of *demens* as distinct from the *furiosus*, see D. 26.5.8.1; C. 5.4.25; C. 5.37.28. Adrien Audibert treats the strict definitions of these terms in his study of madness and prodigality, *Études sur l'histoire du droit romain: La folie et la prodigalité* (Paris: L. Larose & Forcel, 1892). See also Siro Solazzi, *Scritti di Diritto Romano* (Naples: Eugenio Jovene, 1957), 2:623–55.

43. In accord with Aristotle, Bartolus believed the rational component of the human soul operated on two levels that corresponded to two different types of knowledge and their respective objects of knowledge. The speculative form of knowledge (*scientia*) allowed a person to reason in abstract ways about concepts that were universal and necessary. By contrast, the practical form of knowledge (*prudentia*) allowed for the consideration of concrete things that were particular and contingent. Provided that the natural course of these operations was not hindered by defect or disease, human beings were naturally judicious, circumspect, and cautious because they possessed memory, intelligence, experience, aptitude, resourcefulness, foresight, and

skepticism. In other words, human beings could reason about the present, the past, and the future and adjust or change their thinking and acting based on particular experiences. Bart. *De test.*, fol. 160v. This treatise is attributed to Bartolus da Sassoferrato. According to Diplovatatio, however, Baldus maintained that Bartolus died before completing it ("morte preventus incompletum reliquit").

44. Shulamith Shahar, *Growing Old in the Middle Ages: "Winter clothes us in shadow and pain,"* trans. Yael Lotan (London: Routledge, 1997); Catherine J. Kudlick, "Disability History: Why We Need Another 'Other,'" *American Historical Review* 108, no. 3 (June 2003): 763–93; Irina Metzler, *Disability in Medieval Europe: Thinking About Physical Impairment During the High Middle Ages, c. 1100–1400* (London: Routledge, 2006); idem, "Disability in the Middle Ages: Impairment at the Intersection of Historical Inquiry and Disability Studies," *History Compass* 9, no. 1 (2011): 45–60; Cordula Nolte, ed., *Homo debilis: Behinderte, Kranke, Versehrte in der Gesellschaft des Mittelalters* (Korb: Didymos-Verlag, 2009); Sally Crawford and Christina Lee, eds., *Bodies of Knowledge: Cultural Interpretations of Illness and Medicine in Medieval Europe* (Oxford: Archaeopress, 2010); Wendy Turner and Tory Vandeventer Pearman, eds., *The Treatment of Disabled Persons in Medieval Europe: Examining Disability in the Historical, Legal, Literary, Medical, and Religious Discourses of the Middle Ages* (Lampeter: Edwin Mellen Press, 2011); Joshua R. Eyler, ed., *Disability in the Middle Ages: Reconsiderations and Reverberations* (Burlington, Vt.: Ashgate, 2010); Patricia A. Baker, Karine van t'Land, and Han Nijdam, eds., *Medicine and Space: Body, Surroundings and Borders in Antiquity and the Middle Ages* (Leiden: Brill, 2012). See, too, the lecture series, "Disabilities and Abilities in the Middle Ages and the Renaissance," http://cmrs.osu.edu/events/lectureseries/2012–13.cfm (accessed September 1, 2012).

45. Stumpo, *I bambini innocenti.*

46. R. A. Houston encountered the same trend in his study of madness in eighteenth-century Scottish courts.

47. Gavitt, *Gender, Honor, and Charity in Late Renaissance Florence,* chap. 2.

48. Herlihy and Klapisch-Zuber, *Tuscans and Their Families,* xxiii.

CHAPTER 1

1. ASF, MPAP 2276, fol. 6r: "Per informatione del suplicato per Monna Francesca donna fu di Ser Filippo di Lotto con somma reverentia si fa noto a Vostra Eccellenza Illustrissima come epsa narrato havere tenuto a sua spese et governo Francesco di Piergiovanni Banchi oggi d'eta xviiii piu anni per ordine de' Signori Offitiali dei Pupilli quale è mutolo et inpedito di sorte che non parla et non intende cosa alcuna et quale ha tractato come proprio figliuolo."

2. ASF, MPAP 2276, fol. 6r: "Desideria che non potendo fare li fatti sua ne regersi da per se Vostra Eccellenza Illustrissima lo confirmassi sotto la cura et protectione del Magistrato non obstante habbi finito anni xviii et non

si dessi ad altri per che uscendo delle sua mani dubita che presto saria finito per il che habbiamo volsuto intendere Lodovico fratello depso quale per cura tenerlo a suo governo et non ci pare persona molto aproposito per stare per la maggior parte del anno in villa et haver donna et figli et haver più tosto diminuto le sua faculta che altrimenti et per evitare ogni sinistra suspitio atteso che occorendo la morte di detto mentecapto epso Lodovico succederia in [tanti] beni et crediti di monte che rendono 34 o 36 ducati l'anno." This return was roughly equivalent to the annual earnings of an unskilled construction worker. See Richard Goldthwaite, *The Economy of Renaissance Florence* (Baltimore: Johns Hopkins University Press, 2009), 577. For an in-depth discussion of Florentine coinage, see Goldthwaite, "Il sistema monetario fino al 1600: Practica, politica, problematica," in *Studi sulla moneta fiorentina (secoli XIII–XVI)*, ed. Richard A. Goldthwaite and Giulio Mandich (Florence: Olschki, 1994), 9–106.

3. Yan Thomas, "La divisione dei sessi nel diritto romano," in *Storia delle donne in Occidente*, vol. 1, *L'antichità*, ed. P. Schmitt, 117–18. See also Calvi, *Il contratto morale*, 19.

4. ASF, MPAP 2276, fol. 6r: "per evitare ogni sinistra suspitione atteso che occorendo la morte di detto mentecapto epso Lodovico succederia in tanti beni et crediti di monte che rendono 34 o 36 ducati l'anno." Lelio Torelli, the Duke's secretary, ordered the Pupilli to assume his care, "alla cura del Magistrato."

5. Although both the Podestà and the Capitano were initially executive as well as judicial offices—the former established in 1193 as an agent of the Roman emperor and promoter of the power of the urban patriciate, and the latter established around 1250 to represent the interests of the guildsmen— by the late fourteenth and early fifteenth centuries, their spheres of operation were strictly judicial. We will not concern ourselves here with the third foreign rector of Florence, the Executor of the Ordinances of Justice, who typically did not deal with guardianship. See Laura Ikins Stern, *The Criminal Law System of Medieval and Renaissance Florence* (Baltimore: Johns Hopkins University Press, 1994), 33–40 and chap. 6.

6. *Statuti della repubblica fiorentina*, ed. Romolo Caggese, vol. 2, *Statuto del Podestà dell'anno 1325*, ed. Giuliano Pinto, Francesco Salvestrini, and Andrea Zorzi (Florence: Olschki, 1999), 19.

7. D. 26.1.1 pr; C. 5.31.

8. See Thomas Kuehn, "'Cum Consensu Mundualdi' Legal Guardianship of Women in Quattrocento Florence," in *Law, Family, and Women*, 212–37.

9. See D. 26.2.

10. See D. 26.5.

11. Max Kaser, *Römisches Privatrecht: Ein Studienbuch* (Munich: C. H. Beck, 1986), 286–88.

12. I. 1.23.3–4.

13. I. 21.1.

14. D. 26.7.7 pr.

15. See Kaser, *Römisches Privatrecht*, 289–92.

16. I. 25.

17. I. 23.

18. D. 27.19.7 pr.

19. *Statuti della repubblica fiorentina*, book 1, rubric 3, *De officio sex iudicum potestatis*, 19–20. See also rubric 49, *De alimentis*, which says that the Podestà and his judges should ensure that widows, wards, and orphans of both sexes should have basic care (114).

20. Nov. 118.5; Nov. 22.50; Nov. 94.

21. I. 1.13.

22. Nov. 118.5. This new assemblage of law included a codification of the writings of select Roman jurists (*Digesta* or *Pandectae*), a primer for students of the law (*Institutiones*), a collection of extant imperial constitutions from the reign of Hadrian through that of Justinian (*Codex justinianus*), and another collection of new legislation from the period of Justinian (*Novellae Constitutiones*).

23. Nov. 118.5; Nov. 22.50; Nov. 94.

24. See Gigliola di Renzo Villata, *La tutela: Indagini sulla scuola dei glossatori* (Milan: A. Giuffrè, 1975); and idem, "Nota per le storia della tutela nell'italia del rinascimento," in *La famiglia e la vita quotidiana in Europa dal '400 al '600: Fonti e problemi*, Atti del convegno internazionale Milano 1–4 dicembre 1983 (Rome: Ministero per i beni culturali e ambientali, 1986).

25. Cited in Di Renzo Villata, "Nota per le storia della tutela," 59.

26. Sir Edward Coke, *Institutes of the Laws of England, Part 1* (Philadelphia: Robert H. Small, 1853), 88b: "quasi agnem committere lupo ad devorandum."

27. See Di Renzo Villata, "Note per la storia della tutela." See also Calvi, *Il contratto morale*, and Calvi, "Widows, the State, and Guardianship of Children in Early Modern Tuscany," in *Widowhood in Medieval and Early Modern Europe*, ed. Sandra Cavallo and Lyndan Warner (London: Longman, 1999), 213–14.

28. Di Renzo Villata, "Nota per le storia della tutela," 72.

29. The statutes of the Magistrato dei Pupilli e Adulti can be consulted in Francesca Morandini, ed., "Statuti e Ordinamenti dell'Ufficio dei pupilli et adulti nel periodo della Repubblica fiorentina, 1388–1534," *ASI* (1955): 521–51; *ASI* (1956): 92–117; and *ASI* (1957): 87–104. Between 1393 and 1534 additions, adjustments, and reiterations were made in 1429, 1431, 1432, 1442, 1448, 1450, 1466, 1472, 1473, 1477, 1478, 1483, 1487, 1494, 1495, 1496, 1531, 1534. For this citation, see Morandini, "Statuti e Ordinamenti," *ASI* (1955): 529.

30. Caroline M. Fisher, "The State as Surrogate Father: State Guardianship in Renaissance Florence, 1368–1532" (Ph.D. diss., Brandeis University, 2003), 106–7. See also Calvi, *Il contratto morale*, 282–83.

31. Calvi, *Il contratto morale*, 23–24.

32. For discussion of minority and majority in Pupilli statutes, see Morandini, "Statuti e Ordinamenti," *ASI* (1956): 102.

33. ASF, AP 340, fol. 116r: "Ioannis olim Amerighi de Bandis de Florentia fratris carnalis e coniuncti domine Tesse sororis sue et filie olim dicti

Amerighi fatue, dementis, et furiose, pro ipsa domina Tessa est demens, fatua, et furiosa et quod se et sua male gerit et administrat." Tessa's case as well as the cases of Pasqua and Niccolòsa to follow came to my attention through the provocative study of madness in Florence from the fourteenth through the eighteenth century by Magherini and Biotti, *L'isola delle Stinche.*

34. If his surname is not sufficient indication of high status, the records of the Tratte, a list of male citizens eligible for communal or guild offices from 1282 to 1530, show Arnaldo to be a man of influence. His name appears in the electoral bags of the quarter of Santa Maria Novella for the Tre Maggiori, the three highest executive office of the city, from 1351 to 1360. In 1356 he was elected to the council of the Gonfalonieri di Compagnia, in 1357 to the Buonuomini, and in 1358 to the priorate. *Florentine Renaissance Resources*, Online Tratte of Office Holders, 1282–1532. machine readable data file, ed. David Herlihy, R. Burr Litchfield, Anthony Molho, and Roberto Barducci (Providence, R.I.: Florentine Renaissance ResourcesSTG, Brown University, 2002).

35. *Statuti della repubblica fiorentina*, book 1, rubric 3, *De officio sex iudicum potestatis*, 19–20. Compare the language of the 1325 statute: "Et possint licite fieri sequestrationes et extagimenta [sic] et pronuntiari et in eis procedi breviter et summarie et sine strepitu et figura iudicii qualibet die, non obstantibus feriis aliquibus," to that of Giovanni's petition: "predicta quidem fieri potest breviter breviter [sic] et sumarie et sine strepitu et figura iudici omni modo via et iure quibus melius potest."

36. ASF, AP 340, fol. 116r.

37. ASF AP 4210, fols. 16v–17v: "Supradictus dominus iudex ut supra pro tribunali sedum ad suum solit[um] iuris banchum pro iure redendo ut moris est auditum et intelectum exponitum et naratum et coram eo facto per Iustum Nardi Iusti populi Santi Nicholi de florentia nepote Pasque sive domine pasque mentecapte et non sane mentis filie olim francisci bartoli vocate de piazza miniatis ad montem communitatis florentie et sororis domine nicholose matris dicti Iusti qui Iustus coram ipso iudice dixit et exposuit et narravit qualiter ipsa pasqua iam est annus et ultra notorie etiam ex loquelis et gestis suis fuit et est mentecapta et non sane mentis nec intelectu et caruit et caret curator [sic] qui ipsam pasquam et eius bona res et iura et actiones regat gubernat et admminstrat defidat et manteneat et nutriri faciat et alia faciat et observet circa predicta requisit[a] vilia et [uestimenta]."

38. ASF, AP 4210, fol. 17r.

39. ASF, AP 4598, n.p.: "In primis quod dicta Appollonia filia olim Marci Georgii de Moncione iam sunt anni viginti et ultra et ab inde et citra et per totum dictum tempus continue fuit et est demens et mentecapta et sine aliquo sensu saltim rationabili, et ita et taliter sensu caret et impedita est quod rebus suis superesse et intendere non valet nec potest nec fuit vel est compos mentis, nec se ipsam gubernare potuit vel potest sed per totum dictum tempus continue fuit et est sine aliquo sensu rationabili et sine sensu tamquam mentecapta et fatua faciebat et loquebatur et facit et loquitur. Et omni intellectu humano et rationabili caret quemadmodum si esset puella minor quinque d'annorum.

Item quod dicta Appollonia non habet patrem vel avuum vel alterum adscendentem in cuius sit potestate et nullum habet agnatum et maxime ydoneum ad predictam curam. Et ipsa Appollonia est maior etate vigintiquinque d'annorum. Et quod eius pater decessit nullo dato curatore eidem Appollonie." See also ASF, AP 4597, n.p., where the case also appears.

40. Julius Kirshner, *Pursuing Honor While Avoiding Sin: The Monte delle doti of Florence*, Quaderni di Studi Senesi 41 (Milan: A. Giuffrè, 1978); Thomas Kuehn, "Women, Marriage, and *Patria Potestas* in Late Medieval Florence," in *Law, Family, and Women*, 197–211.

41. Julius Kirshner, "Encumbering Private Claims to Public Debt in Renaissance Florence," in *The Growth of the Bank as Institution and the Development of Money-Business Law*, ed. Vito Piergiovanni (Berlin: Duncker & Humblot, 1993), 40.

42. Christiane Klapisch-Zuber, "The 'Cruel Mother': Maternity, Widowhood, and Dowry in Florence in the Fourteenth and Fifteenth Centuries," and "The Griselda Complex: Dowry and Marriage Gifts in the Quattrocento," in *Women, Family, and Ritual in Renaissance Italy*, trans. Cochrane, 117–31, 213–46.

43. For a translation of Morelli's *ricordanze*, see Richard C. Trexler, "In Search of Father: The Experience of Abandonment in the Recollections of Giovanni di Pagolo Morelli," in *Dependence in Context in Renaissance Florence* (Binghamton, N.Y.: Center for Medieval and Early Renaissance Studies, SUNY Binghamton, 1994), 171–202. Trexler also comprehensively analyzes the content of this *ricordanze* in his *Public Life in Renaissance Florence* (Ithaca, N.Y.: Cornell University Press, 1980, 1991), 159–86.

44. ASF, AP 4598, n.p.: "Item quod dictus Cristoforus Antonii Rossi de Molina communis Montirigioni frater uterinus dicte Appollonie fuit et est ydoneus et persona legalis et bone oppinionis vite et fame et ydoneus ad curam regimentum et gubernationem dicte Appollonie."

45. ASF, AP 4598, n.p.: "Ac etiam publicum palam et alta voce in plateis et apud plateas Sancti Johannis Baptiste Orti Sancti Michaelis fori novi et veteris civitatis florentie et ianue et apud ianuam palatii communis florentie residentie domini potestatis civitatis florentie et apud ianuam dicti palatii dimisisse infixam et applicatam cedulam dicte citationis secundum formam statutorum communis Florentie." The statute invoked here came from the 1325 statutes of the Podestà regarding the election and duties of communal heralds or *nuntii*. The *nuntius* was required to promulgate the mandates of the rectors, namely the Podestà, the Capitano, and the Executor of Justice, by going to the house of those to whom requisitions or citations were directed and making known their contents. He was to affix the document (*cedula*) publicly to the door of the house of the people who had been summoned. If they did not have a house or residence in Florence, that is, if they were vagabonds or living outside of the city and district of Florence, then the parties were summoned publicly in the piazzas of San Giovanni Battista, Or' San Michele, and the old and new markets. The *cedula* was affixed to the entrance of the communal palace and was to be left there openly and publicly by the *nuntius* in order to be accessible to all people. See *Statuti della*

repubblica fiorentina, vol. 2, book 1, rubric 12, *De electione nuntiorum communis Florentie officio et securitate*, 41.

46. In the Florentine context, the term "family" meant several things. In the limited sense it referred to a domestic residential unit and therefore the various family relations existing among people living under the same roof. The household could include, for example, the nuclear family of parents and children, the patriarchal family of elderly parents, their grown children, and their minor children, or a joint fraternal family of brothers and their respective families. Among the elite, the term "family" could refer to those who shared surnames and were therefore part of a larger agnatic lineage or patriline limited to the branches who shared descent from a common ancestor. Within this group, sometimes referred to as the *casa* or *consorterie*, there could be a deep sense of solidarity as well as social recognition and a group identity. Florentines also acknowledged the importance of cognatic and affinal kin. See Francis William Kent, *Household and Lineage in Renaissance Florence: The Family Life of the Capponi, Ginori, and Rucellai* (Princeton, N.J.: Princeton University Press, 1977).

47. See Julius Kirshner, "Storm over the 'Monte Comune': Genesis of the Moral Controversy over the Public Debt of Florence," *Archivum Fratrum Praedicatorum* 53 (1983): 219–76. For a comprehensive bibliography, see Lawrin Armstrong, *Usury and Public Debt in Early Renaissance Florence: Lorenzo Ridolfi on the "Monte Comune"* (Toronto: Pontifical Institute of Medieval Studies, 2003), 28n1.

48. Caroline M. Fisher has conducted an in-depth study of this magistracy from its first incarnations in the mid-fourteenth century until the creation of the Florentine duchy in 1530. See Fisher, "Guardianship and the Rise of the Florentine State, 1368–93," in *Famiglie e poteri in Italia tra medioevo ed età moderna*, ed. Anna Bellavitis and Isabelle Chabot (Rome: École française de Rome, 2009), 265–67. Similarly, Giulia Calvi has mined the records of the Pupilli to explore the contours of female empowerment strategies in Tuscan society. See Calvi, *Il contratto morale* and Calvi, "Widowhood and Remarriage in Tuscany," in *Marriage in Italy, 1300–1650*, ed. Trevor Dean and Kate J. P. Lowe (Cambridge: Cambridge University Press, 1998), 275–96.

49. Caroline M. Fisher argues in "The State as Surrogate Father" and "Guardianship and the Rise of the Florentine State" that despite increasing government involvement in the private and public lives of Florentines through the creation of magistracies dedicated to uncovering political conspiracy, regulating prostitution, forbidding sodomy, and helping families provide dowries for their daughters, the creation of the Pupilli actually shows the government's resistance to taking on the guardianship of orphans, seeing it first and foremost as a familial obligation.

50. Morandini, "Statuti e Ordinamenti," *ASI* (1955).

51. Ibid., 535. See also Anthony Molho, "The State and Public Finance," in *The Origins of the State in Italy, 1300–1600*, ed. Julius Kirshner (Chicago: University of Chicago Press, 1995), 115; and Molho, *Marriage Alliance in Late Medieval Florence*, 39.

52. Julius Kirshner, "The State Is 'Back In," in *The Origins of the State in Italy*, ed. Kirshner, 8.

53. Molho, "The State and Public Finance," 113–14.

54. Fisher, "The State as Surrogate Father," 308–19.

55. Ibid., 190–99, 258–63, 375. See also Calvi, *Il contratto morale*.

56. Fisher, "The State as Surrogate Father."

57. Morandini, "Statuti e Ordinamenti," *ASI* (1956): 97–98. See also a reiteration of this statute in ASF, MPAP 2279, fol. 470rv.

58. ASF, MPAP, 2281, fol. 668rv: "sono 14 anni in circa che more detto Francesco lasciati due suoi figliuoli Jacopo minore oggi in età d'anni 34 et Pandolfo altro maggiore et per che questo Jacopo è assai bene scemo di cervello, et non ha saputo mai ne sa fare i fatti suoi, è stato governato sempre et è dal detto Pandolfo suo fratello il quale l'ha sempre molto mal trattato. Però la supplicante madre dell'uno et dell'altro per sgravio della sua conscientia, visto il mal procedere di Pandolfo et dubitando che doppo la sua morte non sia mal trattato, et sia constretta andar accattando o capitar male suplica V.A.S. che le piaccia farle gratia che detto Jacopo sia ricevuto sotto la cura et governo del Magistrato nostro et facci render i conti à Pandolfo et restituirli quel che habbi in mano di suo et provederli per l'avenire secondo il bisogno suo come nella sua suplica sopra la quale la supplicante produce piu fedi de' parenti del mal essere et necessità di detto Jacopo et del mal governo di Pandolfo et così vecchia come ell'è, è venuta in persona avanti il Magistrato a esporre il bisogno di questo suo povero figliuolo et il mal governo di detto Pandolfo. Il qual citato confessa che detto Jacopo suo fratello è di non sana mente et ha bisogno di chi lo governa, et nell'altro cose va fuggendo rendere i conti et dare il suo a detto suo fratello; Noi crederemo per quanto habbiamo visto et inteso che fussi bene che questo Jacopo mentecatto fussi posto sotto la cura del Magistrato, si rivedessero i conti à Pandolfo et si provedesse che detto suo fratelli havessi quello che seli perviene et fussi custodito tanto nella sua persona [668v] quanto ne suoi beni, accio che col suo potessi vivere quietamente. [Reply] il Magistrato ne pigli la cura lui."

59. ASF, MPAP 2277, fol. 237r: "hoggi d'anni 30 ma debile di cervello et impedito del parllare di sorte che ha bisogno di reggimento et la madre per trovarsi vechia et inferma non puo piu aiutarllo [Reply] Concedesseli."

60. ASF, MPAP 2274, fols. 230v–231v: "uno Stefano suo fratello è in modo vexato da humori maninconici che il più del tempo [fol. 231r] lo cavano del cervello et percio lo ha messo nello spedale di Santo Pagolo col quale saria d'acordo di conmetterlo dandoli lo subsidio et faculta depso Stefano et per non ci essere persona habile a fare tale conventione et rescuorere et pagare per fare quello occorressi desierria che per v. Excellentissima fussi commesso del Magistrato dei pupilli o chi altri paressi a V. Excellentissima . . . non havendo epso Stefano altri che detto suplicante suo fratello e religioso quale non puo attendere alla cura . . . è necesso che Vostra Excellentissima li provegha commettere decto Stefano sotto la cura del Magistrato dei Pupilli o dare autorita al altro che in nome depso si possa riscuorere pagare et fare tale commisso in decto spedale di santo pagolo o in altro luogo

dove si pensera sia per stare bene et essere bene trattato. [Reply] Il Magistrato ci provegga come gli parra che stia meglio."

61. For communications about this estate, see ASF, MPAP 2654, fol. 607r. For the formal inventory in the Pupilli records, see ASF, MPAP 2712, fols. 193v–196v. For a genealogy of the Passerini family, see Luigi Passerini, *Storia e genealogia delle famiglie Passerini e De' Rilli* (Florence: M. Cellini, 1874), 35–37 and Table IV.

62. ASF, MPAP 2654, fols. 603r–614v.

63. ASF, MPAP 2279, fol. 506r: "Fulvio et Valerio figli del Capitano Niccolò Passerini da Cortona supplicono Vostra Altezza Serenissima che Girolamo uno dei figli di detto Capitano ben che maggior d'anni 18 per gratia di Vostra Altezza Serenissima sia sotto posto come mentecatto alla cura et protectione del magistrato nostro come nella loro supplica. Per informatione della quale con ogni riverentia le diciamo che et li supplici suoi fratelli et il Prior Silvio altro loro fratello desiderano questa gratia essendo detto Girolamo inhabile et havendo bisogno di curatore non solo circa la sua persona ma circa le facultà. [Reply] Veggasi prima bene, se è veramente inhabile, o non."

64. ASF, MPAP 2279, fol. 506r: "non havendo possuto parlarli per essere riserrato dalli fratelli come mentecatto in una stanza d'un lor palazzo lontano da Cortona."

65. ASF, MPAP 2279, fol. 506r: "quali lo trovarne riserrato solo in detto palazzo et facendo aprire l'uscio et parlandogli di varie cose stette sempre spaventato tremandolo di continuo le mani et parlando quasi forzato; et se bene per allora non fece alcuno segno di pazzo, per quanto potessero conoscere referirne haverlo trovato del tutto inhabile al governo di se stesso et dette sue substantie; per esser balordo et insensato; et tutto riferiscano essere proceduto da humori malenconici non sendo per l'adietro stato tale et che è d'eta d'anni 24 in circa. [Reply] Concedessi."

66. ASF, MPAP, 2654, fol. 592r.

67. See Salvator Battaglia, *Grande dizionario della lingua italiana*, vols. 4 and 10 (Turin: Unione tipografico-editrice torinese, 1961–2008).

68. ASF, MPAP 2280, fol. 32r: "Però oggi supplicono unitamente V.A. che si degni far Loro gratia di confirmare l'elettione dalla supplicata fatta del detto Signore Montino et commettere al Magistrato nostro che l'accetti, et elegga per attore; et curatore della persona del detto Signore Girolamo. Al Magistrato non occorre altro, dependendo questo dalle mera gratia et volontà di V.A. se non mertterle in considerate che piacendole far Loro la gratia che domandano; saria bene come ricercano gli ordini del Magistrato nostro che desse idonea sicurtà in Firenze di render buon conto di sua amministratione al Magistrato come son soliti li altri attori."

69. ASF, MPAP 2280, fol. 60r: "il Signore Montino Lor zio de Marchesi del Monte Santa Maria fusse attore et governatore della personal del Ser Girolamo uno delli figli del detto Signore Niccolò sottoposto alla cura del Magistrato nostro come mentecatto; per gratia di V.A.S. purche detto Ser Montino desse idonea sicurtà in Firenze di rendere buon conto di sua amminstratione al Magistrato come sono soliti li altri attori."

70. ASF, MPAP, 2280, fol. 60r: "detto ser Montino offerisce per mallevadore il ser Pirro uno de figli et heredi del detto Ser Niccolò Passerini et fratello carnale del detto Ser Girolamo, dependendo questa attoria dalla gratia di V.A. il Magistrato non si è risoluto ad accettarlo ne repudiarlo senza il beneplacito che quella; col metterle in consideratione che sono questi fratelli una medesima cosa. [Reply] Non pare ragionevole."

71. ASF, MPAP 2280, fol. 103r: "Il Signore Montino de Marchesi del Monte Santa Maria; supplica V.A.S. che la si degni farli gratia di commettere al Magistrato nostro che si contente che dia sicurtà idonea à Cortona secondo il solito delli altri attori essendo stato eletto attore del Signore Girolamo Passerini da Cortona suo nipote mediante la gratia fatta da V. Alt. per il Magistrato nostro sotto la cura del quale detto Ser Girolamo si retrova. Noi per informatione con ogni riverentia le diciamo che il Magistrato gli ha fatto difficultà di pigliare questa sicurtà in Cortona perche la gratia fatta che di poter esser attora era conditionata dando la sicurtà in Firenze et non poteva il Magistrato senza la gratia di V. A. alterare il suo rescritto. [Reply] Concedessi."

72. ASF, MPAP 2280, fol. 190r: "Hoggi il Magistrato nostro ha aviso dal Comune di Cortona che le cose del detto Signore Girolamo vanno male."

73. ASF, MPAP 2280, fol. 190r: "à principio fu fatto attore il Cavalier suo fratello et dovendo detto Cavalier andare à Roma in servitio del Illustrissimo et reverensissimo Cardinal de Medici renuntio questa attoria benche non habbia mai reso conto di sua aministratione."

74. The Pupilli tried to remedy this situation by having an inventory of his holdings made in May 1581. The record states in brief that he had a house in Cortona of unspecified worth.

75. ASF, MPAP 2281, fol. 125r. Gondi's debt is mentioned in the 1579 arbitration as well in ASF, MPAP 2654, fols. 604v, 610v.

76. Passerini, *Storia e genealogia*, 35–37, Tables IV and V.

77. ASF, MPAP 2278, fol. 134r: "Per informatione del supplicato per Jacopo di Bartolomeo Barbelli quale desideria nella sua prece ottener per gratia da Vostra Altezza che Antonio suo fratello fussi messo sotto la cura et protectione del Magsitrato nostro come di non sana mente per la infermita incurabile che tiene adosso quale lo chava del sentimento come ne produce certe fede in questo alligate . . . bene diciamo a quello che per non havere alcuno attinente se non il supplicate quale dice non posser attender alli negotii occureli alla giornata. Le faculta di epso Antonio et maxime li mobili portano grande pericolo per havessi assidare di servitori . . . in grave danno suo et delli creditori che vi pretendessino interesse. [Reply] Habbine cura loro medesimi."

78. ASF, MPAP 2280, fol. 33r: "Filippo di Francesco Martelli espone all'A.V. come doppo la morte di monna Margherita sua madre quale teneva conto di lui et delle sue facultà è stato alla custodia di Andrea et Giovanni Martelli suoi fratelli come quello che è inhabile à governarsi da se stesso; mediante una ferita che li fù data nel capo che li impedi la memoria: et perche li pare esser mal trattato da questi suoi fratelli si inalimentarlo et investirlo; Supplica V.A.S. si degni farli gratia che sia accettato sotto la cura del

Magistrato nostro; et datoli uno attore che tenga conto di lui et delle sue
facultà si come nella sua supplica. Noi per informazione habbiamo inteso
li detti Andrea et Giovanni; quali dettero intentione d'accomodare questo
negotio amichevolmente ma da Novembre in qua che esso Filippo supplicò
s'è aspettato se seguiva concordia alcuna infra detto fratelli; ma poi che non
è seguita; et il supplicato ha fatto piu volte instantia per l'infomazione Le
diciamo con ogni riverentia che per l'aspetto suo et per quanto si vede dalli
vestimenti et dal parlare non è troppo ben trattato da fratelli et ha bisogno
che qualch'uno ne tenga cura particolare insieme con le sue facultà. [Reply]
Il Magistrato ne pigli la cura et provegga col suo a suoi bisogni."

79. ASF, MPAP 2280, fol. 33r: "ma da Novembre in qua che esso Filippo
supplicò s'è aspettato se seguiva concordia alcuna infra detto fratelli; ma poi
che non è seguita; et il supplicato ha fatto piu volte instantia per l'infomazione Le diciamo con ogni riverentia che per l'aspetto suo et per quanto si
vede dalli vestimenti et dal parlare non è troppo ben trattato da fratelli et ha
bisogno che qualch'uno ne tenga cura particolare insieme con le sue facultà.
[Reply] Il Magistrato ne pigli la cura et provegga col suo a suoi bisogni."

80. ASF, MPAP 1580, fol. 9r: "Monna Maria vedova et donna gia d'A-
lamanno Martelli essendo in età d'anni settanta et trovandosi un figliuolo
chiamato Francesco d'età d'anni 52 mentecatto sotto posto alla cura del
Magistrato nostro et del quale ella è stata et è attrice et governatrice;
dubitando che doppo la sua morte detto suo figliuolo [non: scribbled out]
sia per venire al governo di qualch'uno che lo trattasse male, e volendo
provedere in vita sua all'indemnità, cura et governo del figliuolo supplica
v.a. che si degni per gratia commettere al magistrato nostro o ad altri à
chi piu Le piace per la promisione et qualche buono ordine sopra questo negotio come nella sua supplica. Noi per informazione Le diciamo
che habbiamo havuto à noi la donna supplicata la quale dichiarando la
sua supplica dice che desidera si desse questa cura a Francesco di Lapo
Vespucci cugino di esso mentecatto et nipote della supplicante huomo
d'età circa 45 anni con conditione che potesse godere et usufruttare i beni
che essa supplicante gode con carico di tenere al servitio del mentecatto
due serve et un servitore et provederlo di vitto et di vestito et d'ogni altra
cosa necessaria durante la sua vita. [Reply] Concedessi con le condizioni
sopradette."

81. For a copy of Sigismondo's will, see ASF, Martelli B 232, no. 14, fols.
20r–21r, 114r–115v, 304v–305r.

82. John Najemy, *A History of Florence, 1200–1575* (Malden, Mass.:
Blackwell, 2006), 313.

83. For historical information on the Martelli including Vasari's comment
about Roberto, see Alessandra Civai, *Dipinti e sculture in casa Martelli:
Storia di una collezione patrizia fiorentina dal Quattrocento all'Ottocento*
(Florence: Opus Libri, 1990).

84. Ugolino di Niccolò Martelli, *Ricordanze dal 1433 al 1483*, ed. Fulvio
Pezzarossa (Rome: Edizioni di Storia e Letteratura, 1989), 166–72, 174–79,
211, 261–62, 271–72; Civai, *Dipinti e sculture in casa Martelli*, 37.

85. ASF, Martelli B 232 10, fol. 111r.

86. ASF, Martelli B 232 14, fol. 304v.

87. ASF, Martelli B 232 14, fol. 115r: "detto Alessandro suo figliolo et da lei come di sopra herede instituto in quantita certa a star tacito et contento alla parte et protione di sopre assegnatali et a non molestare et inquietare detti altri suoi fratelli per conto della heredita di detta testatrice o altre delle cagioni soprascritte." There are copies of this will at fols. 20rv and 304rv.

88. ASF, Martelli B 232 14, fols. 2r, 115v. According to the census of 1561, the Martelli rented the entire property at Canto alla Paglia for eighty scudi a year. In other words, they would have had to pay Maria Corsi roughly a third of what the property was worth on the rental market.

89. I extend special thanks to Colin Rose and the DECIMA Project at the University of Toronto for supplying all data pertaining to the Martelli from the 1561 census records.

90. ASF, Martelli 232, B 27, fol. 23r.

91. ASF, Martelli 232, B 27, fol. 26v.

92. ASF, Martelli 232, B 27, fol. 27r.

93. ASF, Martelli 232, B 27, fol. 27v.

94. ASF, Martelli 232, B 27, fols. 28r, 29r.

95. ASF, Martelli 232, B 27, fol. 28rv.

96. ASF, Martelli 232, B 27, fol. 29r.

97. ASF, Martelli 232, B 27, fols. 29v–30r: "la cura delli predetti vengha et venire vole nelli Spetiali Signori de Pupilli della Citta di Firenze per li tempi esisenti li quali detta testatrice prega per l'amor [30r] di Dio che si degnino di pigliare la protettione tutela et cura di tali poveri impediti et de loro beni et faculta facendo l'uno et l'altro delle loro facultà custodire et governare come parra loro a proposito perche confidata nelle prudenza et bonta di quelli Signori non vuole dar loro alcuna regola o ordine particulare prohibendo pero per espresso in perpetuo che mai Alessandro suo figliolo non possa havere ne possa cercare o gli possa etiam Dio essere data da detto magistrato la tutela et cura di detti Lorenzo et Filippo o di alcuno di loro o di loro beni perche in fatto non vuole che venghino sotto sua cura. Et se detto Andrea o Giovanni fussino negligenti o (il che non crede) non usassero verso detti poveri loro fratelli impediti quella cura che si conviene et al manco come Andrea ha fatto insino a hora di che se non faranno si debba stare alla dichiaratione di detti Signori Offitiali de Pupilli."

98. ASF, Martelli B 232 39, fol. 373r.

99. The record specifies that each of these fiorini was equal to seven lire.

100. ASF, MPAP 2281, no. 416, fol. 981rv: "allegando parte de beni [981v] del mentecatto esser lasciateli dalla madre et esser grave peso il custodire un mentecatto."

101. ASF MPAP 2281, no. 416, fol. 981v: "Li sono piu prossimi et li succedano, et non par loro ragionevole che quello che s'avanzi delle sue entrate l'habbi a godere et guadagnare il Vespucci in pregiuditio loro . . . per concludano che non deve esser udito il Vespucci come estraneo nella sua domanda ma lore come piu prossimi et della famiglia de Martelli al detto mentecatto, sebene il Vespucci contradice et insta per la confirmatione del rescritto con la dichiaratione che domando; atteso la mente della madre del mentecatto et

le fatiche sue da durarsi nella custodia di quello. [Reply] Al Granduca pare molto piu conveniente che questo mentecatto sera a custodia di questi Martelli et il Magistrato [tenga] conto che sia bene trattato conforme alle cose."

102. ASF, Martelli B 232 39, fol. 432r.

103. ASF, Martelli B 232 39, fol. 433r.

104. ASF, Martelli B 232 39, fol. 459r: "Prima che si dichiari il detto Francesco Martelli non dovere ne potere essere altrimenti attore di Filippo ne continuare nella sua attoria et governo et questo non solo perche di ragione il pupillo o adulto non deve essere alimentato ne ritenuto da chi et appresso a chi le succede ma ancora per che il detto Filippo e assai mal trattato et mal governato et Filippo stesso si chiama malsadisfatto da detto Francesco et altra volta e stato dichiarato che detto Francesco non possa ritenere appresso di se detto Filippo et prohibito expressamente nel testamento di Monna Margherita loro avola paterna. Et se avanti detto Francesco fussi deputato in attore e in governo di detto Filippo fusse venuto a notitia di detto comparente in detti nomi che egli cercava di essere fatto attore e deputato al governo di detto Filippo si sarebbe comparso a dire et opporre le medesime cose et perche e stato creato senza citare nessuno et non puo essere come di sopra si e detto si domanda che questa cura et governo di Filippo si dia a una terza persona non interessato et idonea."

105. ASF, Martelli B 232 39, fol. 454r.

CHAPTER 2

ASF, OGP 2229, fol. 159rvr: "Hora Signore nostro felicissimo e clementissimo sono tanti i benefitii che io hauto da quella in questi miei affanni che non so quale altra persona piu di me gli sia obbligata, et massime che con l'aiuto suo, mi pare che dove havevo una insensata per donna, adesso haverla sana di mente et d'intelletto, che certamente quel suo si crudele accidente venne che parturendo non si attese, et in corse in quelle crudele furori al presente ne stiamo in buona speranza mai piu habbi a fare un'errore; et mosso da questa speranza fondata in la gratia di Idio. Vorrei piacendo a V.E.I. lei mi fussi liberamente restituita, che la potessi menare a casa mia Dando sicurtà allo offitio de Magnifici Signori Otto, che lei non offendera persona et se questo offerò dalla clementia di quella mi parrà uscire d'uno inferno, et consumamento di spese, et desagi."

1. ASF, MS 1121, no. 332 specifies that Monna Piera "was confined in the Stinche in perpetuity *per pazzo* for having in her *pazzia* killed one of her daughters of seven and a young boy of four."

2. ASF, OGP 2226, fol. 386r: "La decta Monna Piera la paza; et fu messa nelle Stinche di Maggio passato 1550, per haver morti due sua figlioli piccoli con una accetta, et se non era tenuta ne amazava un altro."

3. Guy Geltner, *The Medieval Prison: A Social History* (Princeton, N.J.: Princeton University Press, 2008), 65.

4. Ibid., 20, 40–44.

5. ASF, MS 1121, no. 332.

6. ASF, OGP 2226, fol. 386r: "Pagolo di Benedetto da Falla vicariato di Anghiari havendo in le carcere delle Stinche della citta di Firenze una Monna Piera sua donna oltre di tempo et non molta sana di cervello ma non furiosa . . . per l'amor di Dio farli gratia di permutarli tal confino in casa del detto suo marito col dare sicurta dell'osservantia overo permutargliene in una stanza di tal sua casa da murarsi et serrata tenersi . . . et dar malleva-dore dell'osservantia: accio la possa nutrire et far governare. [Duke's reply] stia pur nelle Stinche."

7. ASF, OGP 2227, fol. 172r: "hora decta sua donna è quasi guarita come ne da segno il recordarse del delicto per lei comesso et di cui assai pentirsi e dolersi et perche a cora esso supplicante è aggravato assai dalla famiglia et non puo tal spesa soportare pero humilmente supplica V.E. si degni conce-derli decta sua donna accio la rimeni a casa sua et fugga tal spesa et non sia causa che li suoi figliuoli vadino attaccando offerendosi dare sufficienti mal-levadori di tenerla con bona custodia. [Duke's reply] Stia la et non propone gratia piu a S.V."

8. ASF, OGP 2228, fol. 495r.

9. ASF, OGP 2229, fol. 124r and following unnumbered: "si offerisce parato dare mallevadori che lei non fara male alcuno o se gli piace la mette-ranno in Arezzo in un monasterio dove lei ha una figliuola et non si conten-tando V.I.E. delle dette cose, lui promette tenerla serrata in una stantia dove almanco la potra governare et lei sara pure contenta di vedere alcuna volta li fligiuoli, il marito et altri suoi parenti ne sara causa di vivere disperata come sta in dette carcere."

10. ASF, OGP 2229, recto following fol. 124r: "la decta Madonna Piera due anni continui stette come insensata et balorda tal che ognuno la giudi-cava mentecatta per che non parlava a nessuno et schifava er sfuggirva ogni conversatione cosi di donne come d'altre persone . . . vivendo come frenetica, et da decti due anni in qua troviamo è ogni di megliorata di tal frenesia in modo che oggi quanti ritra questo luogho che la praticono l'hanno per tor-nata bene in cervello et che la parla a proposito et se alcuno gli raprresenta il delitto per che e in carcere non si ricorda haver mai fatto tal cosa, ma si vuole della sua misera sorte et ogni ora si ricorda del suo marito de figliuoli et de parenti piangendo et lamentandosi con chi gli parla non dimeno fila lavora et sa vita [n]e sta ociosa o sonnolenta et sopratutto dicono queste guardie che l'è molto costumata di bocca et che quando alcuna meretrice di quelle che la entro sono incarcerate dicono alcuna cosa disonesta le riprende et exortale ad esser costumate et a lavorare et a far bene."

11. ASF, OGP 2229, fol. 159rvr.

12. ASF, OGP 2230, fol. 479r: "detto exponente ottene gratia di cavarla [Francesca] delle Stinche et menarsela a casa, dove è stata mesi venti senza uscirne mai, ne in detto tempo ha fatto pazzia alcuna, talche al tutto è ritor-nata et guarita, Pero detto exponente ricorre alli piedi di Vostra Illustrissima Eccellenza quella humilmente supplicando si degni per sua innata bonta farli gratia che detta sua donna possa uscire di detta casa per andare alla messa et altre sua faccende sendo lei del tutto guarita et tornata in cervello. [Duke's reply] Possa."

13. See Dean, *Crime and Justice in Late Medieval Italy*; Susanna Burghartz, *Leib, Ehre, und Gut: Delinquenz in Zürich Ende des 14 Jahrhunderts* (Zurich: Chronos, 1990); Peter King, *Crime, Justice and Discretion in England, 1740–1820* (Oxford: Oxford University Press, 2000); Herman Roodenburg, "Social Control Viewed from Below: New Perspectives," in *Social Control in Europe, 1500–1800*, ed. Herman Roodenburg and Pieter Spierenburg (Columbus: Ohio State University Press, 2004), 1:145–58; and, in the same volume, Martin Dinges, "The Uses of Justice as a Form of Social Control in Early Modern Europe," 1:159–75.

14. D. 1.18.14.

15. D. 48.12.

16. D. 1.18.14; D. 9.2.5.2.

17. D. 9.2.5.2.

18. D. 1.18.14.

19. Dean, *Crime and Justice in Late Medieval Italy*, 18; Laura Ikins Stern, "Inquisition Procedure and Crime in Early Fifteenth-Century Florence," *Law and History Review* 8, no. 2 (1990): 297–308; idem, *The Criminal Law System of Medieval and Renaissance Florence*.

20. For the pursuit of enmity in medieval courts, see Daniel Lord Smail, *The Consumption of Justice: Emotions, Publicity, and Legal Culture in Marseille, 1264–1423* (Ithaca, N.Y.: Cornell University Press, 2003).

21. John Henderson, *The Renaissance Hospital: Healing the Body and Healing the Soul* (New Haven, Conn.: Yale University Press, 2006), 313.

22. John K. Brackett, *Criminal Justice and Crime in Late Renaissance Florence, 1537–1609* (Cambridge: Cambridge University Press, 1992).

23. Ibid., 42.

24. Geltner, *The Medieval Prison*, 50–51.

25. Ibid., 17; Brackett, *Criminal Justice*, 47.

26. ASF, GA 98, fols. 15r–16v.

27. ASF, GA 98, fol. 15rv: "Margaritam uxorem Lotti habitantis in Porta Fugia in terra Prati de sancte florentie mulierem insanam furiosam et incendrariam male conditionis vite et fame contra quam per modum et viam et formam inquistionis ex nostro nostreque curie offitio arbitio et Ballia [formatis] processimus. . . . Quod de anno presenti [1406] et mensi octobre prout parte ipsa Margarita in suo solito furore et insania existente eundo de nocte cum quadam sua lucerna quam habebat in manum. Iniit et adcessit ad domus donne mee uxore Stefani de Prato et dictam monnam meam lumen petiit et tunc dicta monna mea dicte Margarite hostium apperuit et eidem de limine dedit in lucerna dicte Margarite dicendo dicte Margarite 'que ora è questa perchè non mandate Lotto per lume senza venire tu?' Et tunc ipsa Margartia respondit, 'Esso non viene perchè ad paura della familgla.' Dicendo dicta Margarita dicte monne mee 'que ora bene?' Et ipsa respondit 'elgle ad presso a die.' Item dicta monna mea, 'Elgle da cinque a stii hore di nocte et subicto cum inde?' dicta Margarita vellet recedere. Dixit dicta monna mea eidem Margarite, 'va sana et [sanamente] che tu non faccie danno perche se dice che dell'anno passato et del mensis di Dicembre del dicto anno metesti fuoco nelle case et nella stalla di Lionardo.'"

28. ASF, GA 98, fol. 15v: "Et immediate post predictam dicta Margarita veniende versus domum suam et transiret ante domus Stefanii Tomasini fornarii de sancto Nicolao di Prato in loco ubi dicitur el forno delle monnache di sancto Nicolao predicto vidit [. . .] dicti fornarii appertam et subicto intravit dictam scipam causa accipiendis lingna et cannaplos per faciendi ingne cum rediret ad domum cause se calofaciendis cum tunc haberet frigus et cum acciperet dictam lingnam et cannaplos causa predictam et haberet dictam lucernam adcensam in manum et ingnis adcensus in dictis cannaplis existente in dicta stipa culpa et defectu dicte Margarite sicut dementis et cum vellet extinguere dictos cannaplos et ingnem sic in dictos cannapulos adcensusm et non posse."

29. ASF, GA 98, fols. 15v–6r: "Item in eo de eo et super eo quod de anno presenti et mensis Octobris predicta dicta Margarita tanquam insana demens et furiosa cum dicto suo furore dementia et insania pervenit de terra Prati ad villam seu castrum Tizzani contadi Pistri nocte tempore et adcessit ad domum Andree Thomasii di Tizzano . . . et petiit ut apperiret sibi domus ut posse ibi stare illa nocte. Et tunc uxor dicti Andree que erat in dicta domo dixit, 'Non ti volglo adprire che tu sei la pierazza pazza di Firenze che vai mettendo fuoco nei palglaia.' Et tunc dicta Margarita respondit cum furore verborum exclamando, 'Io non so la pierazza pazza anche io so la Magarita di Prato madre dela cuita che sta in casa di monna Ciosa apprime che io mi volglo scaldare.' Et tunc uxor dicti Andree respondit et dixit '[6r]va et scaldati che qui non ti volglo apperire che tu sei una pazza et non volglo pazze in casa.'"

30. ASF, GA 98, fols. 15v–16v.

31. ASF, AP 2605, fol. 6r: "clarum notorium et manisfestum sit quod tempore dicti conmissi homicidii sive paricidii et satis ante et postea dictus Anastaxius fuit erat et hodie est furiosus et maximum furore adstractus et adeo quod de fure eximitur et eximiretur apena tamen it in simile nefas amplius re adiurare non valeat et ut in corpis suum penam luat."

32. ASF, AP 2605, fols. 5v–6r.

33. ASF, PR 119, fols. 100r–v.

34. ASF, PR 119, fol. 100v: "Quod etiam absque aliqua fide vel probatione depredictis vel preditorum aliquo facienda seu aliter requisita seu alia solepnitate servanda dictus Anastasius in die sesti nativitatis beati Iohannis batipste que erit dies vigesima quarta presentis mensis iunii possit et debeat offerri ad ecclesiam sancti Iohannis batipste in civitate florentie et in ore solito duci capite discoperto et cum torchietto in manibus et horis consuetis et cum tubis precedentibus ad oblationem publicam et maxime per benedictum de morellis qui carceratis dicitur deservare."

35. Geltner, *The Medieval Prison*, 77–79; Brackett, *Criminal Justice*, 43, 54.

36. ASF, AP 1652, fols. 2r–13v.

37. ASF, AP 1652, fols. 2r, 4r, 5v, 10r: "Suo iuramento testificando dixit se tantum scire de contentis et dicto articulo videlicet quod Blaxius in dicto capitulo nominatus iam sunt xviii mensis et ultra et a dicto tempore citra et per ipsum tempus et ultra fuit et hodie est notorie furiosus et insanus, et in furore continuo constitutus et extra omnem bonam memoriam."

38. ASF, AP 1652, fols. 4r, 5v: "Super secundo articulo quod incipit item quod inter etc. Suo iura[men]to dixit se tantum scire videlicet quod dum dictus Blaxius sparsisset pecuniam prout dici audivit tunc vidit eum tamquam insanum super dicta platea fortiter exclamare 'chi vole venire a ciurmare?'"

39. ASF, AP 1652, fol. 2r: "Respondit quod nunc sunt xviii mensis vel circa quod dictus Blaxius quod tamquam furiosus et insanus propter actus quos exercebat Messer Antonio Phylippi Cronetti Bastagni tunc temporis potestatis dicte terre prati per matrem et alios et actinentes incarceratus fuit et in conpedibus ferreis et ligneis alligatus in quibus a dicto tempore citra continuo permansit exceptis quibusdam vicibus et diebus quibus fregit catenas vincula [. . .] et eximit." See also fols. 4r, 5v, 10r.

40. ASF, AP 1652, fol. 3r: "Super octavo qui incipit item quod postea etc. Suo iura[men]to testificando dixit se tantum scire videlicet quod dum dictus Blaxius stetisset per plures menses sic inceppatus et ferratus prout supra super quodam solaro in quadam camera vidit eum deduci in quadam camera terrena et ibi stabat ligatus ad quadam catenam ferream secundum cippis prout faciunt canes."

41. ASF, AP 1652, fol. 4v: "Super otavo qui incipit item quod postea etc. Suo iura[men]to testificando dixit se tantum scire videlicet quod immediate postea vidit dictum Blaxium furiosum et in alienatione mentis constitutum extrahi de supradictis cippis et incatenari cum quadam catena ferrea et sic incatenatus teneri in quadam camera terrena per plures menses."

42. ASF, AP 1652, fol. 5r.

43. ASF, AP 1652, fol. 4v.

44. ASF, AP 1652, fol. 6r: "Super octavo qui incipit item quod postea etc. Suo iura[men]to dixit quod dum dictus Blaxius sic fuisset detemptus et ferratus prout supra vidit eum reduci in quandam cavernam terrenam et ibi fuit ligatus cum quadam catina ferrea ad quam catenam stetit per sex menses vel circa et quodam semel dum sic staret ligatus posuit ignem in sacchone super quo dormiebat et nisi fuisset gentes qui traxerunt et cum securibus hostium camera fregerunt se et domum conbursisset tamquam furiosus qui nesciebat quid faceret.Interrogatus quomodo scit dixit quia vidit et fuit unius ex illis qui fregere hostium."

45. ASF, AP 1652, fol. 2v.

46. ASF, AP 1652, fol. 3v: "Super xii qui incipit quod dictus B item quod plures et plures suo iura[men]to testificando dixit quod tempore in capitulo contento plures et plures vidit dictum Blaxium existentum in furore predicto percutere matrem et ei dilaniare pannos quod habebat in dorso." See also fol. 6v.

47. ASF, AP 1652, fol. 6v: "Super xii quod incipit item quod plures etc. Suo iura[men]to testificando dixit quod dicto tempore dum dictus Blaxius staret sic incatenatus et detemptus vidit eum plures capere matrem et ei dilamiare pannos de dorso et eam percutere cum pugnis. Ac etiam dicebat matri et sorori quod volebat eas subponere et levabat sibi pannos et ostendebat eis res suas pudibundas dicendo 'fatene in qua fatene in qua.'"

48. ASF, AP 1652, fol. 2v.

49. ASF, AP 1652, fol. 7v.

50. ASF, AP 1652, fol. 13r.

51. ASF, AP 1652, fols. 8r–v: "Sed stabat tamquam homo insensatus qui prospiciebat quid faciebant. Sed eo ligato cepit proferre multa verba insania nam quandoque dicebat io fui figliuolo de messer Pietro di Bardi quandoque dicebat io sono consorte del pievano [schiacta] quandoque dicebat io son di freschobaldi. Postea incipiebat canerè et multa alia verba et actus dicebat et exercebat prout faciunt furiosi et insani que enarrare longum esset et predicta omnia dictus testis dixit se vidisse et audivisse."

52. ASF, AP 1652, fol. 9v: "Interrogatus quid dicebat et quid faciebat dictus Blaxius illo medio tempore quo sic stetit ligatus antequam esset dies dixit quod multos ei infinitos actus faciebat prout faciunt furiosi et mentecapti nam quandoque exclamabat fortiter tamquam si esset rabiatus postea stabat unum modicum et canebat et udebat nec firmus stabat super uno proponito sed continuo proferebat verba insania sine capite et sine cauda. Mane vero sequenti ipse testis init Pratum pro familia potestatis et ei cum dicta familia venere obviam et ipsum invenere quod ducebatur per alios prope portam dicte terre Prati."

53. ASF, AP 1652, fols. 11v–12r: "Finaliter ipse testis una cum quodam alio init Pratum ad notificandum predictam potestati terre Prati qui potestas subito mane sequenti dictam nocte misit familiam suam pro eo que familia una cum ipso teste invenit eum in via quod ducebat ad dictum potestatem interrogatus quid dicebat et quid faciebat dictus Blaxius dum sic duceretur dixit quod conabatur se dissolvui et eum duxere usque ad [12r] portam sicte terre ubi eum dimisere in fortiam familie et dum sic eum conduxisset ligatum et quasi nudum audiebat omnes trahentes dicentes, 'ecco el paçço, ecco el paçço de biagio.'"

54. ASF, AP 1652, fol. 3r: "Suo iura[men]to dixit se tantum scire videlicet quod dum esset in contrata habitatus ipsius testis et dicti Blaxii vidit dictum Blaxium qui reducebatur a civitate Pistorii super quodam equo una cum Phylippo Ser Iohannis eius consorte qui eum tenebat super dicto equo ne se proiceret in terram et quidam Iohannes ser Pauli etiam eius consors stabat vix equum suum ad iuvando ut rediceretur et tunc ipse testis vidit et audivit eum tamquam insanum et furiosum fortiter exclamare et verba insania proferre quemadmodum ipse habuisset diabolum in corpore ac etiam vidit eum tunc personas trahentes signare prout faciunt episcopi."

55. Magistrates of Florentine counties and districts like Prato were required to denounce serious crimes that took place in their domains to the rectors of Florence; such denunciations are ubiquitous in the records of the Florentine Podestà and the Capitano del Popolo.

56. ASF, SS 85, fol. 13v.

57. Magherini and Biotti, "Madness in Florence in the 14th–18th Centuries."

58. Martines, *Lawyers and Statecraft*, 137–40.

59. Giovanni Antonelli, "La magistratura degli Otto di Guardia a Firenze," *ASI* 92, no. 402 (1954): 4–5; see also Brackett, *Criminal Justice*, 8.

60. Brackett, *Criminal Justice*; Antonelli, "La magistratura degli Otto di Guardia a Firenze"; Marvin E. Wolfgang, "Crime and Punishment in

Renaissance Florence," *Journal of Criminal Law and Criminology* 81, no. 3 (1990): 567–84.

61. Brackett, *Criminal Justice*, 42.

62. Marvin B. Becker, "Changing Patterns of Violence and Justice in Fourteenth- and Fifteenth-Century Florence," *Comparative Studies in Society and History* 18, no. 3 (1976): 281–96.

63. Martines, *Lawyers and Statecraft*, 135–36; Zorzi, *L'amministrazione della giustizia penale nelle repubblica fiorentina.*

64. Historians have noted that centralization was more effectively achieved in Florence than in the localities of the Tuscan dominion. Brackett, *Criminal Justice*, 96.

65. Brackett, *Criminal Justice*, 11, 16. Centralization was not uniform throughout Tuscan domains. Cosimo had a much firmer hold on Florence itself. Elena Fasano Guarini, whose research has addressed the relative success of failure of centralization of Cosimo's ducal state by studying the relationship between the center and Florence and its Tuscan domains, has shown that centralization was not total or uniform throughout his dominion. Cosimo rather sat at the top of a pyramid of competing power blocs. Elena Fasano Guarini, *Lo stato Mediceo di Cosimo I* (Florence: Sansoni, 1973); and "Potere centrale e comunità soggette nel granducato di Cosimo I," *Rivista Storica Italiana* 89, Fasc. 3–4 (1977): 490–538.

66. Brackett, *Criminal Justice*, 14.

67. Ibid., 73–74.

68. Ibid., 16.

69. Ibid., 29.

70. Ibid., 15.

71. Ibid., 20.

72. Luigi Monga, trans. and ed.., *The Journal of Aurelio Scetti: A Florentine Galley Slave at Lepanto, 1565–1577* (Tempe: Arizona Center for Medieval and Renaissance Studies, 2004), 14.

73. Andrew C. Hess, "The Evolution of the Ottoman Seaborne Empire in the Age of the Oceanic Discoveries, 1453–1525," *American Historical Review* 75, no. 7 (December 1970): 1892–1919; Hess, "The Ottoman Conquest of Egypt (1517) and the Beginning of the Sixteenth-Century World War," *International Journal of Middle East Studies* 4, no. 1 (January 1973): 55–76.

74. ASF, OGP 2247, n.p.

75. ASF, MS 1121, no. 332, titled, "prigioni offerti delle stinche."

76. ASF, OGP 2247, no. 398rv; 2253, no. 41rv.

77. Brackett, *Criminal Justice*, 62, 67.

78. ASF, OGP 2247, no. 2253, no. 41rv.

79. ASF, OGP 2247, no. 398rv; 2249, nos. 102r, 309r.

80. ASF, OGP 2249, no. 102r, no. 309r.

81. ASF, OGP 2253, no. 41r: "si come ancora nelle dette Stinche egli fece varie et diverse pazzie et particolarmente si gitto nel pozzo di detto luogo: la onde essendo hoggi di eta d'anni sessanta o meglio et essendo stato nelle dette carcere otto anni."

82. ASF, OGP 2245, no. 131rvr; 2247, no. 168r; 2254, no. 422r.

83. ASF, OGP 2254 nos. 75r, 180r.

84. ASF, OGP 2250, nos. 27rv, 139r; 2251, no. 414rvrv.

85. ASF, OGP 2250, no. 414r: "Bernardo di Michele Ulivi. . . . uno anno passato fu trovato di notte da la guardia del Bargello con una forchetta di fero."

86. ASF, OGP 2250, no. 27v: "Questo supplicante fu messo nelle Stinche per pazzo pericoloso ad instantia del fratello, hora dicono che e tornato [27v] sanio et che lo voglion mandare di fuora sul una nave, el fratello mostra contentarsene pero domanda gratia di esser ne liberato. Io credo che sara tal volta un poco appassito et se va sulla nave a mio giuditio non tornera piu nelle Stinche."

87. ASF, OGP 2250, no. 139r: "et per che la notificatione che mi ha fatto detto Magistrato dicie che io debba subito doppo la mia relassatione andare in su la detta nave et intendendo hora che la nave non e in paese che io possa cosi subito andarvi, non sono voluto uscire di prigione per non contaffare al precepto di tale notificatione: che voglio essere buon figliuolo di obbedientia et pero la vengho di nuovo a supplicare che la mi faccia gratia di potere uscire di carcere sanza mio priuditio con farmi dare tanto tempo che ci sia la nave et che io possa transferirmi a quella sperando che havendomi lei per suo begnignità fatto gratia della liberatione."

88. ASF, OGP 2250, no. 414: "Questa è la seconda volta che questo supplicante e stato messo nelle Stinche per pazzo et quando la prima volta si cavò haveva fede che era rinsanato et in consenti el fratello auctorità, ma in capo di pochi giorni la guardia lo trovo una notte a X hor in uno sportello la dalla miseracordia . . . et veduto el Magistrato che l'humore non era ben digestato. Dice hora che et tornato sanio et ne fanno fede e buon homini et piu persone che sono nella Stinche che egli e di sanamente che buon discorso et intelletto."

89. ASF, OGP 2257, fol. 308rv.

90. ASF, OGP 2257, fol. 308r: "Francesco di Tommaso . . . per due anni in Galea in permuta delle su condennationi di 50 scudi et confino di due anni nelle Stinche et di y 300."

91. ASF, OGP 2241, no. 104v. Florentine braccia measured 58.4 centimeters. See Angelo Martini, *Manuale di metrologia ossia misure, pesi e monete in uso attualmente e anticamente presso tutti i popoli* (Rome: E.R.A., 1976).

92. ASF, OGP 2241, no. 104r: "lei possa ritenerlo in casa sua dove che eli habbia amurrare una stanza la migliore e piu forte vi sia dove che lei lo governera con quello per che substantia che hara detto Barone et detto Giovanbatista suo marito." When Corbolo inspected the room he found Barone chained: "con una catena al piede." He described the room as: "è in casa di lei medesima per piu comodo e manco spesa et farli miglior governo che è una camera terrena larga 5 braccia, lunga 6½ et buone mura et dico che la rassette vanno a uso di prigione con uscio basso et forte et la fenestra altra et ferrata con uno sportello per porgirli el magnari. Et a me par che in possa stare con piu comodita assai del uno et dell'altro." The Duke responded: "Se è luogo sicuro mettisi."

93. ASF, OGP 2237, fol. 170rv: "il decto suo marito vexato da humori maninchonici uscito di se faccendo cose di pericolo alla vita sua et alla famiglia e stato incarcerato nelle Stinche tre mesi dove al presente si trova et per la tanta poverta havendo decta sua moglie a sostenarlo e riducta in modo che piu non puo sanza l'aiuto . . . li piaccia farli gratia che sia accettato nello spedale di Santa Maria Nuova dove secondo li ordini di epso spedale sara medicato et governato et per gratia de Dio et di V.E.I. potra ritornare nella sua valitudine et stando nelle Stinche e la expressa rovina di decta povera donna et in casa non lo puo in modo alcuno tenere." The Otto reported: "Questo Domenico Barbier marito della supplicante fu ad instantia del suocero et altri parenti facto mettere nelle Stinche per pazzo per che avanti che el Magistrato volessi deliberare di mettervelo lo feciono legar in casa."

94. ASF, OGP 2237, fol. 170rv: "Lo spedalingo li faccia curare se si puo se non nel resto si mettanno al ordine dello spedale."

95. Henderson, *The Renaissance Hospital*, 265–71. Henderson demonstrates that the term "poor" described a larger group than one might think. It included the minor employees of the city's main magistracies, the servants and slaves of private families, and a variety of artisans in addition to beggars and vagrants. He points out that members of the Florentine elite were also able to secure beds though not in great numbers. Families were on occasion able to house their mentally disordered relatives in hospitals if they were willing to pay for their upkeep, though it was not common practice. In general, the mad were without a hospital until the foundation of Santa Dorotea.

96. ASF, OGP 2253, no. 437rv: "Madonna Alessandra di Manno degl'Albizi et moglie di Giovanni del Mare, havendo in casa detto Giovanni suo marito da cinque mesi in qua impazzato di pazzia pericolosa à tutta la famiglia, et noiosa, et insopportabile à vicini i quali per la verità sotto scriveranno, et essendo povera con dua figliuoli anchora fanciulli se che non può per la poverta ne governare il marito ne vivere ella con suo figliuoli."

97. ASF, OGP 2253, no. 437rv: "Io Zanobi di Mattheo da Montauto fo fede come si vede il detto Giovanni da Mare far' molti gesti extraordinarii et il giorno et la notte gridare et dir' molte cose adproposito; talche si puo tenere per certo che questo povero homo sia impazzato et à noi vicini è di non poco travaglio haverlo per vicino; quale è pericoloso di non fare qualche scandolo et male vedendolo giettare dalla sua finestra mattoni et tutto quello che li puo venire alle mani et però ho scripto di mia propria mano a die ultimo di Marzo 1570 in Firenze."

98. ASF, OGP 2253, no. 437rv: "Però supplica a V.Al. che si degni di far dare al detto Giovanni un luogo in Santa Maria Nuova dove egli sia governato, come già altri simili sono stati ricevuti in detto spedale et di questo humilmente prega V.Alt. per la molta necessità et dell'infermo, et sua, et per la sodisfazione di tutti i vicini." The Duke replied: "Santa Maria Nuova non ricever pazzia se non [miserabili] et s'ella vuol mandarlo alle Stinche lo può fare ma bisogna pensare di darli le spese."

99. Brackett, *Criminal Justice*, 74.

100. Ibid., 103.

101. Ibid., 108.

102. ASF, OGP 2218, n.p.: "Fu preso alli giorni passati Illustrissimo et eccellentio Signore Duca Antonio di Paulo della Villa di Camprena giovane d'anni 17, mendico di robba et scemo di cervello, per essere stato trovato con uno pugnaletto a canto, non per nemicitia che lui habbia ma per sua dapacaggine et leggerezza, et ha havuto tre tratti di corda, et di piu e minacciato della pena di 20 scudi che se ne vanno in 35 scudi. Onde per essere lui povero et privo di ogni sustantia Agnolo suo zio servigiale dello spedale di Bibbiena confidando nelle infinita clementia et humanita di V. S. Et mosso dalla compassione di una poverina sorella di decto Antonio supplica a quella che per lo amore di Dio gli vogli perdonare tale trasgressione di legge et si degni farlo rilasciare come giovane d'anni mendico di robba, et di poca consideratione et intellecto che tale punitione dalla corda havuta gli sara granfreno di non incorrere un'altra volta in simile errore et egli incambio della gratia ottenuta preghera Dio che esalti et mantegha V.E. in grande feliciss stato."

103. ASF, OGP 2233, fol. 89rv: "Lorenzo di Tommaso Giacomini humile servitore di V.E.I essendo suto preso un suo figliuolo d'età d'anni 21 per esser stato trovato con l'arme el quale in pero è ricorso in tal disubidienza et errore per il poco cervello, che ha sempre havuto come di tutto ne potranno a pieno dar relatione a V.E.I. I Magnifici Signori Otto et per che il povero esponente non solo non ha da poter pagare la condennatione ma muor di fame con tre figliuole che ha da marito in casa et la sua donna: come ne fanno fede a quella e buon' huomini di San Martino et il cavalier Rosso el quale piu volte li ha dato la limosina per ordine della Illustrissima Signora Duchessa Pero quella prega per l'amor de Dio che sia contenta che la sua condennagio ne li sia permutata in un confino dove piu piacera a quella insieme con la pena della fune. Il che facendo ne seguira che con le limosine li sono fatte potra aiutare le sua povere figliuole." The Duke replied: "Dia degli la fune secondo il bando et del resto habbi gratia."

104. ASF, OGP 2249, no. 406rv: "Matteo di Giuliano Pasani humilissimo servitore di V.E.I. con reverentia le expone come la sera di Santo Jacopo un suo figliuolo chiamato Giuliano d'età d'anni 17 et debole di cervello fu trovato dalle guardia con una spada la quale portava come scrocho et fanciullaccio senza havere nimicitie o altro ma solo per mera pazzia et per che il detto povero suo padre dubita che non habbia havere la fune la quale potrebbe forse guastarlo . . . faccia gratia a detto suo figliuolo di detta fune atteso che e si fanciullaccio et privo di cervello." The Otto reported: "Giuliano figliuolo del supplicante la notte di 29 del passato fu dal Magistrato condennato in 10 scudi et tratti due di fune per essere stato trovato dalla guardia con la spada da Sant' Ambrogio et per questo si trova nelle carcere del Bargello. El padre supplicante ricorre et dice che egli e in fan[verso]ciullaccio et scemo di cervello et che ha 17 anni pero domanda sol gratia della fune. Che egli sia giovane si vede che non arriva a 20 anni et dello scroccho el Magistrato se ne accorse nelle examine et tenevalo per tale et il maestro di bottega dove sta all'arte della lana e ha fatto fede che egli e l'uccello di bottega."

105. Brackett, *Criminal Justice*, 67–68.

106. ASF, OGP 2283, fol. 34rv: "Taddeo suo figliuolo per mancamento di cervello sin da piccolo crescendo la pazzia et furor suo con il tempo che

gia e nelli 26 anni e andato facendo molte bestialita et pazzia, et sino l'anno passato il di di Pasqua mosso dalla sua pazzia et furore sparo al suplicante suo padre una archibusata, ch'in contumacia stando nel suo furore fu condennato in 3 anni in Galea et cosi pazzo si sta con di prediudicio dando et per contendo hor questo hor quel a[tto] senza causa come fanno li pazzi. Onde il povero padre supplicante conoscendo il periculo grave che non amazzi qualch'uno et volendo remediare al instante periculo. Supplica humilmente l'Alt. V.S. che li facci gratia cometere che detto Taddeo suo figlio, sia messo nelle Stinche a bene placito et sino che piaccia alla bonta d'Iddio restituirli il cervello, et in detto loco delle Stinche s'intende permutata la pena sopradetta della galea, accioche ne in Galera ne for di Galea non nochi ad alcuno, et sendo pazzo habbi la pena e remedio che si da a pazzi di star carcerato, la qual pazzia e notoria, come mostra la publica testimonianza del detto comune."

107. ASF, OGP 2283, fol. 34rv: "Noi consiglieri . . . rapprensentati detto come per queste nostre lettere testimoniali facciamo—indubitata fede a chiunque sia et a qual si voglia iudice, o, magistrato come Taddeo di Guglielmo dal Onda parte di Casentino podestaria di Prato vecchio et sottoporta alla nostra comunita et universita di San Larino è come si dice furioso et spessisime volte fuora di suoi sensi et bene spesso senza causa grida con questo e con quello; et darebbe se potessi et è molto pericoloso se si lassa star cosi et nel borgo di L'onda et in San Larino et per tutto dove è conosciuto e hauto per furioso et pazzo, et per tale tenuto publicamente in detto luoghe et quando ogni hora grida ad altra voie con questo et con quello ogni homo dice eglie quel pazzo di Taddeo lassalo dire che e pazzo et briaco che oltre la pazzia naturale l'odor del vino solo li piusce di torre il cervello essendo cosi la verita ne haviamo fatto fare queste lettere testimoniali et fatteli sigillare con il nostro sigillo questo di 28 di Aprile 1589." [recto] "Fede per me notaio infrascripto come da Magistrato Signori Soprastanti delle Stinche della Citta di Firenze fu approvato per mall[vadore] Alessandro di San Lad[eo] fumati per il vitto e vestito di Taddeo di Gugliemmo dall'Onda nelle carcere delle Stinche."

108. ASF, OGP 2251, no. 185r: "è stato messo nelle Stinche sotto pretexto che sia diventato pazzo; onde tutta la sua povera famiglia è necessitata et egli insieme per non si potere quivi aiutare à morirsi di fame. Et perche la verità che è gli non è pazzo se bene ogni mese o ogni sei settimane egli entra in certe albagie di cicalare qualche cosa fuora di proposito, et non ha fatto ne fa damno à persona, et non gli dura la detta albagia di cicalare come di sopra, più che duoi giorni o al più lungo tre; il quale tempo di tre giorni passato egli ritorna alla sua bottega del legnuolo e lavora del continuo come se mai havesse havuto l'accidente soprascripta, si come tutto questo anno ha lavorato in quardaroba et in via maggio alla bottega di Bernardo Legnaiuolo et è così cosa notissima à tutti li vicini dove ha habitato nella via del Palagio del Podestà."

109. ASF, OGP 2258, fol. 48r: "come si trova confinato nelle Carcere delle Stinche per un anno da Signori Otto di Balia per un poco di rissa che hebbe con la Ginevra sua cognata, del qual confino ne ha osservato mesi sette, et per trovarsi malato."

110. ASF, OGP 2258, fol. 48r: "havendo presentito da dua giorni in qua che lui ha dato una mallevadore et promesso al Magistrato de Signori Otto di non l'offendere sotto pena di 200 scudi."

111. ASF, OGP 2258, fol. 48v: "La Ginevra Aquilanti de Chelli humil servitrice di V.A. a quella con reverentia expone, come piu mesi fa lei fu ferita da Piero Chelli suo cognato, fratello di Francesco suo marito, di dua colpi mortali nella testa innocentemente, et senza causa, et occasione alcuna, ma solo per la sua mattia e poca religione che ha in se decto suo cognato; dove in sul rapporto dal medico che la curo; ex offitio fu formato una quella avanti a Signori Otto di Balia contro al detto Piero, et sendo capturato per esser lui stato tenuto, et reputato mentecapto fu confinato dal Magistrato per un anno nelle Stinche."

112. ASF, OGP 2258, fol. 48v.

113. Ibid.: "fu confinato dal Magistrato per un anno nelle Stinche, senza che la parte offesa fussi examinata, e potessi dire le sua ragioni et monstrare la innocentia sua, e l'assasinamento factogli a detti Signori e parendogli che il Magistrato gli havessi dato un lieve gastigo rispecto al gran delicto, non havendo detta povera supplicante alcuno che dicessi una parola per lei sopporto tante offese il meglio che potette, et approximandosi alla fine del confine, dubitando di nuovo non esser offesa da detto cognato matto, et informandosi con certi suoi vicini che via lei dovessi tenere per possere vivere sicuramente gli fu detto che il detto Piero non uscirebbe di carcere in sino a tanto che non havessi assicurata la parte o accordatola a tale che detta povera oratrice come donna semplicemente selo credette dove aspectando lei l'occasione d'esser chiamata dal Magistrato pensando di potere condemandare una sicurta conveniente a uno huomo tale in aspectamente et senza che detta supplicante ne havessi notitia alcuna, la mattina di Pasqua di Ceppo detto suo cognato insolentemente ando a picchiare l'uscio a detta supplicante non che una volta dua, quantunque la prima volta dalla [. . .]gli fussi risposto che il marito di detta supplicante non era in casa, et vedendo et sentendo [. . .]tto cio detta oratrice apena credeva a ce medesima parendogli di esser agitata et aggiuniendo di nuovo sospecto al suo gran humore sendo maxime che giornalmente detto suo cognato il quale veramente e mentecapto come V.A.S. degnandosi potra vedere per le introcluse fede facte per mano di gentil'homini che lo cognoscano di non cessa di passare per la sua contrada minacciando di volerla amazzare."

114. ASF, OGP 2258, fol. 48v: "la povera donna e confinata in casa e non puo per il timore et gran sospecto che ha di lui andare pure a una messa o aconfessarsi dubitando sempre di non l'havere dietro come in vero gli riuscirebbe et havendo presentito da dua giorni in qua che lui ha dato una mallevadore et promesso al Magistrato de Signori Otto di non l'offendere sotto pena di 200 scudi tutto senza saputa di detta supplicante o che lei sia stata citata e parendogli questa pena quantoque se gli dessi mallevadore per dumila scudi non che questo lei sarebbe et si sarebbe sicura havendo lei a tractare con un matto che non si puo dire che sia huomo per che doppo la data per lui sicurta ha picchiato l'uscio a detta supplicante et cercha di minacciarla non tenendo conto del magistrato tanto maggiormente non tenga conto d'una donna."

The Duke responded: "Gl'Otto provegghino che questa povera donna possa vivere sicura."

115. ASF, OGP 2258, unnumbered recto following fol. 48: "In virtu della presente Io dico a V.S. come io sono contenta che Mess Francesco Lapini come mio procuratore presentila supplica avanti a V.S. circa alla cosa del confino di Piero Chelli mio cognato sendo che io non mi assicuro a andar fuori et tanto maggiormente che io non voglio che Francesco mio marito lo sappia et se non havessi volsuto che la cosa andassi secreta non sarei ricorsa a sua A[ltissima] ma di prima botta sarei ricorsa avanti al Magistrato di V.S. per che non mi sono mai diffidata della buona iustitia di V.S. ma tutto ho facto per che il mio marito non lo sappia sendogli fratello come li e et prego V.S. che si degnino farmi questa gratia di acceptare tutto quello che dira a V.S. il detto mio procuratore come se fussi la persona mia propria per che sono risolutissima di non comparire costa accio che la cosa non si divulgassi per tutta er se bene e paressi a V.S. che nella supplica io havessi offeso il Magistrato non l'ho facto per offendere, ma per mostrare a S.A. l'innocentia mia per che ho detto la mera verita et se bene il mio marito havessi risposto quando mi trovavo il lecto ferita et ammalata in nome mio va [. . .] cosa piu che un'altra è stato veramente senza mia saputa et accioche il suo fratello havessi minore pena."

116. ASF, OGP 2258, fol. 48v.

117. Butcher, Mineka, and Hooley, *Abnormal Psychology.*

CHAPTER 3

For the Italian, see Leon Battista Alberti, *I libri della famiglia*, ed. Ruggiero Romano and Alberto Tenenti (Turin: Einaudi, 1969), 197 (book 3).

1. I have based this brief account of Francis's life on St. Bonaventure's "Major Legend of Saint Francis," in *Francis of Assisi—The Founder: Early Documents*, ed. Regis J. Armstrong, J. A. Wayne Hellmann, and William J. Short (New York: New City Press, 2000), 2:530–38.

2. ASF, MPAP 2281, fol. 100r: "Messer Andreuolo Niccolini Supplicante: Atteso che alli giorni passati Zanobi suo fratello carnale uscito del sentimento; come lui dice si spoglio nudo in Piazza, et fece alcune altre pazzie publiche con sua vergogna et de suoi parenti; dando li suoi vestimenti et altra roba sua a diverse persone." The Duke's secretary replied: "Il Magistrato ne pigli la cura."

3. Patricia Allerston, "Consuming Problems: Worldly Goods in Renaissance Venice," in *The Material Renaissance*, ed. Michelle O'Malley and Evelyn Welch (Manchester: Manchester University Press, 2007), 11–46 at 13.

4. Goldthwaite, *The Economy of Renaissance Florence*, 481; see also Tim Carter and Richard A. Goldthwaite, *Orpheus in the Marketplace: Jacopo Peri and the Economy of Late Renaissance Florence* (Cambridge, Mass.: Harvard University Press, 2013), 349–58.

5. Dante Alighieri, *La Commedia secondo l'antica vulgata*, ed. Giorgio Petrocchi (Milan: Mondadori, 1966–68), 7.27–63.

6. Peter Brown beautifully captures how these tensions were expressed from the mid-fourth to sixth century CE in his most recent volume, *Through the Eye of a Needle: Wealth, the Fall of Rome, and the Making of Christianity in the West, 350–550 AD* (Princeton, N.J.: Princeton University Press, 2012).

7. Matthew 19:21–26 (RSV).

8. 1 Cor. 1:18–25, 3:19, 4:10.

9. See the introduction to Goldthwaite, *The Economy of Renaissance Florence*. Scholars call this period the "commercial revolution." Robert Lopez associated this with the search for new markets while Raymond de Roover believed that it was not expansion that constituted revolution but the transformation of the structure of business from itinerant merchants to the sedentary firm.

10. See Luke 6:35, which exhorts followers of Jesus to "Lend freely, hoping for nothing thereby," and Luke 14:26.

11. Lawrin Armstrong, "Law, Ethics and Economy: Gerard of Siena and Giovanni d'Andrea on Usury," in *Money, Markets and Trade in Late Medieval Europe: Essays in Honour of John H. A. Munro*, ed. Lawrin Armstrong, Ivana Elbl, and Martin Elbl (Leiden: Brill, 2007), 41–42.

12. Dante, *La Commedia Divina: Inferno*, 17.48–78.

13. Armstrong, "Law, Ethics and Economy."

14. Goldthwaite, *The Economy of Renaissance Florence*, 110.

15. Antonella Astorri, *La mercanzia a Firenze nella prima metà del Trecento: Il potere dei grandi mercanti* (Florence: Olschki, 1998).

16. Armstrong, *Usury and Public Debt in Early Renaissance Florence*. See also Raymond de Roover, "The Commercial Revolution of the Thirteenth Century," in *Enterprise and Secular Change in Economic History*, ed. Frederic C. Lane (Homewood, Ill.: R. D. Irwin, 1953), 80–85; Lester K. Little, *Religious Poverty and the Profit Economy in Medieval Europe* (London: Pail Elek Ltd., 1978); Kirshner, "Storm over the 'Monte Comune'"; idem, "Encumbering Private Claims to Public Debt in Renaissance Florence"; Armstrong, *Usury and Public Debt in Early Renaissance Florence*; Welch, *Shopping in the Renaissance*; Goldthwaite, *The Economy of Renaissance Florence*.

17. Kirshner, "Storm over the 'Monte Comune,'" 228. See also Kirshner, "'Ubi est ille?' Franco Sacchetti on the Monte Comune of Florence," *Speculum* (July 1984): 556–84.

18. Kirshner, "Storm over the 'Monte Comune,'" 257.

19. Molho, *Marriage Alliance in Late Medieval Florence*.

20. Goldthwaite, *The Economy of Renaissance Florence*, 447.

21. Carol Bresnahan Menning, *Charity and State in Renaissance Italy: The Monte di Pietà of Florence* (Ithaca, N.Y.: Cornell University Press, 1993), 15.

22. Goldthwaite, *The Economy of Renaissance Florence*, 471.

23. Menning, *Charity and State*, 1–2.

24. Ibid., 28–29.

25. Goldthwaite, *The Economy of Renaissance Florence*, 375.

26. Menning, *Charity and State*, 9.

27. Goldthwaite, *The Economy of Renaissance Florence*, 425.

28. Ibid., 424.

29. See Little, *Religious Poverty and the Profit Economy*. See also Goldthwaite, *Wealth and the Demand for Art in Italy*, 27. This groundbreaking work inspired a rich and extensive scholarship. See, for example, Marta Ajmar, ed., *Approaches to Renaissance Consumption* (Oxford: Oxford University Press, 2002); Welch, *Shopping in the Renaissance*; and Michelle O'Malley and Evelyn Welch, eds., *The Material Renaissance* (Manchester: Manchester University Press, 2007).

30. Goldthwaite, *Wealth and the Demand for Art in Italy*, 178; Little, *Religious Poverty and the Profit Economy*, 213.

31. A. D. Fraser Jenkins, "Cosimo de' Medici's Patronage of Architecture and the Theory of Magnificence," *Journal of the Warburg and Courtauld Institutes* 33 (1970): 162–70.

32. Louis Green, "Galvano Fiamma, Azzone Visconti and the Revival of the Classical Theory of Magnificence," *Journal of the Warburg and Courtauld Institutes* 53 (1990): 98–113.

33. Both Bruni and Poggio are cited in Patricia Rubin, "Magnificence and the Medici," in *The Early Medici and Their Artists*, ed. F. Ames-Lewis (London: Birkbeck College, University of London, 1995), 43.

34. Peter Howard, "Preaching Magnificence in Renaissance Florence," *Renaissance Quarterly* 61 (2008): 356–57. See also Rubin, "Magnificence and the Medici," 37–50.

35. Richard Goldthwaite, "The Empire of Things: Consumer Demand in Renaissance Italy," in *Patronage, Art and Society in Renaissance Italy*, ed. F. W. Kent and Patricia Simons (Oxford: Oxford University Press, 1987), 155–75.

36. For a thorough study of literature on household management, see Daniela Frigo, *Il Padre di Famiglia: Governo della Casa e Governo Civile nelle Tradizione dell'Economica' tra Cinque e Seicento* (Rome: Bulzoni, 1985). For studies on magnificence, see Jenkins, "Cosimo de' Medici's Patronage of Architecture and the Theory of Magnificence"; Green, "Galvano Fiamma, Azzone Visconti and the Revival of the Classical Theory of Magnificence"; and Rubin, "Magnificence and the Medici."

37. In 1574, an archiepiscopal synod in Florence denounced all usury. Moreover, the seventeenth century opened with the canon lawyer Girolamo Confetti's staunch objection to the practice particularly by the Monte di Pietà. In the first case the Duke successfully enjoined the pope to soften his position. In the second case, the Duke created a commission that circumvented canonical disapproval through carefully crafted reforms. Menning, *Charity and State*, 265.

38. Craig Muldrew, "Interpreting the Market: The Ethics of Credit and Community Relations in Early Modern England." *Social History* 18, no. 3 (May 1993): 163–83.

39. Francis Fukuyama, *Trust: The Social Virtues and the Creation of Prosperity* (New York: Free Press, 1995), 20.

40. Fukuyama, *Trust*, chap. 4.

41. Goldthwaite, *Wealth and the Demand for Art in Italy*, 211.

42. Frigo, *Il padre di famiglia*.

43. Little, *Religious Poverty and the Profit Economy*, 217.

44. Alistair Smart, *The Assisi Problem and the Art of Giotto: A Study of the Legend of St. Francis in the Upper Church of San Francesco, Assisi* (Oxford: Clarendon Press, 1971), 4.

45. In his *Le Vite de' più eccellenti pittori, scultori, ed architettori* (Lives of the most eminent painters, sculptors, and architects) first published in 1550, Giorgio Vasari attributed this fresco cycle to Giotto. That claim has been hotly disputed ever since. I have tried to remain neutral in this debate by referring to the "Master(s) of the St. Francis Cycle." For relevant bibliography, see Donal Cooper and Janet Robson, *The Making of Assisi: The Pope, the Franciscans and the Painting of the Basilica* (New Haven, Conn.: Yale University Press, 2013).

46. Smart, *The Assisi Problem*, 164; Diane Cole Ahl, *Benozzo Gozzoli* (New Haven, Conn.: Yale University Press, 1996).

47. Cooper and Robson, *The Making of Assisi*, 154; Smart, *The Assisi Problem*, 164.

48. Smart, *The Assisi Problem*, 21 and plate 49.

49. It was once thought that access to high altar pieces in mendicant churches was restricted to friars and families who commissioned chapels in the liturgical east end of churches. The presence of *tramezzi*, large architectural fixtures that placed formidable boundaries between the space surrounding the high altar and the rest of the church, seemed to support this view. More recently scholars have argued for greater access to these sites. In particular, Machtelt Israëls has argued that it is too constraining to envision high altars, choirs, and presbyteries of male mendicant and monastic houses as purely liturgical spaces. Outside of Mass and Offices, these places were open to the laity, men and women alike. They played an important role in lay rituals like burial. Also, notarial acts were sometimes drawn up and witnessed in mendicant choirs as a way of adding divine sanction to secular acts. The Borgo San Sepolcro altar piece had the dual role of decorating the altar and marking the shrine of a Franciscan saint. It thus served a religious and lay audience. See Machtelt Israëls, "Painting for a Preacher: Sassetta and Bernardino da Siena," in *Sassetta: The Borgo San Sepolcro Altarpiece*, ed. Machtelt Israëls (Leiden: Primavera Press, 2009), 121–46. For an excellent review of the current state of the question, see Donal Cooper, "Access All Areas? Spatial Divides in the Mendicant Churches of Late Medieval Tuscany," in *Ritual and Space in the Middle Ages: Proceedings of the 2009 Harlaxton Symposium*, ed. Frances Andrews (Donington: Shaun Tyas, 2011), 90–107.

50. Bart. *De test.*, fol. 160v. In Walter Bagehot's formulation, it is the base level of intelligence and judgment expected of the "bald-headed man at the back of the Clapham Omnibus." This principle is not unlike the "prudent man rule," the fundamental standard for money management, laid down by Judge Samuel Putnum in a celebrated 1830 decision, *Harvard v. Amory*, 9

Pick. (26 Mass.) 446 (1830): "Those with responsibility to invest money for others should act with prudence, discretion, intelligence, and regard for the safety of capital as well as income."

51. ASF, AP 340, fol. 116r.

52. ASF, AP 4866, fols. 170v–171r.

53. ASF, MPAP 2274, fol. 12v: "Costanza Loro madre quale non essendo di sana mente et havendo a intervenire in certi acti et instrumenti consideredono venissi sotto la cura del Magistrato dei pupilli . . . et per tale conto si sta Honorabile munistero del Bigallo et e tale che ha bisogno di reggimento et di essere governata da altri non si possendo col suo cervello governare."

54. ASF, MPAP 2279, fol. 293r: "la supplicante narrata un infermità del suo marito per la quale è di maniera uscito di cervello; che non fa cosa che stia bene, ma con evidentissimo danno di quattro poveri figli; da qualche tempo in qua atteso tal sua dementia, ha mandato male alienato beni per pochissimo prezzo; et altre cose in grave preiudicio di detta supplicante et figli. Onde desiderand' ella rimedio a tanto disordine. Supplica che per gratia Vostra Altezza Serenissima di degni commettere che questo magistrato pigli la cura di detto suo marito come pazzo et inhabile a poter reggere a governare se et la famiglia sua et che li sia provisto di attore; et sieno riviste l'alienatione da lui fatte precipitosamente et fuor di dovere. A noi consta per quattro fedi di persone publiche et private molto degne di credenza che il supplicato è vero: et che detto Piero è mentecatto et pazzo et che manda per mala via se et la casa sua."

55. Watkins, 159–60; Romano and Tenenti, 199.

56. Watkins, 160; Romano and Tenenti, 200.

57. *Statuti della repubblica fiorentina*, ed. Romolo Caggese, rev. ed. (Florence: Olschki, 1999), 95–96, 114.

58. *Statuta populi et communis Florentiae: publica auctoritate, collecta, castigata et praeposita anno salutis MCCCCXV* (Freiburg: M. Kluch, 1778–83), vol. 1, book 2, rubric 118, *De contracto prohibio fieri cum male gerentibus*, 208.

59. *Statuta populi et communis Florentiae*, 96.

60. For a historical study of the development of the institution of prodigality in Roman law, consult Audibert, *Études sur l'histoire du droit romain*.

61. D. 27.10.1 pr; D. 27.10.15 pr; C. 5.70.1.

62. D. 12.1.9.7; 27.10.10 pr; 45.1.6.

63. Kaser, *Römisches Privatrecht*, 295–96.

64. D. 27.10.7.

65. ASF, AP 805, fols. 44r–45v: "Guido iam fuit plures menses ellapsos et ab ipso tempore citra gessit et hodie gerit turpem et inhonestam vitam ludendo et utendo tabernis cum inhonestis personis et fuit et est male conditionis et vite et male usus fuit et utitur substancia sua ac eciam patitur per maiorem partem temporis furorem et tamquam fatuus et vagans extra mentem ducit vitam suam in periculum verecundiam et iacturam non modicam sui et dicti sui fratris."

66. ASF, AP 805, fols. 44r–45v.

67. Lorenzo Cantini, *Legislazione Toscana* (Florence: S. Maria in Campo, 1800–1808), 5:288–355.

68. ASF, MPAP 2278, fol. 225r: "un Bernardo lor fratello carnale di poco sentimento e discorso qual va dilapidando il suo in grave detrimento della roba e faculta sue et dell'honor della casa facendo ogni giorno debiti per contratti o per scritte private procedenti tutti da scrocchi talche se non si va provedendo va a manifesta rovina e si ridurra a morire allo spedale o nelle stinche."

69. For the problems *scritte private* generated in marriage contracts, see Molho, *Marriage Alliance in Late Medieval Florence*, 308. In marriage contracts, fathers sometimes used *scritte private* to underreport the full value of a dowry.

70. See Molho, *Marriage Alliance in Late Medieval Florence*. See also Cantini, *Legislazione Toscana*, 6:14–15, 99–101.

71. Cantini, *Legislazione Toscana*, 7:56.

72. Ibid., 7:57.

73. ASF, MPAP 2279, fol. 311r: "Monna Guglielmina di Maso delli Albizi vedova et gia moglie d'Antonio di Lorenzo Cambi; nella sua supplica espone come Lorenzo et Tommaso suoi figli per non esser habile a fare le loro faccende et custodir i loro beni doppo la morte del padre hanno mandato male buona summa di danari dilapidando et distruggendo le loro sustanti con pratiche dishoneste et huomini di mala vita, er per via di molti scrocchi."

74. ASF, MPAP 2279, fol. 311r: "havendo Lorenzo il maggiore d'anni 30; come prodigo fatto debito da poco tempo in qua, con Giudei et altri, che attendono alli scrocchi di piu di mille scudi; et Tommaso il minore benche maggiore d'anni 18 è di poco giuditio et inhabile a governarsi. Pero supplica a Vostro Altissimo Signore che si degni farlo gratia che sieno messi sotto la cura del magistrato nostro come prodighi et inhabili al governo loro et delle loro sustante . . . veduto il debito di detto Lorenzo ascendere alla somma di piu mille scudi in poco tempo; fatti con scrocchi et baroccoli et habbiamo udito in persona lui stesso; et conosciuto che è talmente debole di cervello; che è inhabile a governare se et la roba sua; et similmente habbiamo havuto fedi di parenti et d'altri che Tomaso altro minore d'età; è piu insensato che il maggiore a inhabile al governo di se stesso et de suoi beni; et per maggiore giustificatione della verità, habbiamo fatto chiamare Bernardo di Lorenzi Cambi loro zio; il quale ci ha affirmato il medesimo che narra et supplica la madre loro; onde essendo vero quanto la supplicate espone; crediamo per beneplacito de detti suoi figliuoli che sia degna d'essere esaudita; non solo per causa d'essi prodighi quanto ancora per potersi cognoscere dal magistrato nostro dinignità delli oblighi."

75. ASF, MPAP 2278, fol. 249r and 2280, fol. 261r. I could find no reference to this case in the Magistrato Supremo, but later iterations of it relate that magistracy's judgments.

76. Marco Boari, *Qui venit contra iura: Il "furiosus" nella criminalistica dei secoli XV e XVI* (Milan: Giuffrè, 1983), 24–25.

77. ASF, MPAP 2278, fol. 249rv: "fu messo sotto la cura et protectione di questo magistrato con autorita di custodire la persona et faculta sua non solo

per l'avenire ma rivedere et ridurre a dovere molti imbrogli che haveva facti
in grave suo priudicio per sua semplicita et per malitia."

78. ASF, MPAP 2280, fols. 261r–262r: "Bernardo Carnesecchi vecchio
nel suo testamento institui suo herede Piero suo figliuolo et prohibi alienarsi
tutti i suoi beni excetto però che per monacare o maritare sue figlie et in caso
di altre necessità precedente prima et ottenuta la licentia di tale alienatione
dalli officiali del Monte."

79. ASF, MPAP 2278, fol. 249r.

80. ASF, MPAP 2281, fol. 548r.

81. ASF, MPAP 2279, fol. 159r: "esser di 32 anni et voler pigliare per donna
la vedova di Francesco Buondelmonti . . . come e convenuto col padre d'ac-
cordo riservatosi da obtener la licentia dalli speciali offitiali dei pupilli sotto la
custodia del quali si trova dice esser stato tratenuto dal magistrato con parole
et che non gli hanno volsuto dare tal licentia a requisitione di Cristofano Carnesecchi suo cugino accio epso supplicante non pigli donna et la linea fini-
scha in lui et che epso Cristofano succeda per vigore del fideicomisso per cio
domanda a V. A. tal licentia accio possa effetuare tal matrimonio al che per
excusatione nostra ci occorre dire a V.A.S. come epso e sotto la cura nostra
per ordine et commissione del consiglieri come persona prodiga et dilapidatore
delle sua faculta et non habile potere reggersi et che mai gli e stata degnata tal
licentia sapendo che li matrimonii non si possono impedire ma bene habbiamo
persuasoli a differire al quanto tal matrimonio o altri condecenti insino non
si mariti la Giana sua sorella d'anni 18 qual essendo etiam lei ne pupilli con
intervento delli interessati habbiamo cercho di maritarla et tutta via habbiamo
inpraticha qualcosa et come havessimo concluso li haremo dato buona licentia
[...] per la parte di Cristofano o d'altri non siamo mai stati ricerchi di dene-
garlli tale licentia immo consento con epsi el desiderio di detto supplicante.
Hanno risposto che non pare loro honesto darlli donna insino non si chava la
sorella di chasa che non sarebbe suo honore."

82. ASF, MPAP 2279, fol. 228r: "donna desiderieno che non facessi tal
passo sanza licentia et intervento del magistro non per impedire el matrimonio ma perche non di getti via et non faccia cosa indegna della chasata loro
et della quale sen habbino a vergognare cognoscendo la deboleza del suo cervello et modi del suo governo."

83. Ibid.

84. ASF, MPAP 2279, fol. 117r.

85. ASF, MPAP 2280, fol. 115r.

86. Ibid.

87. Ibid.

88. ASF, MPAP 2280, fol. 115v.

89. ASF, MPAP 2280, fol. 115r.

90. ASF, MPAP 2281, fol. 152r.

91. Ibid.

92. Ibid.

93. ASF, MPAP 2281, fol. 153rv.

94. ASF, MPAP 2280, fol. 261r: "Il che volse il testatore prohibire per che
li heredi con la loro volontà et dichiaratione non sovvertissero et annullassero

tutto il fidei come la seconda per che non penso il testatore dover havere un nipote mentecatto il qual dovesse esser sottoposto alla cura di questo."

95. ASF, MPAP 2280, fol. 261v: The Duke's secretary replied: "à S.A pare che ogni [conto] delli Magistrati faccia quello che li tocca non volendo privar gli officiali di loro Autorità."

96. See ASF, MPAP 2280, fols. 307rv, 359rv, 393r, 413r–414r, 548r; MPAP 2281, fols. 47rv, 152r–153v, 165r–166r. For testimony pertaining to the properties in question, see ASF, MPAP 2407 beginning at fol. 1r.

97. ASF, MPAP 2281, fol. 418r.

98. ASF, MPAP 2281, fol. 418rv.

99. ASF, MPP 2280, fol. 505r: "Giovanni Domenico Buonaccorsi zio; et Zanobi Acciauolo cognato di Vincento di Bartolomeo Micceri espongono à V.A.S. come havendo detto Vincento da quattro anni in qua dilapidato et mandato male la metà o piu di quello haveva; per esser prodigo et non saper fare i fatti sua, et accio non habbia a mandar male il restante. Supplicono V.A.S. che si degni commettere che detto Vincento come prodigo sia messo sotto la cura del Magistrato nostro. Et à giustificaione del disordinato et stravagante modo di spendere anche gittar via che ha fatto et fa; producono molte fedi di varie persone et di gentilhuomini; che dicono che detto Vincento è publicamente tenuto prodigo; et che spesso per prezzi esorti tantissimi compra cavalli, cani, et uccelli; quali poi o rivende con grandissima perdita."

100. ASF, MPP 2280, fol. 505r: "Le amazza si come fecce d'un astore che compro 3 scudi et con l'archibuso l'amazzo."

101. ASF, MPAP 2731, fol. 238.

102. ASF, MPAP 2281, fol. 16r: "ha procurato una cautela per la quale per scritte private si riconosce debitore per denari prestati et robe di preti et frati et altre persone religiose che non sono sottoposte alla jurisditione del Magistrato nostro et quelche è peggio benche non si possa provare, crediamo che siano apposti i giorni alle scritte di qual tempo che non leva sotto la nostra cura."

103. ASF, MPAP 2281, fol. 16r: "et con queste scritte se ne vanno alla corte dell'Arcivescovado et qui vi n'ottengono sententie commandati executivi tanto contro la persona quanto contro li beni del detto prodigo."

104. ASF, MPAP 2281, fol. 16r.

CHAPTER 4

1. ASF, MPAP 2284, fol. 158rv: "nove anni e mezzo sono Domenico Galetti figliuolo della supplicante vivente Girolamo suo padre cadde in una indispositione, mediante la quale egli diventò inhabile da fare li fatti suoi dimostrandose tanto fuor di cervello che bisognò legarlo, et fattolo medicare ritorno in se per sette anni et 30 mesi sono ricadde nella medesima malattia."

2. ASF, MPAP 2284, fol. 158rv: "asserisce la madre hebbe origine dalle multiplicità de negotii che egli haveva havuto per la morte del padre; et per che detto Girolamo trattò di dargli moglie la quale egli prese non con molta libera volontà et per esserli stati tolti circa 400 scudi in Lucca in una hosteria

qual non ha potuto recuperare per via di iustitia; et parendole che la state per i caldi in certi tempi dell'anno esca di maniera di sentimento che inconsideratmente s'imbarazza con in[c]ette con danno suo et de suoi figliuoli." "Il Magistrato ne pigli la cura lui."

3. ASF, MPAP 2284, fol. 158rv: "è reputato per huomo di poco discorso parendoli che ogni anno quando vengano li caldi cominci à girare et alcuni di parenti suoi credono che sia bene che non sia messo sotto la cura nostra, parendo loro che non sia talmente inhabile, che non possa negotiare da perse se bene in qualche tempo dell'anno patisce d'humori malinconici." Compare the case of Domenico with a case of St. Vitus's dance described by Midelfort in *A History of Madness*, 39–40.

4. This arrangement was mentioned in a petition filed in 1607 and refers to an earlier petition of 1590. For the petition of 1607, see ASF, MPAP 2286, fol. 261r. I have not found the 1590 petition.

5. See Jerome Bylebyl, "Medicine, Philosophy, and Humanism in Renaissance Italy," in *Science and the Arts in the Renaissance*, ed. John W. Shirley and F. David Hoeniger (Washington, D.C.: Folger Shakespeare Library, 1985), 27–49; Nancy Siraisi, *Taddeo Alderotti and His Pupils: Two Generations of Italian Medical Learning* (Princeton, N.J.: Princeton University Press, 1981); and Jole Agrimi and Chiara Crisciani, *Edocere Medicos: Medicina Scolastica nei Secoli XIII–XV* (Naples: Guerini e associati, 1988).

6. The classic study is Michael R. McVaugh's *Medicine Before the Plague: Practitioners and Their Patients in the Crown of Aragon, 1285–1345* (Cambridge: Cambridge University Press, 1993). See also Joseph Shatzmiller, *Médecine et justice en Provence Médiévale: Documents de Mansoque, 1262–1348* (Aix-en-Provence: Université de Provence, 1989); and Nancy G. Siraisi, *Medieval & Early Renaissance Medicine: An Introduction to Knowledge and Practice* (Chicago: University of Chicago Press, 1990).

7. In *Dürer's "Melencolia I" eine quellen und typengeschichtliche Untersuchung* (Leipzig: B. G. Teubner, 1923), Erwin Panofsky and Fritz Saxl first turned to the study of melancholy in the course of tracing the sources behind Albrecht Dürer's iconic engraving, *Melancholia I*—a study that would eventually expand into the book *Saturn and Melancholy*, coauthored with Raymond Klibansky.

8. Respectively, Midelfort, *A History of Madness*, 20; Jean Starobinski, *A History of the Treatment of Melancholy from Earliest Times to 1900* (Basle: Geigy, 1962), 38.

9. See Hippocrates, *De aëre aquis et locis, Oeuvres complètes d'Hippocrate*, ed. Emile Littré (Paris: Baillière, 1839–61), 2:12–92; idem, *Epidemics, Oeuvres complètes d'Hippocrate*, ed. Emile Littré (Paris: Baillière, 1839–61), 5:260–342; idem, *De natura hominis, Oeuvres complètes d'Hippocrate*, ed. Emile Littré (Paris: Baillière, 1839–61), 6:29–69.

10. Katharine Park, *Doctors and Medicine in Early Renaissance Florence* (Princeton, N.J.: Princeton University Press, 1985), 116–17. See also Per-Gunnar Ottosson, *Scholastic Medicine and Philosophy: A Study of*

Commentaries on Galen's "Tegni," ca. 1300–1450 (Naples: Bibliopolis, 1984); and McVaugh, *Medicine Before the Plague*, 150.

11. The primer of the medical syllabus was the *ars medicine* or the *articella*, a collection of short treatises that underwent changes in content depending on time and place. The vicissitudes of the *articella* tradition are addressed in the series Articella Studies. See Jon Arrizabalaga, *The Articella in the Early Press, c. 1476–1534* (Cambridge: Cambridge Wellcome Unit for the History of Medicine, 1998); Cornelius O'Boyle, *Thirteenth- and Fourteenth-Century Copies of the Ars Medicine: A Checklist and Contents Descriptions of the Manuscripts* (Cambridge: Cambridge Wellcome Unit for the History of Medicine, 1998); *Papers of the Articella Project Meeting, Cambridge, December 1995* (Cambridge: Cambridge Wellcome Unit for the History of Medicine, 1998); and Fernando Salmón, *Medical Classroom Practice: Petrus Hispanus' Questions on Isagoge, Tegni, Regimen Acutorum and Prognostica (c. 1245–50): (MS Madrid B.N. 1877, fols 24rb–141vb)* (Cambridge: Cambridge Wellcome Unit for the History of Medicine, 1998).

12. For a list of works that constituted this large collection of medical texts, see Luis García-Ballester, "The *New Galen*: A Challenge to Latin Galenism in Thirteenth-Century Montpellier," in *Galen and Galenism: Theory and Medical Practice from Antiquity to the European Renaissance* (Aldershot: Ashgate/Variorum, 2002), 55–83. The four-year course of medical study is outlined in Carlo Malagola, *Statuti delle Università e dei Collegi dello Studio Bolognese* (Bologna: Zanichelli, 1988), 274–77.

13. In the twelfth century, Gerard of Cremona (d. 1187) and his pupils in Spain translated a number of ancient medical works into Latin including the *Canon*. To get a sense of its impact on medieval medical learning, there was one Hebrew and eleven Latin editions of it by 1500. See Siraisi, *Medieval & Early Renaissance Medicine*; and idem, *Avicenna in Renaissance Italy: The Canon and Medical Teaching in Italian Universities After 1500* (Princeton, N.J.: Princeton University Press, 1987). Medical students read Hippocrates and Galen and a good deal of those ancient authors at that, but they were introduced to the bulk of their works through an Avicennic lens. Avicenna, known among physicians as the "prince of physicians," was also the subject of numerous fourteenth- and fifteenth-century commentaries by such notable physicians as Gentile da Foligno (d. 1348), Giacomo da Forlì (d. 1414), and Ugo Benzi. See Nancy Siraisi, "The Changing Fortunes of a Traditional Text: Goals and Strategies in Sixteenth-Century Latin Editions of the *Canon* of Avicenna," in *The Medical Renaissance of the Sixteenth Century*, ed. Andrew Wear, Roger K. French, and I. M. Lonie (Cambridge: Cambridge University Press, 1985), 20.

14. A complete Latin edition of the Hippocratic corpus was printed in 1525 at Rome followed a year later by a complete Greek edition published in Venice under the auspices of the printer Aldo Manuzio (1449–1515). In the 1490s the Aldine press teamed up with the famous professor of medicine, doctor to the Este court, and humanist Niccolò Leoniceno (1428–1524) to produce a complete Greek edition of Galen's works, a project that only came to full fruition in 1525.

15. Avicenna's *Canon,* for example, endured as a key text in medical education. It appeared in fourteen editions before 1500, followed by fifty-one editions printed in the sixteenth century alone. Siraisi, "The Changing Fortunes of a Traditional Text," 20. See also Malagola, *Statuti,* 274–77.

16. For a more detailed discussion of challenges to classical medical authority, see Roger K. French, *Medicine Before Science: The Rational and Learned Physician from the Middle Ages to the Enlightenment* (Cambridge: Cambridge University Press, 2003), primarily chaps. 5, 6.

17. Luis García-Ballester, "*Artifex factivus sanitatis*: Health and Medical Care in Medieval Latin Galenism," in *Galen and Galenism,* 127–50.

18. Mario Vegetti, "Metafora politica e immagine del corpo nella medicina greca," in *Tra Edipo e Euclide: Forme del sapere antico* (Milan: Il Saggiatore, 1983), 46; Pomata, *Contracting a Cure,* 132–33.

19. Barbara Duden, *The Woman Beneath the Skin: A Doctor's Patients in Eighteenth-Century Germany* (Cambridge, Mass.: Harvard University Press, 1991), 127.

20. Pomata, *Contracting a Cure,* 135.

21. Aristotle located the seat of reason in the heart rather than the head.

22. See Gianna Pomata's illuminating discussion of the obstructed body in her *Contracting a Cure,* beginning on 129.

23. See Marilyn Nicoud, *Les régimes de santé au moyen âge* (Rome: École Française de Rome, 2007); Donatella Lippi, *Díaita: The Rules of Health in the Manuscripts of the Biblioteca Medicea Laurenziana* (Florence: Mandragora, 2010); and Cavallo, "Secrets to Healthy Living." These studies owe a great deal to Heikki Mikkeli's excellent work, *Hygiene in the Early Modern Medical Tradition* (Helsinki: Finnish Academy of Science and Letters, 1999).

24. Nicoud, *Les régimes de santé au moyen âge.*

25. Louis Landouzy and Roger Pépin, *Le "Régime du Corps" de Maitre Aldobrandin de Sienne: Texte français du XIIIe siècle* (Paris: H. Champion, 1911); Rosella Baldini, "Zucchero Bencivenni, *La santé del corpo,* Volgarizzamento del Régime du corps di Aldobrandino da Siena (a. 1310) nella copia coeva di Lapo di Neri Corsini (Laur. Pl. LXXIII 47)," *Studi di lessicografia italiana* 15 (1998): 21–300; Sebastiano Bisson et al., "Le Témoin Gênant: Une version latine du *Régime du corps* d'Aldebrandin de Sienne," *Médiévales* 42 (2002): 117–30.

26. Aldobrandino wrote his *Régime* for Beatrice of Savoy, but it enjoyed great success beyond the royal court of Provence. It survives in seventy-four complete or abridged French manuscripts and at least fifty Italian translations. See Bisson, "Le Témoin Gênant," 119; Baldini, "Zucchero Bencivenni," 25; Nicoud *Les régimes de santé au moyen âge,* 953–88; and Lippi, *Díaita,* 80–81.

27. Nicoud, *Les régimes de santé au moyen âge,* Annexe, 1.

28. Ibid., 690.

29. Pedro Gil Sotres, "The Regimens of Health," in *Western Medical Thought from Antiquity to the Middle Ages,* ed. Mirko D. Grmek (Cambridge, Mass.: Harvard University Press, 1998), 291–318.

30. William Eamon, *Science and the Secrets of Nature: Books of Secrets in Medieval and Early Modern Culture* (Princeton, N.J.: Princeton University Press, 1994). Eamon brings this world vividly to life in his most recent book, *The Professor of Secrets: Mystery, Medicine, and Alchemy in Renaissance Italy* (Washington, D.C.: National Geographic, 2010).

31. New scholarship on domestic medicine is incredibly rich. For a comprehensive and current bibliography, see Leong and Rankin, *Secrets and Knowledge in Medicine and Science.* See also Alisha Rankin, "Duchess, Heal Thyself: Elizabeth of Rochlitz and the Patient's Perspective in Early Modern Germany," *Bulletin of the History of Medicine* 82, no. 1 (2008): 109–44; and Sharon T. Strocchia, "The Nun Apothecaries of Renaissance Florence: Marketing Medicines in the Convent," *Renaissance Studies* 25, no. 5 (2011): 627–47.

32. McVaugh, *Medicine Before the Plague.* See also Shatzmiller, *Médecine et justice en Provence Médiévale*; and Siraisi, *Medieval & Early Renaissance Medicine.*

33. For a discussion of salaried physicians in Italy, see Vivian Nutton, "Continuity or Rediscovery? The City Physician in Classical Antiquity and Mediaeval Italy," in *The Town and State Physicians in Europe from the Middle Ages to the Enlightenment,* ed. Andrew W. Russell (Wolfenbüttel: Herzog Aug. Bibliothek, 1981), 9–46. For the role of the guild in regulating medical practice in Florence, see Park, *Doctors and Medicine,* 99. For the influence of regulatory bodies, Protomedicati in particular, on medical practice in several Italian cities, see David Gentilcore, *Medical Charlatanism in Early Modern Italy* (Oxford: Oxford University Press, 2006). For a history of hospitals and their place in Florentine society, see Henderson, *The Renaissance Hospital.*

34. See Andrew Wear, Robert K. French, and I. M. Lonie, *The Medical Renaissance of the Sixteenth Century* (Cambridge: Cambridge University Press, 1985), xiv; Katharine Park, "Medicine and Society in Medieval Europe, 500–1500," in *Medicine in Society: Historical Essays,* ed. Andrew Wear (Cambridge: Cambridge University Press, 1992), 60; idem, "Medicine and Magic: The Healing Arts," in *Gender and Society in Renaissance Europe,* ed. Judith C. Brown and Robert C. Davis (London: Longman, 1998), 133; Matthew Ramsey, *Professional and Popular Medicine in France, 1770–1830: The Social World of Medical Practice* (Cambridge: Cambridge University Press, 1988); Laurence Brockliss and Colin Jones, *The Medical World of Early Modern France* (Oxford: Clarendon Press, 1997); Pomata, *Contracting a Cure*; David Gentilcore, *Healers and Healing in Early Modern Italy* (Manchester: Manchester University Press, 1998); Andrew Wear, *Knowledge and Practice in English Medicine, 1550–1680* (Cambridge: Cambridge University Press, 2000); Gentilcore, *Medical Charlatanism.*

35. David Gentilcore has shown this to be true throughout Italy for medical practitioners recognized officially as charlatans especially in the sixteenth century in *Medical Charlatanism.*

36. See A. Chiappelli, "Gli Ordinamenti Sanitari del Comune di Pistoia contro la Pestilenza del 1348," *ASI,* ser. 4, 20 (1887): 8–22.

37. Cavallo, "Secrets to Healthy Living," 193–94. This article is based on a much larger digital project, which explores households as key sites of healing, medical experimentation, and exchange, "Healthy Homes, Healthy Bodies in Renaissance and Early Modern Italy," Royal Holloway, University of London: Department of History, http://www.rhul.ac.uk/history/Research/HealthyHomes/index.html (accessed June 30, 2013).

38. Joseph Ziegler, *Medicine and Religion c. 1300: The Case of Arnau de Vilanova* (Oxford: Clarendon Press, 1998), 184–90.

39. Cited in Pomata, *Contracting a Cure*, 134.

40. Park, "Medicine and Society in Medieval Europe," 80–82.

41. Mikkeli, *Hygiene in the Early Modern Medical Tradition*, 73.

42. Bartolomeo Montagnana, *Consilia* (Venice, 1514, fols. 71r–v; 1525, fol. 91v): Consilium 47, *De melancholia a materia melancholica fecali*: "Baptista Vincentinus adolescens de honoranda familia Cripie condolendum est: laborat egritudine que proprie melancholia dici debet: eo quia est corruptus in operationibus virtutis imaginative et cogitative: imaginatur enim corrupte se esse prelatum et servum dei devotissumum et catholice legistatorem magnum cum neque habeat dispositionem ad hoc neque ingenium neque exercitium ad talia potentem promovere ipsum."

43. Montagnana, *Consilia* (1525), fol. 91v: "Quod autem dispositio ipsius dependeat a materia melancholica fecali ex membris apparere potest. Primo ex permutatione coloris ad lividitatem quasi plumbeam. Secundo ex habitudinis extenuatione que eversa est in marasmum vel consumtionem totius corporis. Tertio ex fixione imaginationem et extimationum corruptarum in quibus continue laborat delusive orando predicando et sic de aliis. Quarto ex ventris stipticitate. Quinto ex superfluitatum prime digestionie transmutatione ad colorem lividum vel opacum. Sexto ex somni paucitate qui tamen profundus est in tempore in quo dormit. Septimo quia urine eius limpide vel aquose cum remissa albedine cum aliquali lividitate apparent et tenues et clare cum contento crinoidali vel cineritio ad lividitatem tendente. Octavo ex diminuta ipsius digestione quacumque hoc videri potest. Nono ex timoris instantia et fixione. Decimo et ultimo ex luctu eius in quo frequenter laborat. Non dico de pulsu quia notum est omnibus quod est parvus tardus et rarus cum duritie et siccitate representatus. Unde ex omnibus coadunatis ad invicem deducitur hanc dispositionem esse verendam satis et ad ipsius curationem transeundum."

44. Giovanbattista da Monte, *Consultationum Medicarum Opus* (Basel: Henricus Petri, 1565), Consilium XXII: "De iudeo delirante calrissimorum doctorum, Petri Navarre, Frisimelicae et Baptistae Montani," 49: "Dixerunt astantes, quod semper fuerit extra rationem. Ante hoc tempus occupatus fuit maximis occupationibus, timebat multum, et irascebatur levibus de causis, exercuit maxima negocia, longa confecit itinera, sub diu multum fuit, exposuit se calori et frigori. Cum rediit in Italiam in haec mala incidit: aderant haec accidentia, vidi stupidum: oculi impotentis moti erant, irato vultu, iracundus verberare voluit astantes, seipsum ex lecto volutavi."

45. Da Monte, *Consultationum Medicarum Opus* (1565), 53: "Primum omnes causae extrinsecae conveniunt et intrinsecae, temperatura, aetas, anni

tempus, omnia contulerunt ad generanda haec symptomata. Fecit longissimum iter, in quo perpessus magnum calorem in capite, deinde post calorem frigus: laboravit plurimum quitando, usus aromatibus et cibis calidis, ut mos est in Polonia et ultra montes, ut plus aromatum uno die consumat, quam nos integro anno. Bibit vina potentia, et omnibus rebus exiccantibus, et calefacientibus usus est."

46. See German E. Berrios, "Classifications in Psychiatry: A Conceptual History," *Australian and New Zealand Journal of Psychiatry* 33 (1999): 145–60.

47. Avicenna, *Liber Canonis* (Hildesheim: G. Olms, 1964), Liber III, Fen I.

48. Ibid.

49. Avicenna, *Liber Canonis*, Liber III, Fen I, Tractatus V, Capitulum xii, *De apoplexia*.

50. Avicenna, *Liber Canonis*, Liber III, Fen I, Tractatus IV, Capitulum xvii, *De signis manie universalibus*.

51. For a similar argument, see Fernando Salmón, "From Patient to Text? Narratives of Pain and Madness in Medical Scholasticism," in *Between Text and Patient: The Medical Enterprise in Medieval and Early Modern Europe*, ed. Florence Eliza Glaze and Brian K. Nance (Florence: Sismel, 2011), 387. See also Rita Mazza, "La malattia mentale nella medicina del cinquecento: Tassonomia e casi clinici," *in Follia, Psichiatria, e Società: Istituzioni manicomiali, scienza psichiatica e classi sociali nell'Italia moderna e contemporanea*, ed. Alberto de Bernardi (Milan: Franco Angeli, 1982), 304–16, and, in the same volume, Carlo Colombero, "Un contributo alla formazione della nozione di malattia mentale: Le *Questioni medio-legali* di Paolo Zacchia," 317–29.

52. Avicenna, *Liber Canonis*, Liber III, Fen I, Tractatus V, Capitulum viii, *De epilepsia*.

53. Salmón, "From Patient to Text?" 389.

54. The famous Ferrarese physician Michele Savonarola (ca. 1385–1466), Giovanni Arcolani (ca. 1390–1458), professor of medicine at Bologna and Padua, and the Florentine physician Niccolò Falcucci treated melancholy and mania as separate but similar defects of the mind. See Michele Savonarola, *Practica medicinae sive de aegritudinibus* (Venice, 1497), 3v–64r; Giovanni Arcolani, *Practica* (Venice, 1493), 3–60; and Niccolò Falcucci, *Sermones medicinales* (Venice: Bernardinus Staginus, 1490/91), 2:2r–82r. The Pavian physician Antonio Guainerio (d. 1440) and Giovanni Concorreggio of Milan (fl. 1404–1438), on the other hand, treated them together under one heading, suggesting that melancholy and mania were not only two manifestations of the same condition but more properly speaking that mania was a kind of melancholy. Guainerio remarked that damage in the brain can be traced to either melancholy or mania and then, rather ambiguously, added that all physicians properly called mania melancholy. See Antonio Guainerio, *Practica* (Venice, 1517), 3r–27v; and Giovanni da Concoreggio, *Practica nove medicine* (Venice, 1501), 10v–24v.

55. ASF, OGP 2225, fol. 137rv: "come essendo stato Marco di Jacopo del Zacheria linaiuolo suo cognato, et fratello carnale della sua donna condennato

dalli Magnifici Signori Otto di Balia . . . essendo decto suo cognato povero compagno et molestato grandemente dal mal caduco che locava del cervello si et in tal modo che sta come fuori della memoria et smemorato."

56. ASF, MPAP 2281, fol. 607r: "Fra Paolo Guasconi cavaliere di Malta; Havendo notitia fino in Napoli dove era a governo d'una galera che Pierantonio suo fratelli minore ha dato nelli humori malinconici."

57. ASF, MPAP 2281, fol. 633r: "come da certi anni in qua li humori malinconici hanno di maniera assalito, Messer Ridolfo et Pierantonio suoi fratelli, che non solo con molte cure, et diversi remedii usati, sono venuti in miglioramento. Ma peggorati di maniera, che è di bisogno provedere. . . . Però essendosi degnata V.A. per altro suo benigno rescritto, mettere il detto Pierantonio sotto la cura del Magistrato de'Pupilli, dove si trova di presente, et dove si hara cura della sua facultà; si degni concedere; per che non segua disordini, che il detto Pierantonio sia ricevuto nelle carcere delle Stinche che à beneplacito di V.A.S. et ritenuto in quelle carcere, dove sarà giudicato stare meglio in una, o in un'altro secondo li suoi portamenti dal Magistrato de' Pupilli servati sempre li ordini delle Stinche circa le malleverie del mallevato o altre, pure che non possa essere cavato fuori di dette carcere per Fiorenza, ne in catena ne in altro modo senza il placito di V.A.S. Et in oltre si degni concedere per la persona del detto Messer Ridolfo che possa essere ritenuto rinchiuso in un Monasterio di frati o in altro luogo comodo et quivi ritenuto et servito fino che piaccia à Nostro Signore Iddio liberarlo da questi humori frenetici nelli quali si trova. Non essendo, ne in cervelli, ne in sua ragione in parte alcuna."

58. ASF, MPAP 2283, fol. 229r: "ma perche l'esponente ha inclinatione di dargli moglie sperando che egli habbia havere figliuoli parendogli ritornato in cervello. . . . Pierantonio è assai ritornato di buon sentimento facendo tutti li atti convenienti à un huomo di sana mente."

59. ASF, MPAP 2287, fol. 137r.

60. ASF, MPAP 2283, fol. 229r; 2286, fol. 293r; 2287, fol. 137r.

61. I have been unable to find Giovanni's original petition to the Otto di Guardia. The report of Michele's incarceration comes second hand through Giovanni and Battista's petition to the Pupilli in July 1563 and in the Otto di Guardia's report of their interview of the Stinche guards. See ASF, MPP 2276, fol. 125r and ASF, OGBP 2588, fol. 29r, respectively.

62. ASF, OGP 2588, fol. 29r: "Fassi fede per noi Soprastanti delle Stinche come il vero o di Michele di Guasparre Delosso quale si trova carcerato in questo carcere delle Stinche dalli 13 di Ottobre 1562 sino ad hoggi per commessio de Signori Otto di Balìa ad instantia di Giovanni suo fratello per mentecatto e che non si debbe rilasciare sanza licentia de' detti Signori Otto per quanto il Magistrato nostro ha ritratto e per informatione delle guardie e delli altri prigioni della sua carcere e etiam per haverlo udito in voce e fatto discorrere in ragionamento e persona che non ci pare si possa dire mentcapto per che non fa pazzie . . . con le opere a persona più presto si può dire e chiamare de debol mente e cervello che altrimenti et e di tal sorte che ci pare si potrebbe cavare di carcere stante le qualita predette in quorum fidei."

63. The Pupilli bumped the case up to the Magistrato Supremo for final judgment. Unfortunately the relevant volumes of this fondo for these years are unavailable.

64. ASF, MPAP 2279, fol. 338r: "Luigi di Guido Capponi insieme con li piu prossimi parenti devotissimi: Servitori di Vostra Altezza Serenissima ricorano da quella significandoli come circa a mesi sei sono Girolamo di Gino Capponi fratello carnale di detto Luigi Podestà d'Empoli, et doppo d'esservi stato, alcuni mesi fu sopragiunto da certi humori maninconici, de quelli ha patito, ancora altra volta, et in Cambio di fermare sono andati tanto avanti che mentre è stato Podestà ne ha mostro segni evidentissimi com'è notorio, et etiam al suo ritorno qui è stato di necessita tenerlo come si fa serrato in casa. Ne quali tempi e prima ha mandato male, et fatto molti debiti senza ocasione alcuna, per il che dette supplicanti pregano Vostra Altezza Serenissima che voglia esser servita per spetialisima gratia che in avenire detto Girolamo non possi far piu oblighi ne altri contratti senza espressa licentia de sanstissimi uficiali de pupilli a fine che non riduca lui, et figliolini piccoli et la donna in extrema miseria si come seguirla se quella non ci provedessi, del che tutti ne terranno perpetuo obligo con quella e le sua figliuolini et consorte saranno tenuti a pregare Nostro Signore Dio per la felicità et prosperità sua."

65. ASF, MPAP 2731, fol. 168r: "Girolamo di Gino Capponi ancora che maggiore d'anni 18 per che andava continuamente dilapidando e consumando le faculta e sustanze sue in grave suo danno e preiuditio . . . et in corso . . . contrare piu debiti con varie e diverse persone che hanno creduto denari giove mercantie cavalli et altro che tutte mediate agittato via . . . con suo danno e dishonore."

66. ASF, OGP 2264, fol. 257r.

67. Ibid.

68. ASF, MPAP 2276, fol. 153r: "che detto Bernardo è vexato spesso dal mal caduco et insipido et ha bisogno di reggimento"; 162r: "Per informatione del suplicato per Luca Giacomini et Charllo Guasconi et dei putati alla cura et reggimento di Bernardo di Beltramo Guasconi inhabile a potersi reggiere et governare da se per qualche difecto di mente"; 200rv: "epso suplicante non era habile a governarsi da perse per qualche impedimento della persona et come vexato dal mal caduco." Cf. ASF, MPAP 2277, fols. 66r, 213r, 219r.

69. I am grateful to Bob Black for sharing all of the references to the 1427 Catasto with me. ASF, Catasto 47, fol. 8r: Portata of Iachopo di Dino di Stefano who was said to be "no' ha buono sentimento [. . .] iscioccho e non è i' suo sentiment";136r: Portata of Mona Lena vedova donna fu di Giovanni Pigiello whose son was "pazzo": 208r: Portata of Marccho di Bernardo whose son was said to be "infermo del corpo et della mente," and "mal maestro" (prone to fits or seizures); 249v: Portata of Matteo di Franciescho whose wife was "fuori di suo sentimento natural"; 676r–v: Portata of Monna Tessa whose mother was "uscita fuori di sentimento" and "rinbambita"; 50, 718r–721r: Portata of Nozzo di Piero di Nozzo, who was said to have lost his mind "perduto la mente"; 56, 371r: Portata of Monna Antonia di Bacco vedova dal Canto al Monteloro whose daughter was "non è in buono sentiment"; 718r–v: Portata of Mona Chaterina donna fu di Piero di

Francho whose son was "pazzo": 59, 387r; Portata of Salvestro di Giunta, who was said to be "fuori d'ogni sentiment"; 63 (Aggiunte), 403r: Portata of Mona Bella vedova di Nofri di Ruggieri, who had a female cognate relative said to be "fuori di sua memoria"; 474r: Portata of Mona Papera donna fu di Iachopo d'Ubaldino Fastagli whose daughter was given over to the spirit "fa si die a lo spirito."

70. ASF, Catasto 47, fol. 208r: Portata of Marccho di Bernardo whose son was said to be "infermo del corpo et della mente" and "mal maestro." Zucchero Bencivenni (fl. 1300–1313), a Florentine notary who translated a number of learned medical texts from Latin into Italian, defined "mal maestro" as an illness beginning in childhood in which one falls to the ground and the limbs convulse. See Salvatore Battaglia's definition in the *Grande dizionario della lingua italiana*. See also *Lessicografia della Crusca in Rete*, http://www.lessicografia.itController?lemma=MAL+MAESTRO (accessed August 4, 2011).

71. Piers Britton, "'Mio malinchonico, o vero . . . mio pazzo': Michelangelo, Vasari, and the Problem of Artists' Melancholy in Sixteenth-Century Italy," *Sixteenth Century Journal* 34, no. 3 (2003): 655.

72. Niccolò Falcucci claimed that melancholy and mania corrupted the moral operations. Falcucci, *Sermones medicinales*, fol. 71r: "quod mania est lesio omnium virtutum moralium corruptiva," and of melancholy, "Et ut sic aliqui auctores corruptionem operationum ipsarum virtutum omnium moralium." Similarly, Giovanni Arcolani (ca. 1390–1458), professor of medicine at Bologna and Padua, claimed that melancholics and manics could not distinguish between right and wrong, enmity or friendship. Arcolani, *Practica*, 50: "cum iudicent melancholici recta et honesta, inhonesta et non recta, eliciantque inimicitiam pro amicitia."

73. Avicenna, *Liber Canonis*, Liber III, Fen I, Tractatus IV, Capitulum xvi, *De mania canina*.

74. Arcolani, *Practica*, 51: "Mania vero est duplex una lupine, aliter dicta daemonium lupinum; videntur enim non hominess sed daemons, et lupi, qui patiuntur hanc maniam."

75. Guainerio, *Practica*, fol. 23r.

76. Ibid.: "est cum se canina autem est species maniae existens cum ira permixta tripudio, et inquisitione corrupta permixta petitioni, quemadmodum est ex natura canum et in hac est associato vehemens, et amicitia cum obedientia, et conuenientia simul."

77. Roberto Caracciolo [Roberto da Lecce], *Quaresimale padovano*, 1455, ed. Oriana Visani (Padua: Edizioni Messaggero, 1983), 100.

78. Tomaso Garzoni, *L'ospidale de' pazzi incurabili*, ed. Stefano Barelli (Rome: Editrice Antenore, 2004).

79. Avicenna, *Liber Canonis*, Liber III, Fen I, Tractatus IV, Capitulum xx.

80. Giovanni da Concorregio, *Practica nova medicine*, fol. 21r: "Galenus facit mentionem quarto de interioribus nam quidam putant se esse dominos quidam lupos quidam gallos unde errigunt brachia tamquam allas et cantant et quibusdam videtur quid deus senescat et quibusdam videtur quid angelus

qui movet celum fatigetur et fugiunt ne super eos cadat celum et quidam putant se esse epos? et volunt conferre prehendas et quibusdam videtur quid sint vasa vitrea vel argilosa et ideo timent tangine frangantur. Aliis videtur quid sint magistri in omni scientia et incipiunt legere et docere et tamen nihil dicunt rationale."

81. Lorenzo Bellini, *De morbis capitis et pectoris*, cited in Alessandro Dini, *Il medico e la follia: Cinquanta Casi di Malattia Mentale nella Letterature Medica Italiana del Seicento* (Florence: Le lettere, 1997).

82. Falcucci, *Sermones medicinales*, fol. 72r.

83. Nalle, *Mad for God*, chaps. 7, 8.

84. ASF, MP 1913. I am grateful to Brett Auerbach-Lynn for sharing the case of Daria Carli with me. I was able to consult ASF, MP 1913 in Florence. But I have relied on Brett's transcription of Biblioteca Casantense, Rome, ms. 3825, fols. 166r, 222r.

85. ASF, MP 1913.

86. Ibid.

87. Biblioteca Casantense, Rome, ms. 3825, fol. 166r.

88. Ibid., 22r.

89. Siegfried Wenzel, *The Sin of Sloth: Acedia in Medieval Thought and Literature* (Chapel Hill: University of North Carolina Press, 1989), 49.

90. Pomata, *Contracting a Cure*, 134.

91. Guainerio, *Practica*, fol. 24r.

92. Ibid.

93. Girolamo Mercuriale, *Responsorum et consultationum medicinalium tomus tertius*, cited in Dini, *Il medico e la follia*, 45–46.

94. Sharon T. Strocchia, "The Melancholic Nun in Late Renaissance Italy," in *Diseases of the Imagination and Imaginary Diseases in the Early Modern Period*, ed. Yasmin Haskell (Turnhout: Brepols, 2011), 139–58.

95. See Wack, *Lovesickness in the Middle Ages*.

96. Ibid., 61. Pseudo-Aristotle, *Problemata* 30.1, 953a, 10–14, cited in Klibansky, Panofsky, and Saxl, *Saturn and Melancholy*. For the reception of the pseudo-Aristotelian *Problemata* and problem literature in the Renaissance, see Ann Blair, "The *Problemata* as a Natural Philosophical Genre," in *Natural Particulars: Nature and the Disciplines in Renaissance Europe*, ed. Anthony Grafton and Nancy Siraisi (Cambridge, Mass.: MIT Press, 1999), 171–204, and in the same volume, John Monfasani, "The Pseudo-Aristotelian *Problemata* and Aristotle's *De Animalibus* in the Renaissance," 205–47.

97. ASF, MPAP 2257, fol. 214r: "Lorenzo del Gabburra Galigaio servitor fidelissimo di V.A. expone come sono finiti quattr'anni che fu messo nelle carcere delle Stinche per pazo, perche gli dettero noia gl'humor maninconici che non tendevano ad altra danno di persona o suo che seguire una donna che gli parea esserli stato promosso da persona grande che la consentirebbe alle sua voglie et fu si grande l'humore, che egli non abbandonava ne giorno ne notte le cura della casa di Lei a tale che chi v'haveva interesso il fece capturare, et metterlo dove di presente si trova, et non dopo troppi mesi al sole scachato purgo talemente l'humore che sdimenticatosi il tutto gli convenne se volea vivere impazare a far le fusa, et conoscendo la libertà essere cara

supplico V.A. ne lo facesso cavare, et ella mandato per informatione a buon
huomini quando pensò ottenere gratia fu trattenuto che non era tornata la
supplica, et dubitando non essere aggirato da qual che suo amorevole, che
il suo si gode, et egli stenta in carcere torna à in fastidir le benigne orecchie
del A.V. et con ogni vivo affetto la supplica che il faccia li liberare da tanto
stento, sotto mettendosi a ogni maggiore supplitio, se mai piu torna nell'humore, perche oltre l'haver spurgato insieme con qualche altro suo peccato,
ha conosciuto, di che sapore sono i duri ferri delle carcere, et ottendendo tal
gratia si offera pregare Dio sempre per Lei."

98. ASF, OGP 2257, fol. 214rv: "Questo supplicante di Gennaio '67 fu
messo nelle Stinche per pazzo per che oltre all'altre pazzie andava tutto el
[verso] intorno alla moglie di Girolamo Giudacci et gli teneva tutto el di asse-
diato la casa et è quello che gia stava tutto el di nel cortile de' Pitti et poi si
attaccava al Cocchio a infestare S.Al.S. che voleva andare a servirla. Hora
dice che è tornato savio et domanda gratia d'esser liberato."

99. Ficino, *De triplici vita*, 117.

100. Sharon Strocchia has argued that women, particularly nuns, did not
invoke melancholy genius. See "The Melancholic Nun in Late Renaissance
Italy," 143.

101. Brann, *The Debate over the Origin of Genius*, chap. 5.

102. Ibid., 249. Cipriano Giambelli, *Il diamerone ove si ragiona della
natura . . .* (Venice: Appresso Giorgio Angelieri, 1589), 10.

103. Magdalena S. Sánchez, *The Empress, the Queen, and the Nun:
Women and Power at the Court of Philip III of Spain* (Baltimore: Johns
Hopkins University Press, 1998), chap. 8. See the section of chapter 4 tit-
led, "Melancholy: 'The Crest of Courtiers' Arms,'" in MacDonald, *Mystical
Bedlam*, 150–60.

104. Strocchia, "The Melancholic Nun in Late Renaissance Italy," 143.

105. Midelfort, *A History of Madness*, 13.

106. Schleiner, *Melancholy, Genius, and Utopia*.

CHAPTER 5

1. Zac. *Quaest. Med. Leg.*, 160.

2. Innocent X (r. 1644–1655) and Alexander VII (r. 1655–1667).

3. Silvia De Renzi, "Witnesses of the Body: Medico-Legal Cases in Seventeenth-Century Rome," *Studies in History and Philosophy of Science* 33
(2002): 219–42.

4. Gregory Zilboorg, *A History of Medical Psychology* (New York: Nor-
ton, 1951); Erwin H. Ackerknecht, "The Early History of Legal Medicine,"
Ciba Symposia 11, no. 7 (1950): 1286–89; J. H. Langbein, *Prosecuting
Crime in the Renaissance: England, Germany, France* (Cambridge, Mass.:
Harvard University Press, 1974), 179–98; Paul Foriers, "La condition des
insensés à la Renaissance," in *Folie et déraison à la Renaissance* (Brussels:
Editions de l'Université de Bruxelles, 1976), 26–40; Boari, *Qui venit contra
iura*, 70; Esther Fischer-Homberger, *Medizin vor Gericht: Gerichtsmedizin
von der Renaissance bis zur Aufklärung* (Bern: Verlag Hans Huber, 1983);

Carol A. G. Jones, *Expert Witnesses* (Oxford: Oxford University Press, 1994), chap. 2.

5. Katherine D. Watson, *Forensic Medicine in Western Society: A History* (New York: Routledge, 2011); Cathy McClive, "Blood and Expertise: The Trials of the Female Medical Expert in the Ancien-Régime Courtroom," *Bull. Hist. Med.* 82 (2008): 86–108; Gianna Pomata, "Malpighi and the Holy Body: Medical Experts and Miraculous Evidence in Seventeenth-Century Italy," *Renaissance Studies* 21 (2007): 568–86; Monica Calabritto, "A Case of Melancholic Humors and Dilucida Intervalla," *Intellectual History Review* 18, no. 1 (2008): 139–54; Alessandro Pastore, *Il medico in tribunale: La perizia medica nella procedure penale d'antico regime (secoli XVI–XVII)* (Verona: Casagrande Bellinzona, 1998).

6. Eugenio Garin published a collection of humanist treatises on this subject in *La disputa delle arti nel Quattrocento* (Florence: Vallecchi, 1947). For a brief analysis of these works, see Lynn Thorndike, "Medicine Versus the Law in Late Medieval and Medicean Florence," *Romanic Review* 17 (1926): 8–31.

7. The absence of England in this narrative is telling. Dozens of monographs pertaining to medico-legal problems circulated throughout the early modern European continent. The English contribution to this debate before 1800 was, in Erwin Ackerknecht's words, "practically nil." See Ackerknecht, "Early History of Legal Medicine." Catherine Crawford has revised this view by showing that homicide trials in the Old Bailey used medical testimony during the eighteenth century. By and large, however, she has argued that the slow development of legal medicine in England relative to the Continent rests wholly on the difference between the two legal systems. The Romano-canonical tradition of law practiced on the Continent encouraged interactions between law and medicine, whereas English common law tended to inhibit it. See Crawford, "Legalizing Medicine: Early Modern Legal Systems and the Growth of Medico-Legal Knowledge," in *Legal Medicine in History*, ed. Michael Clark and Catherine Crawford (Cambridge: Cambridge University Press, 1994), 89–116.

8. Ambroise Paré published *Traicté des rapports, et du moyen d'embaumer les corps morts* in his collected works at Paris in 1575. This text has been digitally reproduced and is available online through the Bibliotèque Interuniversitaire de Médecine e d'Ondotologie. For works of Parè, see http:web2.bium.univ-paris5.frlivancindex.las (accessed August 16, 2008); Giovanni Filippo Ingrassia published *Methodis dandi relationes pro mutilavis torquendis, aut a tortura excusandis* in Venice in 1578. No copies of this edition are extant. A manuscript of the work survived in Palermo, however, and was published in 1938; Giovanni Battista Codronchi published *Methodus testificandi* in Frankfurt in 1597; and Fortunato Fedele published his work *De relationibus medicorum* around 1602 although the actual date of first publication is the occasion for some debate. Debates about the connection between death and pregnancy also generated lively discussion at the turn of the seventeenth century, especially in Rome. On this subject, see Silvia De Renzi, "Women's

Deaths in the Law Courts of Seventeenth-Century Rome," *Bull. Hist. Med.*
84 (2010): 549–77.

9. See Michael Clark and Catherine Crawford, eds., introduction to *Legal Medicine in History* (Cambridge: Cambridge University Press, 1994).

10. Carlo Colombero, "Il medico e il giudice," *Materiali per una storia della cultura giuridica* 16 (1986): 363–81, and idem, "Un contributo alla formazione della nozione di malattia mentale."

11. ASF, MPAP 2276, fol. 242r: "Allegando quella essere vexata da humori malinconici et altri accidenti et non essere habile a reggersi et governersi da perse et allegando etiam quella havere fatto certa donatione in Roma a un Piero Mellini di Fulto il suo."

12. ASF, MPAP 2276, fol. 242r: "Et per quanto conosciamo ci pare detta monna Maria essere di buona et sana mente ne troviamo in lei qualita che ci parve conforme al supplicato et in effetto la troviamo nel discorso del parlare assai experta et cosi nel tractare del sua negotii allegando quella di havere piati a Roma et volersi transferire la et non havere bisogno che la sorella si intrometta ne suoi affarri et che se ha fatta la donatione l'ha fatta per doppo la morte sua et reservatosi l'usufructo et essere vedova et poter dispore del suo." The Duke's secretary replied: "non occorre altro."

13. ASF, MPAP 2277, fol. 25r: "Per informatione del suplicato per Monna Maria figliuola fu de Thommaso Placiti . . . come quella narrato sua prece essere di certa provecta et essere spesso vexata da humori malenconici et non essere habile a a [sic] reggiersi ne a governare et custodire e sua beni desideria per gratia obtenere da Vostra Excellentissima Illustrissima che il magistrato nostro pigli la administratione dei suoi beni et reggimento depsa a cio in breve non habbi a mendicare."

14. ASF, MPAP 2277, fol. 25r: "et ci pare assai instabile et homorosa et male apta a reggiersi o governare li sua beni." The Duke replied: "Concedessi quando la donna non habbia parenti che possino pigliare di lei simil cura et governo."

15. ASF, MPAP 2277, fol. 84r: "si degni commettere a tal magistrato o a chi quella piaceva la annullatione di tal donatione costui facta in suo danno et della sorella et dona sua nipote di fratello che si trova innupta et sanza padre."

16. ASF, MPAP 2277, fol. 84r: "detta Monna Maria insiste nel medesimo et a justificatione di cio produce piu fede di private persone attestanti della sua mente non sana et quella dice essere [facta] indocta a fare tale donatione con le grandi promissioni factegli."

17. ASF, MPAP 2277, fol. 84r: "Non solo gli di poi observate con per decto Pietro si replica quella essere assai prudente et havere facta tal dispositione come conveniente a ciascuna persona di sano intellecto per essersi reservato l'usufructo et haverlli dati certi [. . .] di pigliare la sua nipote per donna et altro et facto in quella certa substitione et havere cosi donato per li benementi et faticha . . . per lei in Roma et per sepse facte in litigare."

18. ASF, MPAP 2277, fol. 84v: "Con che altra volta epsa Monna Maria quando non si intendeva con Monna Thommasa sua sorella Donna di Vicento Rucellai apparso la quale hoggi si trova diceva el contrario cioe di

essere savia et prudente et havere agitato piu cause avanti quanti tribunali haveva Roma et non havere bisogno di reggimento et che voleva che la donatione valessi come facta pensatamente con decreto del Giudica di Campidoglio et giurato et con tutte le solemnita requisite con essere sula rimessa alla gabella come piu volte affermo in persona avanti al magistro de' pupilli." The Duke's secretary replied: "I pupilli rivegghino questa donatione perche essendo mentecatta non e ragionevole che habbi luogo."

19. Testimony relating to Maria's case can be found in ASF, MPAP 2402, fols. 679r–763r, 852r–911r and 2404, fols. 556r–593v.

20. C. 6.36.5. In an undated *consilium*, the celebrated jurist Filippo Decio (1454–1535) upheld the provision stated in the *Codex* that sanity should be presumed in cases where there is doubt. See Decio, *Consilia*, vol. 4 (Lyon: Iacobus Giunta, 1546), Consilium 448, fol. 9r. The Sienese jurist Mariano Sozzini (1401–1467) similarly upheld the claim that proof of mental incapacity was incumbent on the accuser. See Mariano Sozzini and Bartolomeo Sozzini, *Consiliorum seu Responsorum Mariani Socini ac Bartholomeaei fili Senensium* (Venice: Franciscus Zilettum, 1579), *Consilium* 42, fol. 88r.

21. Bart. *De test.*, fols. 156v–163v at 161v: "furiosus probatur ex actibus: et si testis dicat quod vidit eum furere et actus furiosum facere satis exprimit sunt enim tales actus communiter noti." Decio cites Bartolus and Angelo Aretino (d. 1472) on this point. See Decio, *Consilia*, 9r: "et ideo si testis dicit quod vidit aliquem fuere et actus furiosorum facere, bene probat, ita Bartolo dicit in tractatu de testibus . . . Bartolo concludit quod in tali casu potius sensus corporis quam iudicium intellectus attendatur: et ad hoc est decisio in terminis Angeli . . . ubi dicit . . . quod furor per visum percipitur."

22. Decio, *Consilia*, fol. 9v: "ad probandum quem esse furiosum requiritur perspicax inquisitio."

23. Bart. *De test.*, fol. 161v: "Quid si dixerit quod viderit eum detineri in carcere vel ligatum funibus ut furiosum: puto hoc non sufficere sed adminiculari sed si adderet quod in vinculis vidi eum insana verba dicere sufficeret si predicta aliquo tempore fecerit sufficit dicere ad hoc ut furiosus etiam hodie presumatur nisi aliud doceatur."

24. Decio, *Consilia*, fol. 9v.

25. Jurists wrote *consilia* to answer nettlesome legal questions both as *exempla* for their students or as formal opinions for courts. They were sometimes written on behalf of one of the parties in a suit (*consilium pro parte*) or at the request of a presiding judge who may or may not have had formal legal training (*consilium sapientis*). In them, jurists constructed seemingly endless chains of precedent beginning with the opinions of Roman jurists and linking them with the most famous contemporary ruminations on the tradition. Although cases in this study did not seem to have generated specific *consilia*, a long legal commentary tradition that dealt with mental incapacity existed.

26. Decio, *Consiliorum sive Responsorum*, 2 vols. (Venice, 1575), 108v. This fiction is outlined in D. 5.2. See also Julius Kirshner, "Baldo de Ubaldo on Disinheritance: Contexts, Controversies, *Consilia*," in *Ius Commune* 27 (2000): 119–85.

27. Decio, *Consilia*, fol. 8v: "In prima consideratione videbatur dicendum quod sic nam in positionibus in xiiii.c.dicitur quod ab eius pueritia usque ad eius mortem fuit, et erat mentecaptus, et quod per vicos, et vias more stultorum, et mentecaptorum ibat, et loquebatur."

28. Decio, *Consilia*, fol. 9r: "Secundo in eodem capitulo dicitur quod si quis eum interrogabat non respondebat ad propositum, et quod habebat continue sermones et gestus et actus mentecaptorum, et nesciebat exprimere quod volebat et quod memoriam non habebat ordinatam."

29. Decio, *Consilia*, fol. 9r: "Tertio in eodem capitulo dicitur quod pro tali semper fuit habitus et reputatus: et de presenti habetur tenetur et reputatur, et in c.xv plenius dicitur quod parentes sui et omnes consanguinei, et omnes qui ipsum cognoscebant semper, et continue reputaverunt et tenuerunt Ioannem pro mentecapto stulto et fatuo."

30. Decio, *Consilia*, fol. 9v: "Primo enim apparet quod capitula super quibus debuerunt testes examinari cum magna et exquisita, insolitaque diligentia formata fuerunt a peritissimis viris, qui voluerunt instruere testes ad probandum dementiam."

31. Decio, *Consilia*, fol. 9v: "Unde ista insolita diligentia suspicionem fraudis inducit. . . . Secunda coniectura videtur: quia dicti tres vestes [sic] videntur deponere per eundem premeditatum et compositum sermonem: quia omnes eodem modo dicunt vera esse contenta in capitulo et eandem reddunt causam et rationem, quo casu redduntur suspecti."

32. Decio, *Consilia*, fol. 9v: "Tertio quia deponunt dictum Joannem ab eius infantia fatuum stultum et mentecaptum fuisse, et hoc videtur impossibile consyderata etate dicti Joannis qui nunc ageret annum septuagesimum si viveret, ut plerique testes attestantur quo casu dicti tres testes qui sunt longe minoris etatis, ut in processu ex ipsorum confessione constat non potuerunt de tempore pueritie dicti Joannis deponere cum nati non essent, et ideo non possunt dicere vera esse contenta in capitulo."

33. Decio cites both Paulo di Castro (ca. 1360–1416) and Aretino on this point. Decio, *Consilia*, fol. 9v: "qui examinati pro parte reorum deponunt dictum Joannem non fuisse stultum, neque mentecaptum: sed sane mentis, licet dicant illum fuisse grossolanum, prout etiam aliqui testes actorum dicunt, et tres presbyteri attestantur illum audivisse in confessione, et quod erat bonus Christianus, et quod erat sane mentis, et quod fatui et dementes non confitentur, et sic in effectu videtur probari quod non esset stultus neque mentecaptus, sed grossolanus, quo casu talis qui sit obtusi et grossi ingenii non prohibetur de bonis suis disponere . . . dicit Paulus de Castro . . . quod post pupilliarem etatem quis testari potest, licet non habeat naturalem vigorem sensus . . . et idem no[tat] Angelus Aretinus . . . non est permissam facere testamentum.ubi post Joan.Fab. dicit de mentecapto qui non potest testari, intelligitur de tali mentecapto, qui non intelligat quid agat nec habeat iudicium, secus si haberet intellectum. . . . Et idem pariter videtur in donatione, que licet a mentecapto facta non valeat quando sit talis mentacaptus qui nihil intelligit. Secus videtur in grossolano, qui cognoscit et intelligit quid agat, prout in casu isto videtur, et ex omnibus supradictis intentio reorum bene fundata videtur."

34. Bart. *De test.*, fol. 162r: "Sed quid si multa verba ordinate proferebant inter que alia fatua interserunt certe in illo actu fatuus presumitur." Bartolus was commenting here on book 21 of the *Digest*, which asked whether a slave who did not always manifest signs of madness and sometimes spoke rationally should still be considered sane. D. 21.1.9.

35. Sozzini, *Consiliorum*, fol. 88v: "Tres testes deponunt qualiter se mente captum volebat appellari."

36. Sozzini, *Consiliorum*, fol. 89r: "Assignant etiam testes deponentes pro sana mente bonas rationes scilicet quod quasi continue exercuit artem lanae, et quod habuit uxorem ex bonis parentibus, et civibus, quae non solent fieri nec haberi nisi ab hominibus sanae mentis."

37. Sozzini, *Consiliorum*, fol. 88v: "Nec probant aliae rationes allegatae per testes, quae videntur magis in specie concludere; quoniam ratio, quod appellebat se mentecaptum vel volebat se appellari, non est concludens imo potius videtur concludere contrarium; cum fatui semper existiment communiter se sapientes."

38. ASF, MPAP 2281, fol. 455r: "Domenico di Girolamo da Starda povero mentecatto e sotto posto alla cura del Magistrato de' Pupilli con ogni debita reverentia le narra come altra volta ricorse à V.A.S. narrandoli come eta stata fatta vendita di alcuni suoi beni, nella quale era stato ingannato oltre la meta del giusto prezzo e la pregava che si degnassi farli gratia si ritrattassi detta vendita e li fussi pagato il giusto prezzo." The Duke replied: "questa non è supplica da mentecatto, et essendo sotto la cura de'pupilli al magistrato tocca a parlare et non altro."

39. Sozzini, *Consiliorum*, fol. 89v: "Et sic ut intelligamus, quod dictus Ioannes Vernelli habuit dilucida intervalla, scilicet quod aliquando fuerit sanae mentis, prout deponunt testes Nicholai: aliquando fatuus prout deponunt testes curatoris: alias enim praedicti testes essent omnino contrarii sunt ergo ita intelligendi . . . quo testes partis adversae deponunt se vidisse ipsum facere multa signa fatuitatis, probent fatuitatem; non tamen sequitur, quod semper fuerit fatuus, quia non semper viderunt eum talia facere."

40. Bart. *De test.*, fol. 161v: "Sed an actus de quo agitur inquiete vel sanitate factus fuerit in dubio ipse actus ostendit."

41. Bart. *De test.*, fol. 161v.

42. I want to thank Jane Black for alerting me to this citation. Prospero Farinacci, *Praxis et theoricae criminalis* (Frankfurt, 1606), 191–92: "Si enim (exempli gratia) quis publice, et palam occiderit alterum, cum quo nullam habebat inimicitiam, nec caussam occidendi, illumque vulneravit, non se abscondidit, nec aufugit aut quid simile fecit, quod illius furorem, vel insaniam prae se ferat, et tunc utique crederem . . . et delictum praesumi patratum, tempore furoris, si caute ex caussa, seu inimicitia, aut saltem rixa praecedente vulneraverit et occiderit et post vulnus se deliquisse agnoscens aufugerit, se latitaverit; aut alias delictum occultare quaesierit, aut quid simile fecerit, quod mentis compotem eum fuisse tunc temporis, demonstrat."

43. ASF, MPAP 2402, fol. 872rv: "Disse che cognosce maddonna Maria de Placiti Piero Mellini nominati nello interrogatorio quali comincio à cognoscere cio è madonna maria del anno 1556 et Piero dell anno 1566 sebene si

ricorda et non sa che servitii precisamente detto Piero habbi fatto à madonna maria ma che bene sa et ha visto che stava in casa di essa et governava et questo lo sa perche stava rincontro alla casa di detta madonna maria et hoggi habita in esso nella quale ha habitato da che si parte in qui et che non sa se le spese fatte da Piero sono [872r] de danari sua o di madonna maria. . . . Disse che piu volte avanti la donatione fatta secondo che li pare ricordarsi dell'anno 1567 il detto Piero ragionando spesso con lui lo disse che l'entrate di detta madonna maria erano confuse sequestrate et interdetteli et che lui era necessitata litigare et spendere per lei de suoi denari tanto nel vitto quanto in ogni altra cosa necessaria et che per questi servitii detta madonna maria gli haveva promesso farli donatione, et che continuamente durava grandissima fatica et che per questo giudica che non obstante detta madonne maria [872v] ma ogni altro che havessi ricevuti simili servitii da lui."

44. ASF, MPAP 2402, fols. 875rv, 877v, 879r, 881rv, 885v, 900r, 910r.

45. ASF, MPAP 2402, fol. 875rv: "disse interrogato singularmente sopra ciascuno che fu presente alla stipulatione della donatione la quale si fece in casa di detta madonna maria con consenso [875v] del giudice et sebene si ricorda fu da mattina ma che non si ricorda del nome del notaro et giudice et che mentre che il notaro la stipulava et scriveva lei gli ricordava di molte cose et che disputava col giudice et era benissimo in cervello come sempre l'ha cognocsiuta et che stipulata che fu lei di sua mano secondo il solito di Roma la sottoscrisse et il simile li testimonii come esso et che non sa giudicare circa il donare tutti li suoi beni et che sene rimette come di sopra sopra il restante disse non sapere deponere et che mai ha inteso dire da nissuno che detta madonna maria non sia stata in cervello et sopra li altri ripose bene."

46. ASF, MPAP 2402, fol. 885v: "disse che fu testimone alla donatione fatta per detta madonna maria dove fu al principio che il notario comincio asirirere in presentia del giudice di campidoglio de nomi de quali disse non si ricordare, et che detta madonna maria stava competendo et disputando con il giudice et il notaro et voleva intendere passo per passo et che faceva replicare quando non intendeva bene et che si cognosceva che era benissimo in cervello et mostrava d'essere una donna savia et sebene si ricorda eredecrede che detta madonna maria sottoscrivessi di sua mano la donation."

47. ASF, MPAP 2402, fol. 879r: "disse sopra il contenuto nel capitolo non sapere depone altro se non che quando si stipulava la donatione la detta madonna maria si fece leggere piu volte dal notaro dicendoli Io voglio intendere bene ogni cosa."

48. ASF, MPAP 2402, fol. 761r: "disse non saper altro sendo che egli ha udito la diversa persone la dicta Madonna Maria esser stata vessata da certi humori di tal sorte che piu presto la pareva haver del pazo che altro et di piu haver inteso dir che era quasi spiritata et esserli durato certo tempo tale influenzia."

49. ASF, OGP 2222, fol. 792rv: "volendo detto Francesco supplicante provare come è la verita che sino l'anno 1546 havendo detto Jacopo a fare certo contratto con uno Marchuccio Pagnini di detto luogo dove detto Marchuccio li haveva a restituire certi danari andorono a piu notai li quali conosciuto et sappiendo la dementia di detto Jacopo non lo volsono rogare et

finalmente fu rogato da un certo Ser. Piero Boldrini notaio giovane et non molto sperimentato."

50. On this subject, see Bylebyl, "Medicine, Philosophy, and Humanism in Renaissance Italy"; Siraisi, *Taddeo Alderotti and His Pupils*; and Agrimi and Crisciani, *Edocere Medicos*.

51. Baldo degli Ubaldi, *Commentaria in quartum et quintum codicis lib* (Venice: Iuntas, 1572), fol. 41v: "Scias quod iudex sicut medicus: medicus enim cognoscit aegritudinem tripliciter, uno modo figuraliter, et improprie per urinam . . . videt enim infirmitatem sicut homo videt aliquid in speculo per quandam umbram sic se habet iudex quando videt speculando, et intra se conferendo per verisimilia, et proxima ad veritatem cognoscendam. Secundo modo videt medicus per tactum pulsi, sic iudex se habet quando (ut ita dixerim) tangit veritatem per aperta testimonia. Tertio modo videt medicus a remotis pronosticando: ita iudex eum annexa suspicatur, quod non pertinet condemnationem in genere." Note the play on *speculum* and *speculare*. Through artful wordplay, Baldo compares the physician's view of disease through urine as if through a mirror (*speculum*) to the judge's use of speculation (*speculare*).

52. For a good discussion of Baldo's analogy between medicine and law and a discussion of medieval and early modern legal medicine, see De Renzi, "Witnesses of the Body," 223.

53. D. 24.3.22.7; C. 5.70.6; C. 6.22.9.

54. Bart., *De test.*, fol. 161v: "si predicta aliquo tempore fecerit sufficit dicere ad hoc ut furiosus etiam hodie presumatur nisi aliud doceatur."

55. Angelo Aretino [Angelo Gambiglioni], *Tractatus maleficiorum* (Mantua: Petrus Adam de Michaelibus, 1472), no foliation, n.p., "et sic antiquus furor transferat onus probandi in adversarium . . . quod semel furiosus semper praesumatur furiosus, quia passiones humori praesumuntur durare, nisi contrarium probetur."

56. BAV, Urb. Lat. 1132, *Consilia Varia*, fol. 289r; 287r modern numeration: "Et sic vult in effectu Bartolo quod si probatum est quem fuisse furiosum certis mensibus presumatur in posterum furiosus."

57. Giulio Claro, fol. 162r: "Sic etiam quaedam Iacobina Ferraria, quae puellam quandam trimam baculo interfecerat, comperto, quod laborabat atrabile, et quod alias uti mentacapta custodita fuerat in hospitali S. Vincentii, fuit absoluta, et ad ipsum hospitale iterum transmissa 24 Februarii 1454."

58. Catherine Crawford, "Medicine and the Law," in *Companion Encyclopedia of the History of Medicine*, ed. W. F. Bynum and Roy Porter (New York: Routledge, 1993), 2:1624.

59. Zac. *Quaest. Med. Leg.*, book 3, title 2, "De morborum simulatione," and Quaestio 5, "De simulata insania," 160.

60. Zac. *Quaest. Med. Leg.*, 160: "intersit inter melancholiam, et furorem, nimirum, quod illa affecti in quiete sint, timidi, tristes, animoque demisso, hoc autem laborantes, in perpetuo motu, sine ulla requie, audaces, et iracundi."

61. Zac. *Quaest. Med. Leg.*, 160: "consideranda enim primo facies, quae in his, qui vere melancholici sunt aut furentes, tendit ad quasi terreum

colorem, vel lividum, aut est ultra consuetum rubicunda, sed cum quadam livedine ob melancholiae admictionem, in furentibus praesertim."

62. Zac. *Quaest. Med. Leg.*, 160: "Si sanguis melancholiae sit admixtus . . . se ipsis fortiores evadunt, iracundi fiunt, minimaque ex caussa excandescunt, clamant vociferantur, absentibus praesentibus minantur, torvo aspectu sunt et violento corporis motu formidabiles."

63. Zac. *Quaest. Med. Leg.*, 160: "Quilibet ergo videt, quod haec omnia simul non tam facile fingi possunt; et si animum prudens medicus adverterit, ex plurimorum supradictorum absentia aut praesentia sine magno negotio deprehendere poterit, quando furor aut melancholia vere fatiget, quando vero simulare."

64. Zac. *Quaest. Med. Leg.*, 160: "Adest insuper praeter haec omnia signum maximopere considerabile, quod est perpetua vigilia, qua tam furentes omnes, quam melancholici magna ex parte perpetuo afflictantur, vel ob humoris ipsius, qui cerebrum obsidet, siccitatem."

65. Zac. *Quaest. Med. Leg.*, 160: "ut recte dixerit Celsus, somnum in his tam difficilem esse, quam necessarium; itaque hoc uno signo considerato, aliquando deprehendere licebit eum, qui furorem simulat impossibile enim est, hunc consueto somno non capi, ac praeter morem per longum tempus vel volentem vigilare, ubi caussa interna eum vigilare non cogat."

66. Zac. *Quaest. Med. Leg.*, 160: "si quando somno indulgere possunt, perturbantur."

67. Zac. *Quaest. Med. Leg.*, 161: "Denique nonnulla ingenia ad insaniam deprehendam proponuntur, scio primum doctissimum et experissimum quemdam Medicum, cuius nomen iustis ex caussis non profero, cum sibi oblatus esset is casus, in quo de simulata insania ambigebatur, insanum illum multis verberibus affici illico iussisse eo sine et intentione, ut si vere insaniret iis verberibus [humores] ad vapulantes partes diverteret, sin vero simularet, eorundem verberum virtute vel nolens resipisceret."

68. ASF, MPAP 2279, fol. 83r: "quello esser matto si al parllare et rispondere come al guardarllo in viso per havere e capelli per insino alle spalle et macilento et di malissimo color et li ochi spaventati."

69. ASF, MPAP 2279, fol. 83r: "et dice havere scoperto parte della chasa havere lasciato goder al lavoratori parechi anni tutti e fructi: per haver compassione di quello come povero et ha 2 botteghine sotto la sua chasa quale tiene spigionate da piu anni in qua et non se ne serve et dice volere e, topi possino ire aspasso et compra zuche et biade per dar mangiare a detti topi et del suo modo di fare et di vivere da pazo."

70. ASF, MPAP 2280, fol. 32r.

71. Darrel W. Amundsen and Garry B. Ferngren, "The Forensic Role of Physicians in Roman Law," *Bull. Hist. Med.* 53, no. 1 (1979): 47.

72. Ibid., 45–46.

73. Osvaldo Cavallar, "Agli arbori della medicine legale: I trattati *De percussionibus* e *De vulneribus*," in *Ius Commune* 26 (1999): 27–89. See also Cavallar, "La *benefundata sapienta* dei periti: Feritori, feriti e medici nei commentari e consulti di Baldo degli Ubaldi," *Ius Commune* 27 (2000): 215–81; Mario Ascheri, "Consilium sapientis, perizia medico, e res iudicata:

diritto dei dottori e istituzioni comunali," in *Proceedings of the Fifth International Congress of Medieval Canon Law (Salamanca 21–25 September, 1976)*, ed. Stephen Kuttner and Kenneth Pennington (Vatican City: Biblioteca Apostolica Vaticana, 1980).

74. Cavallar, "Agli arbori della medicine legale," 38.

75. Cited in ibid., 40: Bartolus, *Tractatus testimoniuroum*, in *Tractatus de testibus* (Venice, 1574), 39n12: "Ned in hiis contradicit quod in hiis, que consistunt in artis peritia, medici, obstetrices et similes de crdulitate deponunt. Non enim sunt proprie tested, des magis ut iudices adsumuntur ad illum cause articulum iudicandum."

76. Gina Fasoli and Pietro Sella, eds., *Statuti di Bologna dell'anno 1288* (Vatican City: Biblioteca apostolica vaticana, 1937), 1:172–74, book 4, post rubric 4, *Quot possint accusari vel denunciari de morte licuius et de medicis mittendis et de vulneribus illatis post mortem.*

77. Severino Caprioli and Attilio Bartoli Langeli, eds., *Statuto del Comun di Peugia del 1279* (Perugia: Deputazione di storia patria per l'Umbria, 1996), 1:98–99, rubric 80: *Qualiter duo medici, unus cirusicus et alius fisicus, habenatur.*

78. Francesco Salvestrini, ed., *Statuti del Comune di San Miniato al Tedesco* (Pisa: ETS, 1994), 140, book II, rubric 14: "*De pena membri debilitati, incisi vel inutilis facti*"; Mario Brogi, ed., *Gli albori del Comune di San Gimignano e lo statuto del 1314* (Siena: Cantagalli, 1995), 284–85, dist. 5, rubric 53, *De pecunia danda madeico cerurgico*; Ackercknecht, "Early History of Legal Medicine," 1288.

79. Decio, *Consilia*, fol. 9v: "tres presbyteri attestantur illum audivisse in confessione, et quod erat bonus Christianus, et quod erat sane mentis, et quod fatui et dementes non confitentur, et sic in effectu videtur probari quod non esset stultus neque mentecaptus."

80. ASF, MPAP 2402, fol. 760v: "Et esse pratico in conoscerla malatia delli humori malinconici essendo lui della professione fisica."

81. ASF, MPAP 2402, fol. 756v: "dixit haver visto la dicta madonna maria far tutti quelli atti da lui detti sopra et altri assai simili da sciocca et balorda et humorista che sarebbe lungho a raccontarli."

82. ASF, MPAP 2402, fol. 756r: "Haver conosciuto da xxv anni in qua in Roma la articolata monna maria placida e sempre haver la vista piena d'humor malinconici, e fare e dire cose da pazze e come sempre haverla vista di volte cavalcare a certe sue vigne fuori di Roma, andando adosso al marito e a figlicoli con l'arme et alle volte stando a tavola voltarsi loro con coltelli e dire delle cose sciochissime dalle volte senza proposito haver'mandato a chiamare barbieri et stufanioli e fatto si cavar sangue senza bisogno, o licenzia di medici, et simile altre cosacce. Et spesso ella esse vessata dal simili humori come dire una volta intrallalto si parte sola di Roma da un Mulattini si fece menar al oreto e altre simil cose che sarebbe lungho a raccontarle, et in somma lei era per tale tenuta conosciuta e reputata da chiunche la conosciuta et haveva sua pratica come haveva esso testimonio."

83. ASF, MPAP 2402, fol. 756v: "come dire stando una notte in terra senza andaresene a letto ne dormire durare gran pazzo a parlare di cose

senza proposito et sgharbate ne tempi da lui detti di sopra in presenza di quelli da lui detti di sopra e di servitori et servo che stavano in casa col maria et co' altri, che disse non si ricordar dei nomi et cio esse stato nella casa che tenevano a Piazza Catinara."

84. ASF, MPAP 2402, fol. 756v: "la stava a Piazza Catinara et in spezie di un certo mess Gisberto Tedesco fisico della medico gran tempo per simili humori et continuando lettura dictorum interrogatiorum dixit haver visto la dicta madonna maria far tutti quelli atti da lui detti sopra et altri assai simili da sciocca et balorda et humorist."

85. ASF, MPAP 2402, fol. 756r: "haver'mandato a chiamare barbieri et stufanioli e fatto si cavar sangue senza bisogno, o licenzia di medici, et simile altre cosaccie."

86. ASF, MPAP 2402, fols. 756v–757r: "Et non esse pratico a conoscere li humori malinconici se non per li effeti come faceva et diceva la decta madonna maria che faceva et diceva cose non convenienti a persona di sana-mente come ha decto di sopra . . . et non haver mai visto alcuna altra per-sona che patisca delli humori malinconici che stia in cervello lungho tempo con cio sia che dicti humori gli tengano alterarla la mente et il cervello et in spezie disse haver conosciuto Agnolo figliolo della madonna maria che pativa di simili humori, che altre volte bisogna tenerlo legato et serrato e . . . et cosi d'un'altra cugina di lei che era [757r] pur vessata e e da tali humori che la ha fatto e fa cose da paze."

87. ASF, MPAP 2402, fols. 757v–758r: "fu chiamato da Francesco Ser-ragli ultimo suo marito a scrivere et copiar certe scritture, et haver praticato in casa delli detti Maria et Francesco quando habitavano in piaza catinara et haver di continuo considerata la dicta madonna maria et haverla hauta et tenuta et tenerla per persona humorista variabile di poco cervello et cio haver conosciuto nella varieta dei gesti che la faceva . . . [758r] disse non esso pra-tico in conoscere la infirmita malinconi che ne credere che quelli di monna maria sopradetta fussino humori malinconici ma piu tosto ramo di leggerezza et sciocheza e spezie di pazo."

88. ASF, MPAP 2402, fol. 758r: "Et non saper per quella che d. m. maria sia stata tenuta in firenze nelli aritcolati anni 65 et 66 per non ci esser lui stato ma saper bene che in Roma ella era tenuta per mezza pazza e sciocha."

89. ASF, MPAP 2402, fols. 758v–759r: "disse che del anno 1540 in qua che egli ha conosciuta la articolata madonna maria placida che fu quando la fu maritata al secondo Francesco Serragli egli la ha tenuta per donna sciocca o senza cervello per havergli visto fare e dire cose che non si sarebbeno ne fatte dette la donna sana et di buon cervello [759r] ma segl'altri la tengano per tale, disse non saper, ma egli disse lui haveva tenuta per detto tempo sem-pre per pazzo."

90. ASF, MPAP 2402, fol. 759r: "et non esse pratico in conoscerli humori malinonici, ma disse che li humori della dicta monna maria erano piutosto di paza et furiosa che di malinconici et non haver tristo ne saper cazioni delli humori malinconici ma non haver mai vista la dicta maria star in cervelli."

91. ASF, MPAP 2402, fol. 760v: "Et esse pratico in conoscerla malatis delli humori malinconici essendo lui della professione fisica . . . disse haver

conosciuta l'articolata Madonna Maria da tre anni fa in circa sebene si ricorda e parerli che la dicta madonna maria fusse vessata da humori malinconici et per tale infirmita ella si faceva medicare et esso testimonio come medico haverla medicata et haverla tenuta per donna di non troppa sana mente."

92. ASF, MPAP 2402, fol. 760v: "disse che nel parlar di lei si conosceva el suo cervello esse vagante e quando era in un proposito et quando in un altro et non si ricordar delle parole che la diceva . . . si conoscano in visione sanguinis aduste humoris collerici petentis cerebrum id est facultatem cogitativam egli segni la dicta madonna maria haveva et non esser dubio che fatto che l'humor malinconico habbia el corso suo efforgato, che'l paziente ritorna et creder che delli interrogari anni 1565 et 66 esso testimonio medicasse la paziente madonna maria impero riferirsi alle sue ricette."

93. ASF, MPAP 2402, fol. 761r: "disse non saper altro sendo che egli ha udito la diversa persone la dicta Madonna Maria esser stata vessata da certi humori di tal sorte che piu presto la pareva haver del pazo che altro et di piu haver inteso dir che era quasi spiritata et esserli durato certo tempo tale influenzia."

94. ASF, MPAP 2402, fol. 761v: "dixit haver conosciuta la dicta madonna maria placido dalli articolati dieci anni e piu per donna di mancamanto di cervello ma de tal difetto sia proceduto da humori malinconici o altri disse non sapere."

95. ASF, MPAP 2402, fol. 762rv: "disse che poi che l'articolata m. maria placida si marito con Francesco Serragli ultimo suo marito che possono essere [762v] da ventianni in circa, essa Madonna non e mai stata in cervello ne donna di buon discorso ne di sana mente e per tale ella e stata di continuo per detti tempi tenuta e reputata da chiunque la conosceva."

96. ASF, MPAP 2402, fol. 866r: "disse che ha cognosciuto madonna Maria et Piero nel interrogatorio nominati qui in Roma et che circa tre o quattro anni sono vidde spessissime volte il detto Piero in casa di Madonna Maria ma non sa gia che servitii seli habbi fatto et che cognosce detta Maddona Maria qui in Roma da detto tempo in qua perche e stata sua parrochiana et l'ha confessata et communicata et molte volte l'ha visitata malata in casa."

97. ASF, MPAP 2402, fol. 866r: "et ha detto un anno per lei ogni sabato continuamente una messa a san cesareo et li dava continuamente l'olio per il sabato per la lampada anzi molte volte."

98. ASF, MPAP 2402, fol. 870v.

99. ASF, MPAP 2402, fols. 869v–870r: "Che esso testimone dal tempo che la conosciuta detta madonna maria l'ha cognosciuta et trovata nel parlare donna prudente et di sana mente."

100. ASF, MPAP 2402, fol. 873v: "come fanno tutte le donne savie et di mente sana, et che l'ha vista spessissime volte andare a detta Chiesa della trinita et in quella udire li offitii et dopo i quelli ancora andava a visitare li convalescenti dello spedale di detta chiesa come fanno tutte le persone sanie et buone christiane et che vivono con il timore di dio et che per tale e sempre stata tenuta da tutti che l'hanno conosciuta et che cosi fu e e vero."

101. ASF, MPAP 2402, fol. 876r: "et che lei se bensi ricorda si confessava dal parrochiano di san paulo all a regola al quale mai de casi de detta madonna maria ha parlato et sopra li altri disse non sapere deponere—"

102. ASF, MPAP 2402, fol. 884r.

103. ASF, MPAP 2277, fol. 84v.

104. ASF, MPAP 2404, fol. 573r.

105. ASF, MPAP 2404, fol. 570v: "Item se Francesco fu et era huomo di cervello o pure mentecapto."

106. ASF, MPAP 2404, fols. 568v, 573r, 577r, 588v, 589rv.

107. ASF, MPAP 2404, fols. 569r, 570r, 577rv, 587v.

108. ASF, MPAP 2404, fol. 571r: "Et non sapere che detto Francesco negociassi con banchi ma si bene sapere che detto Francesco faceva mercantia de Mortella compagnia di Corami con certi vaccinari et faceva un magazzino grossissimo di vino di campagna quale vino faceva condurre dalli suoi muli et suoi mulattieri particulari."

109. ASF, MPAP 2404, fol. 569v: "quando detto Francesco la prese per moglie piglio tutti li affitti robbe mercantie vini mortelle et altro che era restato del primo marito di detta Madonna Maria insieme con le massaritie et bestiami et che di tutto sborso incontanti li dinari et che di detti danari li figlioli della detta Maria." See also fols. 580v, 577r, 588v, 589rv.

110. ASF, MPAP 2404, fol. 586v: "post mortem dicti sui primi viri ipsa domina Maria dum stetit in viduitate percepit fructus hereditatis eius Francesci sui viri qua era 4000 scutorum nempe duarum vinearum diversorum afficiorum domorum et aliorum qua erant in dicta hereditate ex quibus similiter potuit acquirere maximam quantitatem pecuniarum et de eis ad suum beneplacitum disponere."

111. ASF, MPAP 2404, fol. 586r: "Francescum de Serragliis qui fuit vir facultosissimus et abbundans pecuniis a quo ipsa domina Maria tempore vite eius de primi mariti habuit multas gemmas margheritas anullos catenas aureas pecunias vestimenta preciosa et quam plura alia ad ornatum mulieris quibus, moruo primo viro eidem domine Maria remanentibus potuit eas vendere ultra pretium mille scutorum et de dictis pecuniis emere stabilia et mobilia ad sui beneplacitum."

112. ASF, MPAP 2404, fol. 570rv: "sapere che la detta Madonna Maria era persona [570v] altiera et che voleva metter le mano in ogni cosa amministrare et governare ogni cosa et che quando Francesco suo marito li opponeva in niente cominciava a gridare bravarlo et dire villania et minacciarlo di sorte che detto Francesco era forzato lassarli fare quello che essa voleva, come piu volte esso testimone per essere huomo di casa disser haver visto sentito et esser stato presente infinite volte. Et pero tiene et giudica che la detta Madonna Maria per la sua mala natura sia stata potissima causa della sua ruina." See also fols. 578rv, 589v–590r.

113. ASF, MPAP 2404, fol. 570r: "et ita prodigaliter se gessit quod in processu temporis dictus Francescus eius maritus pauper et senex affectus fuit propter malam administrationem et protamenta dictae donnae Mariae communiterque reputabatur quod dicta domina Maria esset causa de paupertate

et ruina dicti Francisci sui viri et quod illa illum in extrema paupertate adduxit." See also fols. 578rv, 588r.

114. ASF, MPAP 2404, fol. 570v.

115. ASF, MPAP 2404, fol. 571r: "detto Messer Francecso lo trovo homo savio et di lettere et giuditio et prudente sino al'ultima sua vecchiezza." See also fol. 578r.

116. ASF, MPAP 2404, fol. 589r: "cognobbe detto Francesco sempre lo trovo huomo di cervello et savio salvo che poco avanti la sua morte convincio piu presto a rimbanbire." See also fol. 590r: "cognobbe detto Francesco per persona di cervello et huomo sano, et che poco avanti sua morte parte per la vecchiezza et parte per la poverta comincio piu presto che non a rimbambire."

117. Lawrence Stone, *Uncertain Unions: Marriage in England, 1660–1753* (Oxford: Oxford University Press, 1992), 5.

CONCLUSION

ASF, SDP, reg. 341, fol. 515r: "La pazzia è un infermita forse la maggior che possa aver l'huomo prima perche privandolo del discorso lo rende simile agli animali irragionevoli non gli lasciando d'umana altro che l'aspetto. Secondo per che ella non gl'induce come fanno tutte l'altre malattie, un desiderio di liberarsene. . . . Perciò . . . per legge d'umanità e di cristiana religione siamo serviti alla compassione e soccorso quanto maggiormente lo dobbiamo fare in un caso ove il paziente non si può aiutare non avendo a sua disposizione la propria volontà."

1. Nalle, *Mad for God*, 159.

2. Roscioni, *Il governo della follia.*

3. Roscioni convincingly argues against reading too much into this literature of folly while Graziella Magherini and Vittorio Biotti tend to see Florence's Stinche and Santa Dorotea dei Pazzarelli in Foucauldian terms. See Magherini and Biotti, eds., *"Un luogo della città per custodia de' pazzi": Santa Dorotea dei Pazzerelli di Firenze nelle delibere della sua congregazione (1642–1754)* (Florence: Casa Editrice Le Lettere, 1997).

4. ASF, SDP, reg. 42, fol. 96r, cited in Magherini and Biotti, *"Un luogo della città,"* 68–69.

5. ASF, SDP, reg. 341, fol. 475r: "Essendo noi informato della necessità che vi è nel nostro Gran ducato di Toscana d'uno spedale idoneo per curare et compassionerli malattie comprese nel genere della mania e che custodirvi quelli che sono incurabili."

6. ASF, SDP,

reg. 341, fol. 475r: "ed ai molti inconvienienti che' innocentemente cagionano nel pubblico i furiosi abbandonati e vaganti per le pubbliche strade."

7. ASF, SDP, reg. 341, fols. 475v–476r: "la fabbrica capace per sessanta malati almeno e opportunamente divisa per servire con la dovuta decenza ai due sessi e alle [476r] diverse condizioni di persone."

8. ASF, SDP, reg. 341, fol. 517v: "I quali 12 governatori siano sempre et in ogni tempo liberi di ricevere sotto il loro governo pazzi di qualsivoglia sorte tanto maschi, come femmine d'ogni paese, nazione, popolo, stato, grado, e condizione."

9. ASF, SDP, reg. 341, fols. 520r–521r.

10. Nalle, *Mad for God*, 158.

11. Roscioni, *Il governo della follia*, 55.

12. Ibid., xv.

BIBLIOGRAPHY

ARCHIVAL SOURCES

Archivio di Stato, Florence (ASF)

Acquisti e Doni

Atti del Podestà (AP)

Capitano del Popolo (CP)

Catasto of 1427

Online Catasto of 1427. Version 1.3. Eds. David Herlihy, Christiane Klapisch-Zuber, R. Burr Litchfield and Anthony Molho. [Machine readable data file based on D. Herlihy and C. Klapisch-Zuber, Census and Property Survey of Florentine Domains in the Province of Tuscany, 1427–1480.] Providence, R.I.: Florentine Renaissance Resources/STG: Brown University, 2002.

Giudice degli appelli e nullità (GA)

Innocenti, Estranei

Magistrato dei pupilli ed adulti avanti il principato (MP)

Magistrato dei pupilli ed adulti del principato (MPP)

Martelli

Magistrato Supremo (MS)

Otto di Guardia e Balia della avanti il principato (OG)

Otto di Guardia e Balia del principato (OGP)

Provvisioni Regstri (PR)

Santa Dorotea dei Pazzerelli (SDP)

Soprastanti alle Stinche (SS)

Online Tratte of Office Holders, 1282–1532. *Florentine Renaissance Resources*, machine readable data file. Ed. David Herlihy, R. Burr Litchfield, Anthony Molho, and Roberto Barducci. Providence, R.I.: Florentine Renaissance Resources/STG: Brown University, 2002.

PRINTED PRIMARY SOURCES

Alberti, Leon Battista. *I libri della famiglia*. Ed. Ruggiero Romano and Alberto Tenenti. Turin: Einaudi, 1969.

Alighieri, Dante. *La commedia secondo l'antica vulgate*. Ed. Giorgio Petrocchi. Milan: Mondadori, 1966–68.

Arcolani, Giovanni. *Practica*. Venice, 1493.

Angelo degli Ubaldi. *Consilia*. Frankfurt: Typis Andreae Wecheli: Sumptibus Sig. Feyrabend, 1575.

Avicenna. *Liber Canonis*. Ed. Aldrea Alpago. Trans. Gerard of Cremona. Basel: Ioannes Hervagios, 1556.

Baldo degli Ubaldi. *Commentaria in quartum et quintum codicis lib*. Vol. 6. Venice: Iunta, 1572.

———. *Consilioum primus-quintus volumen et repertorium*. Vol. 3. Venice, 1526.

Bartolus da Sassoferrato. *De testibus* in *Commentaria: Cum additionibus Thomae Diplovatatii*. Ed. G. Polara. Rome, Istituto giuridico Bartolo da Sassoferrato: Il cigno Galileo Galilei, 1996.

Benzi, Ugo. *Consilia*. Venice, 1518.

St. Bonaventure. "Major Legend of Saint Francis." In *Francis of Assisi— The Founder: Early Documents*, ed. Regis J. Armstrong, J. A. Wayne Hellmann, and William J. Short, 2:530–38. New York: New City Press, 2000.

Cantini, Lorenzo. *Legislazione Toscana*. Florence: S. Maria in Campo, 1800–1808.

Caracciolo, Roberto [Roberto da Lecce]. *Quaresimale padovano, 1455*. Ed. Oriana Visani. Padua: Edizioni Messaggero, 1983.

Da Monte, Giovanbattista. *Consultationum medicarum opus*. Basel: Henricus Petri, 1565.

Decio, Filippo. *Consilia*. 5 vols. Lyon: Iacobus Giunta, 1546.

———. *Consiliorum sive Responsorum*. 2 vols. Venice, 1575.

Falcucci, Niccolò. *Sermones medicinales*. 4 vols. Venice: Bernardinus Staginus, 1490/91.

Farinacci, Prospero. *Praxis et theoricae criminalis*. Frankfurt, 1606.

Ficino, Marsilio. *De triplici vita*. Trans. Carol V. Kaske and John R. Clark. Binghamton, N.Y.: Medieval & Renaissance Texts & Studies, 1989.

Giambelli, Cipriano. *Il diamerone ove si ragiona della natura . . .* Venice: Appresso Giorgio Angelieri, 1589.

Hippocrates. *De aëre aquis et locis, Oeuvres complètes d'Hippocrate*. Ed. Emile Littré, 2:12–92. Paris: Baillière, 1839–61.

————. *Epidemics, Oeuvres complètes d'Hippocrate*. Ed. Emile Littré, 5:260–342. Paris: Baillière, 1839–61.

————. *De natura hominis, Oeuvres complètes d'Hippocrate*. Ed. Emile Littré, 6:29–69. Paris: Baillière, 1839–61.

Galen, *Claudii Galeni opera omnia*. 20 vols. Ed. Karl Gottlob Kühn. Leipzig: Knobloch, 1821–33.

Gambiglioni, Angelo [Angelo Aretino]. *De maleficiis*. Venice: Dominicus Lilius, 1558.

————. *Tractatus maleficiorum*. Mantua: Petrus Adam de Michaelibus, 1472.

Garzoni, Tomaso. *L'ospidale de' pazzi incurabili*. Ed. Stefano Barelli. Rome: Editrice Antenore, 2004.

Giovanni da Concoreggio. *Practica nove medicine*. Venice, 1501.

Guainerio, Antonio. *Practica*. Venice, 1517.

Landouzy, Louis, and Roger Pépin. *Le "Régime du Corps" de Maitre Aldobrandin de Sienne: Texte français du XIIIe siècle*. Paris: H. Champion, 1911.

Martelli, Ugolino di Niccolò. *Ricordanze dal 1433 al 1483*. Ed. Fulvio Pezzarossa. Rome: Edizioni di Storia e Letteratura, 1989.

Montagnana, Bartolomeo. *Consilia*. Venice, 1514.

Savonarola, Michele. *Practica medicinae sive de aegritudinibus*. Venice, 1497.

Sozzini, Mariano, and Bartolomeo Sozzini. *Consiliorum seu Responsorum Mariani Socini ac Bartholomeaei fili Senensium*. Venice: Franciscus Zilettum, 1579.

Statuta populi et communis Florentiae: Publica auctoritate, collecta, castigata et praeposita anno salutis MCCCCXV. 3 vols. Freiburg: M. Kluch, 1778–83.

Statuti della repubblica fiorentina. Ed. Romolo Caggese. Vol. 2, *Statuto del Podestà dell'anno 1325*. Ed. Giuliano Pinto, Francesco Salvestrini, and Andrea Zorzi. Florence: Olschki, 1999.

Statuti della repubblica fiorentina. Ed. Romolo Caggese. Rev. ed. Florence: Olschki, 1999.

Statuti delle Universita e dei Collegi dello Studio Bolognese. Ed. Carlo Malagola. Bologna. 1st ed. 1888; reissued, 1988.

Tartagni, Alessandro. *Consilia Varia*. Fabius Bartholinus D. Honofrii iussus obtulit Bibliotheca huius Serenissimi Urbini Ducis. Consilium, 249. BAV Urb. lat. 1132.

————. *Primum-quintum volumen Consiliorum*. Venice: Baptista de Tortis, 1510–11.

Zacchia, Paolo. *Quaestiones Medico-Legales*. Amsterdam: Johanne Blaeu, 1651.

———. *Quaestionum Medico-Legalium Tomus Prior[-Posterior]*. 2 vols. Lyon: Joannes-Antonius Huguetan, & Marcus-Antonius Ravaud, 1661.

SECONDARY SOURCES

Ackerknecht, Erwin H. "The Early History of Legal Medicine." *Ciba Symposia* 11, no. 7 (1950): 1286–89.

Agrimi, Jole, and Chiara Crisciani. *Edocere Medicos: Medicina Scolastica nei Secoli XIII—XV*. Naples: Guerini e associati, 1988.

Ahl, Diane Cole. *Benozzo Gozzoli*. New Haven, Conn.: Yale University Press, 1996.

Ajmar, Marta, ed. *Approaches to Renaissance Consumption*. Oxford: Oxford University Press, 2002.

Alexander, Franz G., and Sheldon T. Selesnick. *The History of Psychiatry: An Evaluation of Psychiatric Thought and Practice from Prehistoric Times to the Present*. New York: Harper & Row, 1967.

Allerston, Patricia. "Consuming Problems: Worldly Goods in Renaissance Venice." In *The Material Renaissance*, ed. Michelle O'Malley and Evelyn Welch, 11–46. Manchester: Manchester University Press, 2007.

Amundsen, Darrel W., and Garry B. Ferngren. "The Forensic Role of Physicians in Roman Law." *Bull. Hist. Med.* 53, no. 1(1979): 39–56.

Andrews, Jonathan, and Andrew Scull. *Customers and Patrons of the Mad-Trade: The Management of Lunacy in Eighteenth-Century London*. Berkeley: University of California Press, 2003.

Antonelli, Giovanni. "La magistratura degli Otto di Guardia a Firenze." *ASI* 92, no. 402 (1954): 3–39.

Anzilotti, Antonio. *La Costituzione Interna dello Stato Fiorentino sotto il Duca Cosimo I de' Medici*. Florence: Francesco Lumachi, 1910.

Aram, Bethany. *Juana the Mad: Sovereignty and Dynasty in Renaissance Europe*. Baltimore: Johns Hopkins University Press, 2005.

Armstrong, Lawrin. "Law, Ethics and Economy: Gerard of Siena and Giovanni d'Andrea on Usury." In *Money, Markets and Trade in Late Medieval Europe: Essays in Honour of John H. A. Munro*, ed. Lawrin Armstrong, Ivana Elbl, and Martin Elbl, 41–42. Leiden: Brill, 2007.

———. *Usury and Public Debt in Early Renaissance Florence: Lorenzo Ridolfi on the "Monte Comune."* Toronto: Pontifical Institute of Medieval Studies, 2003.

Arrizabalaga, Jon. *The Articella in the Early Press, c. 1476–1534*. Cambridge: Cambridge Wellcome Unit for the History of Medicine, 1998.

———. "The Death of a Medieval Text: The *Articella* and the Early Press." In *Medicine from the Black Death to the French Disease*, ed. Roger French et al., 184–220. Burlington, Vt.: Ashgate, 1998.

Ascheri, Mario. "Consilium sapientis, perizia medico, e res iudicata: diritto dei dottori e istituzioni comunali." In *Proceedings of the Fifth International Congress of Medieval Canon Law (Salamanca 21–25 September, 1976)*, ed. Stephen Kuttner and Kenneth Pennington. Vatican City: Biblioteca Apostolica Vaticana, 1980.

———. *Tribunali, giuristi e istituzioni dal medioevo all'età moderna.* Bologna: Il Mulino, 1989.

Astorri, Antonella. *La mercanzia a Firenze nella prima metà del Trecento: Il potere dei grandi mercanti.* Florence: Olschki, 1998.

Audibert, Adrien. *Études sur l'histoire du droit romain: La folie et la prodigalité.* Paris: L. Larose & Forcel, 1892.

Baker, Patricia A., Karine van t'Land, and Han Nijdam, eds. *Medicine and Space: Body, Surroundings and Borders in Antiquity and the Middle Ages.* Leiden: Brill, 2012.

Baldini, Rosella. "Zucchero Bencivenni, *La santé del corpo*, Volgarizzamento del Régime du corps di Aldobrandino da Siena (a. 1310) nella copia coeva di Lapo di Neri Corsini (Laur. Pl. LXXIII 47)." *Studi di lessicografia italiana* 15 (1998): 21–300.

Baruchello, François. *La folie de la Renaissance: Analyse de "L'hospital des fols incurables" de Garzoni, 1549–1589.* Evrecy: Association France-Italie, 1998.

Basile, Bruno. *Poëta melancholicus: Tradizione classica e follia nell'ultimo Tasso.* Pisa: Pacini, 1984.

Battaglia, Salvator. *Grande dizionario della lingua italiana.* Vols. 4 and 10. Turin: Unione tipografico-editrice torinese, 1961–2008.

Becker, Marvin B. "Changing Patterns of Violence and Justice in Fourteenth- and Fifteenth-Century Florence." *Comparative Studies in Society and History* 18, no. 3 (1976): 281–96.

———. "Economic Change and the Emerging Florentine Territorial State." *Studies in the Renaissance* 13 (1966): 7–39.

———. *Florence in Transition.* Baltimore: Johns Hopkins University Press, 1967.

———. "The Republican City-State in Florence: An Inquiry into Its Origin and Survival (1280–1434)." *Speculum* 35, no. 1 (1960): 39–50.

Berrios, German E. "Classifications in Psychiatry: A Conceptual History." *Australian and New Zealand Journal of Psychiatry* 33 (1999): 145–60.

Biotti, Vittorio, ed. *"È matto e tristo, pazzo e fastidioso": I saperi sulla fol-*

lia, magistrati, medici, e inquisitori a Firenze e negli stati italiani del '600. Florence: Nicomp, 2002.

Bisson, Sebastiano, et al. "Le Témoin Gênant: Une version latine du *Régime du corps* d'Aldebrandin de Sienne." *Médiévales* 42 (2002): 117–30.

Blair, Ann. "The *Problemata* as a Natural Philosophical Genre." In *Natural Particulars: Nature and the Disciplines in Renaissance Europe*, ed. Anthony Grafton and Nancy Siraisi, 171–204. Cambridge, Mass.: MIT Press, 1999.

Boari, Marco. *Qui venit contra iura? Il "furiosus" nella criminalistica dei secoli XV e XVI*. Milan: Giuffrè, 1983.

Brackett, John K. *Criminal Justice and Crime in Late Renaissance Florence, 1537–1609*. Cambridge: Cambridge University Press, 1992.

Brann, Noel L. *The Debate over the Origin of Genius During the Italian Renaissance*. Leiden: Brill, 2002.

Britton, Piers. "'Mio malinchonico, o vero . . . mio pazzo': Michelangelo, Vasari, and the Problem of Artists' Melancholy in Sixteenth-Century Italy." *Sixteenth Century Journal* 34, no. 3 (2003): 653–75.

Brockliss, Laurence, and Colin Jones. *The Medical World of Early Modern France*. Oxford: Clarendon Press, 1997.

Brogi, Mario, ed. *Gli albori del Comune di San Gimignano e lo statuto del 1314*. Siena: Cantagalli, 1995.

Brown, Patricia Fortini. *Private Lives in Renaissance: Venice Art, Architecture, and the Family*. New Haven, Conn.: Yale University Press, 2004.

Brown, Peter. *Through the Eye of a Needle: Wealth, the Fall of Rome, and the Making of Christianity in the West, 350–550 AD*. Princeton, N.J.: Princeton University Press, 2012.

Burghartz, Susanna. *Leib, Ehre, und Gut: Delinquenz in Zürich Ende des 14 Jahrhunderts*. Zurich: Chronos, 1990.

Butcher, James N., Susan Mineka, and Jill M. Hooley. *Abnormal Psychology*. 14th ed. Boston: Allyn & Bacon, 2010.

Bylebyl, Jerome. "Medicine, Philosophy, and Humanism in Renaissance Italy." In *Science and the Arts in the Renaissance*, ed. John W. Shirley and F. David Hoeniger, 27–49. Washington, D.C.: Folger Shakespeare Library, 1985.

Bynum, W. F., Roy Porter, and Michael Shepherd, eds. *The Anatomy of Madness: Essays in the History of Psychiatry*. London: Tavistock Publications, 1985–88.

Calabritto, Monica. "A Case of Melancholic Humors and Dilucida Intervalla." *Intellectual History Review* 18, no. 1 (2008): 139–54.

Calvi, Giulia. *Il contratto morale: Madri e Figli nella Toscana Moderna*. Rome: Laterza, 1994.

————. "Widowhood and Remarriage in Tuscany." In *Marriage in Italy, 1300–1650*, ed. Trevor Dean and Kate J. P. Lowe, 275–96. Cambridge: Cambridge University Press, 1998.

————. "Widows, the State, and Guardianship of Children in Early Modern Tuscany." In *Widowhood in Medieval and Early Modern Europe*, ed. Sandra Cavallo and Lyndan Warner, 209–19. London: Longman, 1999.

Caprioli, Severino, and Attilio Bartoli Langeli, eds. *Statuto del Comun di Perugia del 1279*. Perugia: Deputazione di storia patria per l'Umbria, 1996.

Carter, Tim, and Richard A. Goldthwaite. *Orpheus in the Marketplace: Jacopo Peri and the Economy of Late Renaissance Florence*. Cambridge, Mass.: Harvard University Press, 2013.

Cavallar, Osvaldo. "Agli arbori della medicine legale: I trattati *De percussionibus* e *De vulneribus*." *Ius Commune* 26 (1999): 27–89.

————. "La *benefundata sapientia* dei periti: Feritori, feriti e medici nei commentari e consulti di Baldo degli Ubaldi." *Ius Commune* 27 (2000): 215–81.

Cavallo, Sandra. "Secrets to Healthy Living: The Revival of the Preventative Paradigm in Late Renaissance Italy." In *Secrets and Knowledge in Medicine and Science, 1500–1800*, ed. Elaine Leong and Alisha Rankin, 191–212. Burlington, Vt.: Ashgate, 201.

Cerquiglini-Toulet, Jacqueline. *La couleur de la mélancolie: La fréquentation des livres au XIVe siècle 1300–1415*. Paris: Hatier, 1993.

Chabot, Isabelle. *La dette des familles: Femmes, lignage et patrimoine à Florence aux XIVe et XVe siècles*. Rome: École française de Rome, 2011.

Chiappelli, A. "Gli Ordinamenti Sanitari del Comune di Pistoia contro la Pestilenza del 1348." *ASI*, ser. 4, 20 (1887): 8–22.

Chojnacki, Stanley. *Women and Men in Renaissance Venice: Twelve Essays on Patrician Society*. Baltimore: Johns Hopkins University Press, 2000.

Civai, Alessandra. *Dipinti e sculture in casa Martelli: Storia di una collezione patrizia fiorentina dal Quattrocento all'Ottocento*. Florence: Opus Libri, 1990.

Clark, Michael, and Catherine Crawford, eds. *Legal Medicine in History*. Cambridge: Cambridge University Press, 1994.

Clarke, Basil. *Mental Disorder in Earlier Britain*. Cardiff: University of Wales, 1975.

Coing, Helmut, ed. *Handbuch der Quellen und Literatur der neueren europäischen Privatrechtsgeschichte*. Munich: C. H. Beck, 1973.

Colombero, Carlo. "Un contributo alla formazione della nozione di malattia mentale: Le *Questioni medico-legali* di Paolo Zacchia." In *Follia, Psichiatria e Società: Istituzioni manicomiali, scienza psichiatrica e classi sociali nell'Italia moderna e contemporanea*, ed. Alberto De Barbardi, 317–29. Milan: Franco Angeli, 1982.

———. "Il medico e il giudice." *Materiali per una storia della cultura giuridica* 16 (1986): 363–81.

Cook, Harold. *The Decline of the Old Medical Regime in Stuart London.* Ithaca, N.Y.: Cornell University Press, 1986.

Cooper, Donal. "Access All Areas? Spatial Divides in the Mendicant Churches of Late Medieval Tuscany." In *Ritual and Space in the Middle Ages: Proceedings of the 2009 Harlaxton Symposium*, ed. Frances Andrews, 90–107. Donington: Shaun Tyas, 2011.

Cooper, Donal, and Janet Robson. *The Making of Assisi: The Pope, the Franciscans and the Painting of the Basilica.* New Haven, Conn.: Yale University Press, 2013.

Crawford, Catherine. "Legalizing Medicine: Early Modern Legal Systems and the Growth of Medico-Legal Knowledge." In *Legal Medicine in History*, ed. Michael Clark and Catherine Crawford, 89–116. Cambridge: Cambridge University Press, 1994.

———. "Medicine and the Law." In *Companion Encyclopedia of the History of Medicine*, ed. W. F. Bynum and Roy Porter, 2:1619–40. New York: Routledge, 1993.

Crawford, Sally, and Christina Lee, eds. *Bodies of Knowledge: Cultural Interpretations of Illness and Medicine in Medieval Europe.* Oxford: Archaeopress, 2010.

Dean, Trevor. *Crime and Justice in Late Medieval Italy.* Cambridge: Cambridge University Press, 2007.

Dean, Trevor, and Kate J. P. Lowe, eds. *Marriage in Italy, 1300–1650.* Cambridge: Cambridge University Press, 1998.

De Renzi, Silvia. "Witnesses of the Body: Medico-Legal Cases in Seventeenth-Century Rome." *Studies in History and Philosophy of Science* 33 (2002): 219–42.

———. "Women's Deaths in the Law Courts of Seventeenth-Century Rome." *Bull. Hist. Med.* 84 (2010): 549–77.

De Roover, Raymond. "The Commercial Revolution of the Thirteenth Century." In *Enterprise and Secular Change in Economic History*, ed. Frederic C. Lane, 80–85. Homewood, Ill.: R. D. Irwin, 1953.

Diaz, Furio. *Il Granducato di Toscana: I Medici.* Turin: UTET, 1976.

Digby, Anne. *Madness, Morality, and Medicine: A Study of the York Retreat, 1796–1914.* Cambridge: Cambridge University Press, 1985.

Dinges, Martin. "The Uses of Justice as a Form of Social Control in Early Modern Europe." In *Social Control in Europe, 1500–1800*, ed. Herman

Roodenburg and Pieter Speirenburg, 1:159–75. Columbus: Ohio State University Press, 2004.

Dini, Alessandro. *Il medico e la follia: Cinquanta Casi di Malattia Mentale nella Letterature Medica Italiana del Seicento.* Florence: Le lettere, 1997.

Di Renzo Villata, Gigliola. "Nota per le storia della tutela nell'italia del rinascimento." In *La famiglia e la vita quotidiana in Europa dal '400 al '600: Fonti e problemi*, Atti del convegno internazionale Milano 1–4 dicembre 1983. Rome: Ministero per i beni culturali e ambientali, 1986.

———. *La tutela: Indagini sulla scuola dei glossatori.* Milan: A. Giuffrè, 1975.

Duden, Barbara. *The Woman Beneath the Skin: A Doctor's Patients in Eighteenth-Century Germany.* Cambridge, Mass.: Harvard University Press, 1991.

Duffin, Jacalyn. "The Doctor Was Surprised; or, How to Diagnose a Miracle," *Bull. Hist. Med.* 81, no. 4 (2007): 699–729.

Eamon, William. *The Professor of Secrets: Mystery, Medicine, and Alchemy in Renaissance Italy.* Washington, D.C.: National Geographic, 2010.

———. *Science and the Secrets of Nature: Books of Secrets in Medieval and Early Modern Culture.* Princeton, N.J.: Princeton University Press, 1994.

Eyler, Joshua R., ed. *Disability in the Middle Ages: Reconsiderations and Reverberations.* Burlington, Vt.: Ashgate, 2010.

Farge, Arlette. *Le goût de l'archive.* Paris: Editions du Seuil, 1989.

Fasano Guarini, Elena. "Potere centrale e comunità soggette nel granducato di Cosimo I." *Rivista Storica Italiana* 89, Fasc. 3–4 (1977): 490–538.

———. *Lo stato Mediceo di Cosimo I.* Florence: Sansoni, 1973.

Fasoli, Gina, and Pietro Sella, eds. *Statuti di Bologna dell'anno 1288.* Vatican City: Biblioteca apostolica vaticana, 1937–39.

Fischer-Homberger, Esther. *Medizin vor Gericht: Gerichtsmedizin von der Renaissance bis zur Aufklärung.* Bern: Verlag Hans Huber, 1983.

Fisher, Caroline M. "Guardianship and the Rise of the Florentine State, 1368–93." In *Famiglie e poteri in Italia tra medioevo ed età moderna*, ed. Anna Bellavitis and Isabelle Chabot, 265–67. Rome: École française de Rome, 2009.

———. "The State as Surrogate Father: State Guardianship in Renaissance Florence, 1368–1532." Ph.D. diss., Brandeis University, 2003.

Foucault, Michel. *Histoire de la folie à l'âge classique: Folie et déraison.* Paris: Plon, 1961.

———. *Madness and Civilization: A History of Insanity in the Age of Reason.* New York: Vintage Books, 1973.

French, Roger K. *Medicine Before Science: The Rational and Learned Physi-*

cian from the Middle Ages to the Enlightenment. Cambridge: Cambridge University Press, 2003.

French, Roger K., Jon Arrizabalaga, Andrew Cunningham, and Luis García-Ballester, eds. *Medicine from the Black Death to the French Disease.* Aldershot: Ashgate, 1998.

Frick, Carole Collier. *Dressing Renaissance Florence: Families, Fortunes, & Fine Clothing.* Baltimore: Johns Hopkins University Press, 2002.

Frigo, Daniela. *Il Padre di Famiglia: Governo della Casa e Governo Civile nelle Tradizione dell'Economica' tra Cinque e Seicento.* Rome: Bulzoni, 1985.

Foriers, Paul. "La condition des insensés à la Renaissance." In *Folie et déraison à la Renaissance,* 26–40. Brussels: Editions de l'Université de Bruxelles, 1976.

Fukuyama, Francis. *Trust: The Social Virtues and the Creation of Prosperity.* New York: Free Press, 1995.

García-Ballester, Luis. *"Artifex factivus sanitatis*: Health and Medical Care in Medieval Latin Galenism." In *Galen and Galenism: Theory and Medical Practice from Antiquity to the European Renaissance,* 127–50. Aldershot: Ashgate/Variorum, 2002.

———. "The *New Galen*: A Challenge to Latin Galenism in Thirteenth-Century Montpellier." In *Galen and Galenism: Theory and Medical Practice from Antiquity to the European Renaissance,* 55–83. Aldershot: Ashgate/Variorum, 2002.

———. "On the Origins of the 'Six Non Natural Things' in Galen." In *Galen and Galenism: Theory and Medical Practice from Antiquity to the European Renaissance,* 105–15. Aldershot: Ashgate/Variorum, 2002.

García Gibert, Javier. *Cervantes y la melancolía: Ensayos sobre el tono y la actitud cervantinos.* València: Edicions Alfons el Magnànim, Institució Valenciana d'Estudis i Investigació, 1997.

Garin, Eugenio. *La disputa delle arti nel Quattrocento.* Florence: Vallecchi, 1947.

Gatrell, V. A. C., Bruce Lenman, and Geoffrey Parker, eds. *Crime and the Law: The Social History of Crime in Western Europe Since 1500.* London: Europa Publications Limited, 1980.

Gavitt, Philip. *Gender, Honor, and Charity in Late Renaissance Florence.* New York: Cambridge University Press, 2011.

Geltner, Guy. *The Medieval Prison: A Social History.* Princeton, N.J.: Princeton University Press, 2008.

Gentilcore, David. *Healers and Healing in Early Modern Italy.* Manchester: Manchester University Press, 1998.

————. *Medical Charlatanism in Early Modern Italy.* Oxford: Oxford University Press, 2006.

Gil Sotres, Pedro. "The Regimens of Health." In *Western Medical Thought from Antiquity to the Middle Ages,* ed. Mirko D. Grmek, 291–318. Cambridge, Mass.: Harvard University Press, 1998.

Goldberg, Ann. *Sex, Religion, and the Making of Modern Madness: The Eberbach Asylum and German Society, 1815–1849.* New York: Oxford University Press, 1999.

Goldthwaite, Richard. *The Economy of Renaissance Florence.* Baltimore: Johns Hopkins University Press, 2009.

————. "The Empire of Things: Consumer Demand in Renaissance Italy." In *Patronage, Art and Society in Renaissance Italy,* ed. F. W. Kent and Patricia Simons, 155–75. Oxford: Oxford University Press, 1987.

————. "Il sistema monetario fino al 1600: Practica, politica, problematica." In *Studi sulla Moneta Fiorentina (Secoli XIII–XVI),* ed. Richard A. Goldthwaite and Giulio Mandich, 9–106. Florence: Olschki, 1994.

————. *Wealth and the Demand for Art in Italy, 1300–1600.* Baltimore: Johns Hopkins University Press, 1993.

Gowland, Angus. *The Worlds of Renaissance Melancholy: Robert Burton in Context.* Cambridge: Cambridge University Press, 2006.

Grassi, Ernesto, and Maristella Lorch. *Folly and Insanity in Renaissance Literature.* Binghamton, N.Y.: Medieval & Renaissance Texts & Studies, 1986.

Green, Louis. "Galvano Fiamma, Azzone Visconti and the Revival of the Classical Theory of Magnificence." *Journal of the Warburg and Courtauld Institutes* 53 (1990): 98–113.

Hacking, Ian. *Mad Travelers: Reflections of the Reality of Transient Mental Illnesses.* Charlottesville: University Press of Virginia, 1998.

————. *Rewriting the Soul: Multiple Personality and the Sciences of Memory.* Princeton, N.J.: Princeton University Press, 1995.

Henderson, John. *The Renaissance Hospital: Healing the Body and Healing the Soul.* New Haven, Conn.: Yale University Press, 2006.

Herlihy, David, and Christiane Klapisch-Zuber. *Tuscans and Their Families: A Study of the Florentine Catasto of 1427.* New Haven, Conn.: Yale University Press, 1985.

Hess, Andrew C. "The Evolution of the Ottoman Seaborne Empire in the Age of the Oceanic Discoveries, 1453–1525." *American Historical Review* 75, no. 7 (1970): 1892–1919.

————. "The Ottoman Conquest of Egypt (1517) and the Beginning of the Sixteenth-Century World War." *International Journal of Middle East Studies* 4, no. 1 (1973): 55–76.

Houston, R. A. *Madness and Society in Eighteenth-Century Scotland.* Oxford: Oxford University Press, 2000.

Howard, Peter. "Preaching Magnificence in Renaissance Florence." *Renaissance Quarterly* 61 (2008): 356–57.

Israëls, Machtelt. "Painting for a Preacher: Sassetta and Bernardino da Siena." In *Sassetta: The Borgo San Sepolcro Altarpiece*, ed. Machtelt Israëls, 121–46. Leiden: Primavera Press, 2009.

Jenkins, A. D. Fraser. "Cosimo de' Medici's Patronage of Architecture and the Theory of Magnificence." *Journal of the Warburg and Courtauld Institutes* 33 (1970): 162–70.

Jones, Carol A. G. *Expert Witnesses.* Oxford: Oxford University Press, 1994.

Jones, Colin. *The Charitable Imperative: Hospitals and Nursing in Ancien Régime and Revolutionary France.* London: Routledge, 1989.

Jones, Colin, and Roy Porter, eds. *Reassessing Foucault: Power, Medicine, and the Body.* London: Routledge, 1994.

Kaiser, Walter. *Praisers of Folly: Erasmus, Rabelais, Shakespeare.* Cambridge, Mass.: Harvard University Press, 1963.

Kantorowicz, Hermann U. "Cino da Pistoia ed il primo trattato di medicina legale." *ASI* (1906): 115–28.

———. *Studies in the Glossators of Roman Law: Newly Discovered Writings of the Twelfth Century.* Cambridge: Cambridge University Press, 1938.

Kaser, Max. *Römisches Privatrecht: Ein Studienbuch.* Munich: C. H. Beck, 1986.

Kent, Francis William. *Household and Lineage in Renaissance Florence: The Family Life of the Capponi, Ginori, and Rucellai.* Princeton, N.J.: Princeton University Press, 1977.

King, Peter. *Crime, Justice and Discretion in England, 1740–1820.* Oxford: Oxford University Press, 2000.

Kirshner, Julius. "Baldo de Ubaldo on Disinheritance: Contexts, Controversies, *Consilia*." *Ius Commune* 27 (2000): 119–214.

———. "Encumbering Private Claims to Public Debt in Renaissance Florence." In *The Growth of the Bank as Institution and the Development of Money-Business Law*, ed. Vito Piergiovanni, 19–75. Berlin: Duncker & Humblot, 1993.

———. *Pursuing Honor While Avoiding Sin: The Monte delle doti of Florence, Quaderni di Studi Senesi* 41. Milan: A. Giuffrè, 1978.

———. "Some Problems in the Interpretation of Legal Texts *RE* the Italian City-States." *Archiv für Begriffsgeschichte* 19 (1975): 16–27.

———. "The State Is 'Back In.'" In *The Origins of the State in Italy, 1300–1600*, ed. Julius Kirshner. Chicago: University of Chicago Press, 1995.

————. "Storm over the 'Monte Comune': Genesis of the Moral Controversy over the Public Debt of Florence." *Archivum Fratrum Praedicatorum* 53 (1983): 219–76.

————. "'Ubi est ille?' Franco Sacchetti on the Monte Comune of Florence." *Speculum* (July 1984): 556–84.

Kitzes, Adam. *The Politics of Melancholy from Spenser to Milton.* New York: Routledge, 2006.

Klapisch-Zuber, Christiane. *Women, Family, and Ritual in Renaissance Italy.* Trans. Lydia G. Cochrane. Chicago: University of Chicago Press, 1985.

Kleinman, Arthur. *Patients and Healers in the Context of Culture: An Exploration of the Borderland Between Anthropology, Medicine, and Psychiatry.* Berkeley: University of California Press, 1980.

Klibansky, Raymond, Erwin Panofsky, and Fritz Saxl. *Saturn and Melancholy: Studies in the History of Natural Philosophy, Religion, and Art.* New York: Basic Books, 1964.

Kromm, Jane. *The Art of Frenzy: Public Madness in the Visual Culture of Europe, 1500–1850.* London: Continuum, 2002.

Kudlick, Catherine J. "Disability History: Why We Need Another 'Other.'" *American Historical Review* 108, no. 3 (June 2003): 763–93.

Kuehn, Thomas. "*Fama* as a Legal Statute in Renaissance Florence." In *Fama: The Politics of Talk and Reputation in Medieval Europe*, ed. Thelma Fenster and Daniel Lord Smail, 27–46. Ithaca, N.Y.: Cornell University Press, 2003.

————. *Law, Family, and Women: Toward a Legal Anthropology of Renaissance Italy.* Chicago: University of Chicago Press, 1991.

————. "Review: Reading Microhistory: The Example of Giovanni and Lusanna." *Journal of Modern History* 61, no. 3 (1989): 512–34.

Langbein, J. H. *Prosecuting Crime in the Renaissance: England, Germany, France.* Cambridge, Mass.: Harvard University Press, 1974.

Lange, Hermann. *Römisches Recht im Mittelalter.* Vol. 1. *Die Glossatoren.* Munich: C. H. Beck, 1997.

Leong, Elaine, and Alisha Rankin, eds. *Secrets and Knowledge in Medicine and Science, 1500–1800.* Burlington, Vt.: Ashgate, 2011.

Lippi, Donatella. *Díaita: The Rules of Health in the Manuscripts of the Biblioteca Medicea Laurenziana.* Florence: Mandragora, 2010.

Little, Lester K. *Religious Poverty and the Profit Economy in Medieval Europe.* London: Pail Elek Ltd., 1978.

Lynch, Katherine A. *Individuals, Families, and Communities in Europe, 1200–1800: The Urban Foundations of Western Society.* Cambridge: Cambridge University Press, 2003.

MacDonald, Michael. *Mystical Bedlam: Madness, Anxiety, and Healing in Seventeenth-Century England*. Cambridge: Cambridge University Press, 1981.

Magherini, Graziella, and Vittorio Biotti. *L'isola delle Stinche et i percorsi della follia a Firenze nei secoli XIV–XVIII*. Florence: Ponte alle Grazie, 1992.

———, eds. *"Un luogo della città per custodia de' pazzi": Santa Dorotea dei Pazzerelli di Firenze nelle delibere della sua congregazione (1642–1754)*. Florence: Casa Editrice Le Lettere, 1997.

———. "Madness in Florence in the 14th–18th Centuries." *International Journal of Law and Psychiatry* 21, no. 4 (1998): 355–68.

Martini, Angelo. *Manuale di metrologia ossia misure, pesi e monete in uso attualmente e anticamente presso tutti i popoli*. Rome: E.R.A., 1976.

Martines, Lauro. *Lawyers and Statecraft in Renaissance Florence*. Princeton, N.J.: Princeton University Press, 1968.

Mazza, Rita. "La malattia mentale nella medicina del cinquecento: Tassonomia e casi clinici." In *Follia, Psichiatria, e Società: Istituzioni manicomiali, scienza psichiatica e classi sociali nell'Italia moderna e contemporanea*, ed. Alberto de Bernardi, 304–16. Milan: Franco Angeli, 1982.

McClive, Cathy. "Blood and Expertise: The Trials of the Female Medical Expert in the Ancien-Régime Courtroom." *Bull. Hist. Med.* 82 (2008): 86–108.

McVaugh, Michael R. *Medicine Before the Plague: Practitioners and Their Patients in the Crown of Aragon, 1285–1345*. Cambridge: Cambridge University Press, 1993.

Menning, Carol Bresnahan. *Charity and State in Renaissance Italy: The Monte di Pietà of Florence*. Ithaca, N.Y.: Cornell University Press, 1993.

Metzler, Irina. *Disability in Medieval Europe: Thinking About Physical Impairment During the High Middle Ages, c. 1100–1400*. London: Routledge, 2006.

———. "Disability in the Middle Ages: Impairment at the Intersection of Historical Inquiry and Disability Studies." *History Compass* 9, no. 1 (2011): 45–60.

Midelfort, H. C. Erik. *A History of Madness in Sixteenth-Century Germany*. Stanford, Calif.: Stanford University Press, 1999.

———. *Mad Princes of Renaissance Germany*. Charlottesville: University Press of Virginia, 1994.

Mikkeli, Heikki. *Hygiene in the Early Modern Medical Tradition*. Helsinki: Finnish Academy of Science and Letters, 1999.

Minio-Paluello, Maria-Luisa. *La "Fusta dei Matti": Firenze giugno 1514*. Florence: F. Cesati, 1990.

Molho, Anthony. *Marriage Alliance in Late Medieval Florence*: Cambridge, Mass.: Harvard University Press, 1994.

———. "The State and Public Finance." In *The Origins of the State in Italy, 1300–1600*, ed. Julius Kirshner, 97–135. Chicago: University of Chicago Press, 1995.

Monfasani, John. "The Pseudo-Aristotelian *Problemata* and Aristotle's *De Animalibus* in the Renaissance." In *Natural Particulars: Nature and the Disciplines in Renaissance Europe*, ed. Anthony Grafton and Nancy Siraisi, 205–47. Cambridge, Mass.: MIT Press, 1999.

Monga, Luigi, trans. and ed. *The Journal of Aurelio Scetti: A Florentine Galley Slave at Lepanto, 1565–1577*. Tempe: Arizona Center for Medieval and Renaissance Studies, 2004.

Morandini, Francesca, ed. "Statuti e Ordinamenti dell'Ufficio dei pupilli et adulti nel periodo della Repubblica fiorentina, 1388–1534." *ASI* (1955): 521–51; *ASI* (1956): 92–117; and *ASI* (1957): 87–104.

Mueller, Reinhold, C. *The Procuratori di San Marco and the Venetian Credit Market*. New York: Arno Press, 1977.

Muldrew, Craig. "Interpreting the Market: The Ethics of Credit and Community Relations in Early Modern England." *Social History* 18, no. 3 (May 1993): 163–83.

Musacchio, Jacqueline Marie. *Art, Marriage, and Family in the Florentine Renaissance Palace*. New Haven, Conn.: Yale University Press, 2008.

Najemy, John. *A History of Florence, 1200–1575*. Malden, Mass.: Blackwell, 2006.

Nalle, Sara Tilghman. *Mad for God: Bartolomé Sánchez, the Secret Messiah of Cardenete*. Charlottesville: University Press of Virginia, 2001.

Neugebauer, Richard. "Mental Illness and Government Policy in Sixteenth- and Seventeenth-Century England." Ph.D. diss., Columbia University, 1976.

Nicoud, Marilyn. *Les régimes de santé au moyen âge*. Rome: École Française de Rome, 2007.

Nolte, Cordula, ed. *Homo debilis: Behinderte, Kranke, Versehrte in der Gesellschaft des Mittelalters*. Korb: Didymos-Verlag, 2009.

Nutton, Vivian. "Continuity or Rediscovery? The City Physician in Classical Antiquity and Mediaeval Italy." In *The Town and State Physicians in Europe from the Middle Ages to the Enlightenment*, ed. Andrew W. Russell, 9–46. Wolfenbüttel: Herzog Aug. Bibliothek, 1981.

O'Boyle, Cornelius. *Thirteenth- and Fourteenth-Century Copies of the Ars Medicine: A Checklist and Contents Descriptions of the Manuscripts*. Cambridge: Cambridge Wellcome Unit for the History of Medicine, 1998.

O'Malley, Michelle, and Evelyn Welch, eds. *The Material Renaissance.* Manchester: Manchester University Press, 2007.

Ottosson, Per-Gunnar. *Scholastic Medicine and Philosophy: A Study of Commentaries on Galen's "Tegni," ca. 1300–1450.* Naples: Bibliopolis, 1984.

Papers of the Articella Project Meeting, Cambridge, December 1995. Cambridge: Cambridge Wellcome Unit for the History of Medicine, 1998.

Park, Katharine. "Country Medicine in the City Marketplace: Snake Handlers and Itinerant Healers." *Renaissance Studies* 15, no. 2 (2001): 104–20.

———. *Doctors and Medicine in Early Renaissance Florence.* Princeton, N.J.: Princeton University Press, 1985.

———. "Medicine and Magic: The Healing Arts." In *Gender and Society in Renaissance Europe*, ed. Judith C. Brown and Robert C. Davis, 129–49. London: Longman, 1998.

———. "Medicine and Society in Medieval Europe, 500–1500." In *Medicine in Society: Historical Essays*, ed. Andrew Wear, 59–90. Cambridge: Cambridge University Press, 1992.

———. "The Organic Soul." In *The Cambridge History of Renaissance Philosophy*, ed. Charles B. Schmitt and Quentin Skinner, 464–84. Cambridge: Cambridge University Press, 1988.

Passerini, Luigi. *Storia e genealogia delle famiglie Passerini e De' Rilli.* Florence: M. Cellini, 1874.

Pastore, Alessandro. *Il medico in tribunale: La perizia medica nella procedure penale d'antico regime (secoli XVI–XVII).* Verona: Casagrande Bellinzona, 1998.

Pastore, Alessandro, and Giovanni Rossi, eds. *Paolo Zacchia alle origini della medicina legale, 1584–1659.* Milan: Franco Angeli, 2008.

Pomata, Gianna. *Contracting a Cure: Patients, Healers, and the Law in Early Modern Bologna.* Baltimore: Johns Hopkins University Press, 1998.

———. "Malpighi and the Holy Body: Medical Experts and Miraculous Evidence in Seventeenth-Century Italy." *Renaissance Studies* 21 (2007): 568–86.

Porter, Roy. *Mind Forg'd Manacles: A History of Madness in England from the Restoration to the Regency.* Cambridge, Mass.: Harvard University Press, 1987.

Porter, Roy, and David Wright, eds. *The Confinement of the Insane: International Perspectives, 1800–1965.* Cambridge: Cambridge University Press, 2003.

Radding, Charles M. *Origins of Medieval Jurisprudence: Pavia and Bologna, 850–1150.* New Haven, Conn.: Yale University Press, 1988.

Radding, Charles M., and Antonio Ciaralli. *The "Corpus Iuris Civilis" in the Middle Ages: Manuscripts and Transmission from the Sixth Century to the Juristic Revival.* Leiden: Brill, 2007.

Ramsey, Matthew. *Professional and Popular Medicine in France, 1770–1830: The Social World of Medical Practice.* Cambridge: Cambridge University Press, 1988.

Rankin, Alisha. "Duchess, Heal Thyself: Elizabeth of Rochlitz and the Patient's Perspective in Early Modern Germany." *Bull. Hist. Med.* 82, no. 1 (2008): 109–44.

Roodenburg, Herman. "Social Control Viewed from Below: New Perspectives." In *Social Control in Europe, 1500–1800,* ed. Herman Roodenburg and Pieter Speirenburg, 1:145–58. Columbus: Ohio State University Press, 2004.

Roscioni, Lisa. *Il governo della follia: Ospedali, medici e pazzi nell'età moderna.* Milan: Bruno Mondadori, 2003.

Roy, Arundati. *The God of Small Things.* New York: Random House, 2008.

Rubin, Patricia. "Magnificence and the Medici." In *The Early Medici and Their Artists,* ed. F. Ames-Lewis, 37–50. London: Birkbeck College, University of London, 1995.

Salmón, Fernando. "From Patient to Text? Narratives of Pain and Madness in Medical Scholasticism." In *Between Text and Patient: The Medical Enterprise in Medieval and Early Modern Europe,* ed. Florence Eliza Glaze and Brian K. Nance, 373–95. Florence: Sismel, 2011.

———. *Medical Classroom Practice: Petrus Hispanus' Questions on Isagoge, Tegni, Regimen Acutorum and Prognostica (c. 1245–50): (MS Madrid B.N. 1877, fols 24rb–141vb).* Cambridge: Cambridge Wellcome Unit for the History of Medicine, 1998.

Sánchez, Magdalena S. *The Empress, the Queen, and the Nun: Women and Power at the Court of Philip III of Spain.* Baltimore: Johns Hopkins University Press, 1998.

Salvestrini, Francesco, ed. *Statuti del Comune di San Miniato al Tedesco.* Pisa: ETS, 1994.

Sass, Louis A. *Madness and Modernism: Insanity in the Light of Modern Art, Literature, and Thought.* Cambridge, Mass.: Harvard University Press, 1992.

Sbriccoli, Mario. "Fonti giudiziarie et fonti giuridiche: Riflessioni sulla fase attuale degli studi di storia del crimine e della giustizia criminale." *Studi Storici* 29 (1988): 491–501.

Schleiner, Winfried. *Melancholy, Genius, and Utopia in the Renaissance.* Wiesbaden: In Kommission bei Otto Harrassowitz, 1991.

Schutte, Anne Jacobson, Thomas Kuehn, and Silvana Seidel Menchi, eds.

Time, Space, and Women's Lives in Early Modern Europe. Kirksville, Mo.: Truman State University Press, 2001.

Shahar, Shulamith. *Growing Old in the Middle Ages: "Winter clothes us in shadow and pain."* Trans. Yael Lotan. London: Routledge, 1997.

Shatzmiller, Joseph. *Médecine et justice en Provence Médiévale: Documents de Mansoque, 1262–1348.* Aix-en-Provence: Université de Provence, 1989.

Siraisi, Nancy. *Avicenna in Renaissance Italy: The Canon and Medical Teaching in Italian Universities After 1500.* Princeton, N.J.: Princeton University Press, 1987.

———. "The Changing Fortunes of a Traditional Text: Goals and Strategies in Sixteenth-Century Latin editions of the *Canon* of Avicenna." In *The Medical Renaissance of the Sixteenth Century*, ed. Andrew Wear, Roger K. French, and I. M. Lonie, 16–41. Cambridge: Cambridge University Press, 1985.

———. *Medieval & Early Renaissance Medicine: An Introduction to Knowledge and Practice.* Chicago: University of Chicago Press, 1990.

———. *Taddeo Alderotti and His Pupils: Two Generations of Italian Medical Learning.* Princeton, N.J.: Princeton University Press, 1981.

Solazzi, Siro. *Scritti di Diritto Romano.* Vol. 2. Naples: Eugenio Jovene, 1957.

Smail, Daniel Lord. *The Consumption of Justice: Emotions, Publicity, and Legal Culture in Marseille, 1264–1423.* Ithaca, N.Y.: Cornell University Press, 2003.

Smart, Alistair. *The Assisi Problem and the Art of Giotto: A Study of the Legend of St. Francis in the Upper Church of San Francesco, Assisi.* Oxford: Clarendon Press, 1971.

Soufas, Teresa Scott. *Melancholy and the Secular Mind in Spanish Golden Age Literature.* Columbia: University of Missouri Press, 1990.

Starn, Randolph. "The Early Modern Muddle." *Journal of Early Modern History* 6, no. 3 (2002): 296–330.

Starobinski, Jean. *A History of the Treatment of Melancholy from Earliest Times to 1900.* Basle: Geigy, 1962.

Stern, Laura Ikins. *The Criminal Law System of Medieval and Renaissance Florence.* Baltimore: Johns Hopkins University Press, 1994.

———. "Inquisition Procedure and Crime in Early Fifteenth-Century Florence." *Law and History Review* 8, no. 2 (1990): 297–308.

Still, Arthur, and Irving Velody, eds. *Rewriting the History of Madness: Studies in Foucault's "Histoire de la folie."* London: Routledge, 1992.

Stone, Lawrence. *Uncertain Unions: Marriage in England, 1660–1753.* Oxford: Oxford University Press, 1992.

Strocchia, Sharon T. "The Melancholic Nun in Late Renaissance Italy." In *Diseases of the Imagination and Imaginary Diseases in the Early Modern Period*, ed. Yasmin Haskell, 139–58. Turnhout: Brepols, 2011.

———. "The Nun Apothecaries of Renaissance Florence: Marketing Medicines in the Convent." *Renaissance Studies* 25, no. 5 (2011): 627–47.

Stumpo, Enrico. *I bambini innocenti: Storia della Malattia mentale nell'Italia moderna (secoli XVI–XVIII)*. Florence: Le Lettere, 2000.

Tanfani, Gustavo. "Il concetto di melancholia nel cinquecento." *Rivista di storia delle scienze mediche e naturali* 39 (1948): 145–68.

Terpstra, Nicholas. *Cultures of Charity: Women, Politics, and the Reform of Poor Relief in Renaissance Italy*. Cambridge, Mass.: Harvard University Press, 2013.

Thomas, Yan. "La divisione dei sessi nel diritto romano." In *Storia delle donne in Occidente*, vol. 1, *L'antichità*, ed. P. Schmitt, 103–76. Bari: Editori Laterza, 1990–92.

Thompson, Edward Palmer. *The Making of the English Working Class*. New York: Vintage, 1966.

Thorndike, Lynn. "Medicine Versus the Law in Late Medieval and Medicean Florence." *Romanic Review* 17 (1926): 8–31.

Trevor, Douglas. *The Poetics of Melancholy in Early Modern England*. Cambridge: Cambridge University Press, 2004.

Trexler, Richard C. "In Search of Father: The Experience of Abandonment in the Recollections of Giovanni di Pagolo Morelli." In *Dependence in Context in Renaissance Florence*. Binghamton, N.Y.: Center for Medieval and Early Renaissance Studies, SUNY Binghamton, 1994.

———. *Public Life in Renaissance Florence*. Ithaca, N.Y.: Cornell University Press, 1991.

Turner, Wendy J., ed. *Madness in Medieval Law and Custom*. Leiden: Brill, 2010.

Turner, Wendy, and Tory Vandeventer Pearman, *eds. The Treatment of Disabled Persons in Medieval Europe: Examining Disability in the Historical, Legal, Literary, Medical, and Religious Discourses of the Middle Ages*. Lampeter: Edwin Mellen Press, 2011.

Vegetti, Mario. "Metafora politica e immagine del corpo nella medicina greca." In *Tra Edipo e Euclide: Forme del sapere antico*. Milan: Il Saggiatore, 1983.

Wack, Mary Frances. *Lovesickness in the Middle Ages: The Viaticum and Its Commentaries*. Philadelphia: University of Pennsylvania Press, 1990.

Wakefield, Jerome. "The Concept of Mental Disorder: On the Boundary Between Biological Facts and Social Values." *American Psychologist* 47, no. 3 (1992): 373–88.

Watson, Katherine D. *Forensic Medicine in Western Society: A History.* New York: Routledge, 2011.

Wear, Andrew. *Knowledge and Practice in English Medicine, 1550–1680.* Cambridge: Cambridge University Press, 2000.

Wear, Andrew, Roger K. French, and I. M. Lonie, eds. *The Medical Renaissance of the Sixteenth Century.* Cambridge: Cambridge University Press, 1985.

Welch, Evelyn. *Shopping in the Renaissance: Consumer Cultures in Italy, 1400–1600.* New Haven, Conn.: Yale University Press, 2005.

Wenzel, Siegfried. *The Sin of Sloth: Acedia in Medieval Thought and Literature.* Chapel Hill: University of North Carolina Press, 1989.

Winroth, Anders. *The Making of Gratian's "Decretum."* Cambridge: Cambridge University Press, 2000.

Wolfgang, Marvin E. "Crime and Punishment in Renaissance Florence." *Journal of Criminal Law and Criminology* 81, no. 3 (1990): 567–84.

———. "A Florentine Prison: Le Carceri delle Stinche." *Studies in the Renaissance* 7 (1960): 148–66.

Ziegler, Joseph. *Medicine and Religion c. 1300: The Case of Arnau de Vilanova.* Oxford: Clarendon Press, 1998.

Zilboorg, Gregory. *A History of Medical Psychology.* New York: Norton, 1951.

———. *The Medical Man and the Witch in the Renaissance.* New York: Cooper Square Publishers, 1969.

Zorzi, Andrea. *L'amministrazione della giustizia penale nelle repubblica fiorentina: Aspetti e problemi.* Florence: Olschki, 1988.

INDEX

ACKNOWLEDGMENTS

While writing this book, I sometimes felt a certain kinship with Dante, who, on his journey through hell, lamented the alienation, sadness, and torment the damned endured there. Many of the families I found in archival documents faced tremendous challenges. Some of them suffered terrible abuse or were themselves abusers. I often had to remind myself that in addition to cases of neglect or exploitation, I also saw what looked like compassion and generosity. I had to remind myself, too, that I was not traveling the path alone. Where Dante had only one guide through that dark place, I was fortunate to have many. I could not have completed this project without the support of institutions, mentors, teachers, colleagues, family, and friends. It gives me great pleasure to thank them here.

Research for this book was made possible by fellowships from the History Department and the Graduate School of Arts and Sciences at Harvard University, the History Department and the College of Liberal Arts at the University of New Hampshire, the Italian Fulbright Commission, the American Historical Association, and Harvard's Institute for Italian Renaissance Studies at Villa I Tatti. I would like to extend special thanks to Jack Eckert, Reference Librarian of Rare Books and Special Collections at the Francis Countway Memorial Library, David Warrington, Head of Special Collections, and David Ferris, Curator of Rare Books and Early Manuscripts at Harvard's Law School Library, and Michael Rocke at the Villa I Tatti Library. I would also like to thank the staffs of Harvard's Houghton Library, Columbia University's Rare Book and Manuscript Library, the New York Academy of Medicine's Historical Collections; in Rome, the Biblioteca Apostolica Vaticana, the Biblioteca Angelica, the Biblioteca Vallicelliana, the Biblioteca Nazionale Centrale di Roma, and the library at the American Academy in Rome; in Florence, the Archivio di Stato, the Biblioteca Nazionale Centrale di Firenze, the Biblioteca Laurenziana, the Biblioteca Riccardiana, and the Istituto Nazionale di Studi sul Rinascimento.

My mentors James Hankins, Katharine Park, and Charles Donahue helped me conceive of this project and begin to give it shape. Jim gave me the critical tools I needed to work with all manner of medieval and early modern documents. Katy introduced me to the history of medicine and Charlie the history of law. Under their tutelage I began to see and firmly to believe that the study of medical and legal ideas is incomplete without a deep understanding of how they work in practice. Many people became important mentors along the way though they may not have known it: Sharon Strocchia, Christopher P. Jones, Monica Calabritto, Giovanna Benadusi, John Henderson, Nancy Siraisi, Kate Lowe, Nicholas Terpstra, Richard Goldthwaite, Matteo Duni, Chris Celenza, Michael McCormick, and Daniel Smail.

Trying to write about a group of people that history tends to forget is not easy. I was fortunate to find a vibrant and generous community of scholars in Florence's libraries and archives who shared with me their ideas, technical expertise, and cases of incapacity they found by chance. Christiane Klapisch-Zuber was kind enough to give me several mentions of madness that she found in *ricordanze*; Robert Black compiled for me a list of mad men and women who appeared in the Catasto of 1427; Brett Auerbach-Lynn gave me his transcriptions and archival references for the fascinating case of Daria Carli; Lorenz Böninger told me about a letter from the vicar of Poppi in 1450 that described a mad monk; Alison Lewin passed on a reference to a mad man in the Carte Strozziane; and Joe Figliuolo sent me his transcription of a case from the Executor of Justice, involving the imprisonment of the violently insane Nero Calvalcanti in 1347. These bits and pieces helped me put my sample of cases in a broader social and legal context.

Two weeks before I finished this manuscript I had the pleasure of attending a spectacular conference organized by Niall Atkinson at the Kunsthistorisches Institut in Florence called "Italia Illustrata: Digital Mapping and Techniques of Visualizing the Pre-Modern Italian City." It was there that I first learned about DECIMA (Digitally Encoded Census Information Mapping Archive), a project supervised by Nicholas Terpstra at the University of Toronto. Colin Rose, a member of that research team, generously worked with me to locate properties and trace movements of select members of the Martelli family from Chapter 1. This simple exercise brought the nature of their struggles into sharper relief. Had there been more time, I would have tried to create a social geography of madness to capture more concretely how incapacity affected the movement of property and the constitution of households in the city of Florence. For now, I eagerly await DECIMA's formal launch; the mapping of madness I leave to another scholar.

I met a number of other people in the Florentine archives whose conversation and humor helped make the long hours spent there fun and productive: Robert Fredona, Brian Sandberg, Ed Goldberg, Dana Katz, Kate Jansen, Tovah Bender, Nic Baker, Brian Maxson, Corey Tazzara, and Mariana Labarca Pinto.

This book came together during a magical year spent as a fellow at the Villa I Tatti under the directorship of Lino Pertile and Anna Bensted. The influence of the art historians, literary scholars, musicologists, and historians who converged there in 2010–11 can be found all over this book. Frances Andrews, Louise Bordua, Machtelt Israëls, Gerardo de Simone and especially Janet Robson helped me see the life of St. Francis in a new light. I am particularly indebted to Janet for spending hours with me in Franciscan churches throughout Tuscany and Umbria, sharing her unparalleled knowledge of St. Francis and the celebration of his life through objects and images. I learned a tremendous amount about Florentine families through Lisa Kaborycha's massive study of *zibaldoni*; Liz Horodowich read and commented on Chapter 1; Catherine Kovesi, Frances Andrews, and Andrea Rizzi read and commented on Chapter 3. But I am indebted to the whole crew for their valuable insights as I struggled to figure out what I was doing over coffee, lunch, or tea and cookies. Thanks go to Déborah Blocker, Seth Coluzzi, Eva Del Soldato, Giovanni Fara, Allen Grieco, Peggy Haines, Eva Helfenstein, Areli Marina, Marcella Marongiu, Nadia Marx, Simona Mercuri, Peta Motture, Jonathan Nelson, Cara Rachele, Diana Sorensen, Marica Tacconi, Joan Thomas, Richard Thomas, Pier Mattia Tommasino, and Blake Wilson. A grant from the Lila Wallace-Reader's Digest publication subsidy at Villa I Tatti generously covered the licensing costs for all images.

I owe a significant debt of gratitude to the people who helped me complete this project. My colleagues at the University of New Hampshire read countless drafts and proposals. Several anonymous readers read the manuscript with great care. The book is better for their thoughtful words of advice, caution, correction, and encouragement. I want to extend special thanks to Jerry Singerman for his enthusiastic and steadfast support of the project and a good dose of humor along the way, to Rachel Taube, Caroline Hayes, Jennifer Backer, who helped me iron out the last of the wrinkles, and to Tim Roberts and the Modern Language Initiative for supporting the book's production.

I could not have dreamed of writing this book without the support of friends who generously lent eyes and ears to the endeavor: Jennifer Davis, Lauren Willig, Clare Gillis, John Ondrovcik, John Gagne, Leah Whittington, Goretti Gonzales, Amanda Dale Smith, Ariane Schwartz, Abigail Fradkin, Brooke Rosenzweig, Angela Rossi, Jim Foley, Christopher B. Krebs, Amy Houston, Tom Zanker, Susan Hamilton, Royal Hansen, Linus Hansen, and Soren Hansen. Evan MacCarthy, Timothy McCall, Douglas Dow, and Anne Leader made the days before final submission manageable. They helped me remember that when Dante emerged from hell at the end of his trying journey he found himself looking at a sky filled with stars.

My deepest and sincerest thanks go to my parents. My father, Kevin Mellyn, nurtured historical interests by sharing freely of his library. Our discussions of books and ideas have enriched my life in so many ways that I cannot imagine a life without them. The unstinting patience and support of my mother, Judith Mellyn, have sustained me from the beginning; she has read this work more times than anyone including myself. I dedicate this work to the memory of her father and my grandfather, who first made me dream of Italy.